Perception
A multisensory perspective

Nicola Bruno and Francesco Pavani

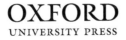
OXFORD
UNIVERSITY PRESS

UNIVERSITY PRESS

Great Clarendon Street, Oxford, OX2 6DP,
United Kingdom

Oxford University Press is a department of the University of Oxford.
It furthers the University's objective of excellence in research, scholarship,
and education by publishing worldwide. Oxford is a registered trade mark of
Oxford University Press in the UK and in certain other countries

First Edition published in 2018
Impression: 1

Published in the United States of America by Oxford University Press
198 Madison Avenue, New York, NY 10016, United States of America

British Library Cataloguing in Publication Data
Data available

Library of Congress Control Number: 2017962125

ISBN 978–0–19–872502–2

Printed and bound by
CPI Group (UK) Ltd, Croydon, CR0 4YY

Oxford University Press makes no representation, express or implied, that the
drug dosages in this book are correct. Readers must therefore always check
the product information and clinical procedures with the most up-to-date
published product information and data sheets provided by the manufacturers
and the most recent codes of conduct and safety regulations. The authors and
the publishers do not accept responsibility or legal liability for any errors in the
text or for the misuse or misapplication of material in this work. Except where
otherwise stated, drug dosages and recommendations are for the non-pregnant
adult who is not breast-feeding

Links to third party websites are provided by Oxford in good faith and
for information only. Oxford disclaims any responsibility for the materials
contained in any third party website referenced in this work.

Perception

Preface

The world is inherently multisensory, and most of us intuitively agree that multisensory experience is more gratifying, longer lasting, and more engaging and capable of attracting attention. Furthermore, multisensory issues have become increasingly fashionable in recent decades. Art is rich in celebrations of the hedonic implications of the senses. Many approaches to marketing stress multisensory experience. In the design of retail stores, of brands, of advertising campaigns, manipulations of sensory aspects often substitute the traditional emphasis on functions and value for products or services. In education, the idea that multisensory experience enhances the learning process and promotes creative solutions to problems is commonplace. Finally, multisensory considerations have become increasingly important in understanding neurological diseases, in designing rehabilitation procedures, and reportedly they will soon become relevant even for weight-loss programmes. Reports of facts about multisensory perception are plentiful in technical journals as well as in the mass media.

Although multisensory approaches permeate a number of endeavours in contemporary culture, few non-specialists are aware that in recent decades empirical work has begun to identify the general principles, the potentials, and the limits of multisensory perception. Experts can access this body of knowledge in specialized journals and in excellent reference works. However, those who have no specific expertise will not find these sources easy to understand. More likely, they will instead stumble upon pseudo-scientific claims, hastily posted on the internet in newsgroups and webpages. Even university undergraduates in psychology or neuroscience, who often take at least one course on perception, do not get much training on multisensory processes. The standard approach of introductory perception textbooks is to discuss each sense separately, usually giving most space to vision, then to hearing, and most often only a couple of chapters to touch, smell, and taste. However, most of our daily dealings with the environment are multisensory. For instance, even a simple task such as judging the location of a light in a dark room depends on vision but also on proprioceptive cues about the position of our body in space. One does not learn much about such multisensory processes from the textbooks adopting a unisensory approach.

In this book, we take a different stance. Rather than discussing each sense separately, we define perception as intrinsically multisensory from the start. This has two consequences that set this book apart from other books about perception. First, we discuss in detail themes such as the perception of one's body, the perception of agency and of action control, the perception of edible objects, and the peculiar condition known as synaesthesia. These are unusual themes for the standard perception textbooks but natural choices for one that adopts a multisensory perspective. Second, we strongly emphasize the active, exploratory nature of perceptual processes and therefore the strong links between perceiving and acting. This is a natural consequence of adopting a multisensory perspective. The sensory control of action is intrinsically multisensory, as movement necessarily requires that information from the external world (most often, coded by visual photoreceptors) be combined with information about the state of our body (most often, coded by stretch receptors in the muscles and joints). But multisensory interactions in the perceptual guidance of actions are much more complex and sophisticated that this obvious point, and have been reported to involve truly surprising effects. Furthermore, internal models of action turn out to be important in understanding other perceptual phenomena that do not require overt movement. The multisensory approach taken by this book leads us naturally to discuss these issues, which are often neglected in standard books on perception.

Writing this book has taken longer than we forecast. The project begun about three years ago, when we decided to adapt our earlier monograph (which appeared in Italian seven years ago; Bruno, Pavani, & Zampini, 2010) to an English readership. However, multisensory perception is a rapidly evolving field, and as we started working on the book we realized that most of the materials needed considerable updating. In addition, we wanted to write a book that could be understandable to the non-specialist while remaining interesting for scientists. The combination of these two features forced us to do much more restructuring and rewriting than we originally deemed necessary, and to add several parts that were not present in the earlier book. Whether we have achieved our two goals successfully is for the reader to decide. On our side, we can only state that we enjoyed writing this book and that we have learned a lot in the process.

Acknowledgments

This book could not have been written without the help of many colleagues and mentors. We are especially indebted to those who introduced us to the study of perception, attention, and the neurosciences at the early stages of our careers: Walter Gerbino, James Cutting, Paul Bertelson, Jon Driver, Charles Spence, Elisabetta Làdavas, and Alessandro Farnè. We owe special thanks to Massimiliano Zampini, who wrote an earlier book on multisensory perception with us. Massimiliano decided not to join us in this new endeavour, but many ideas especially in Chapters 5 and 8 of this book originated with him, and we are grateful for his generosity in letting us re-use them. Michael Kubovy, William Simpson, Leonardo Fogassi, and Leonardo Capanni read and provided advice on some of the chapters. Charlotte Holloway provided editorial assistance at all stages of the project, as well as several friendly reminders that we were late in submitting the book. Finally, we are grateful to our families for their patience when this book interfered with the time they deserved.

Contents

List of Figures and Boxes

Figures

Table

Boxes

Chapter 1

A Multisensory Perspective

1.1 Perception

Perception is how we know what is out there. At this very moment, I am (my body is) sitting on a soft flat object. This is part of a regular arrangement of other identical objects, neatly aligned within a large, narrow, and long enclosure. The enclosing walls are partly opaque and partly transparent. The box, and my body with it, are travelling at high speed relative to the environment outside. On my lap is a flat, hard surface with small black squares I can press with my fingers to make things appear and disappear on a luminous surface. I know that these soft flat objects have a certain size and shape and colour, that they allow sitting, and that they are train seats; that the squares are small and black, that they allow pressing, and that they are part of my laptop's keyboard; that I am in a train and that outside are houses, trees, fields, and many other things. These are very far from me, whereas my coat and my backpack are on a nearby seat and are within the reach of my arm; somewhat farther away are the door of the compartment, with its handles for opening and closing, and the bodies and other belongings of fellow passengers. All this I know immediately and effortlessly. How does it happen?

In the traditional view, perception is described as a chain of events. The senses are stimulated by physical energy and this stimulation, within each sense, generates *sensations,* the raw data that are passed on to higher order processes of interpretation. The interpretation combines elemental sensations first within and then between the senses, using constraints from internalized knowledge about objects, the environment, and our body. The final products are *percepts,* the conscious experiences of objects and events in the environment. This view is captured by the time-honoured model of the *psychophysical chain* (Figure 1.1). In this model, perception happens in three stages. In the first stage, an external object interacts with some form of energy that can travel from the external environment to a sense organ. This object is called the *distal stimulus.* In the second stage, the energy from the distal stimulus is coded by the sense organ, generating the *proximal stimulus.* In the third stage, finally, several internal processes interpret the proximal stimulus, generating a conscious *percept.* The three stages are often exemplified by considering vision. Distal objects reflect light to the eye, where a proximal 'image' is formed. A network of light-sensitive cells build a neural representation of this image which is sent to the brain for further processing, which eventually produces percepts. A similar scheme can be applied to hearing. A distal event causes a body to vibrate. The vibration generates

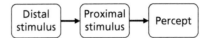

Figure 1.1 The psychophysical chain. The distal stimulus is any physical property of the environment. The proximal stimulus is the pattern of energy that becomes available at the receptors for that property. The percept is the corresponding mental conscious experience.

a periodic change of pressure in the air molecules, a travelling wave, which eventually stimulates a network of cells that build a neural representation of the frequency spectrum of the incoming wave. This is sent to the brain for further processing, which eventually produces a percept. And so on.

The view of perception as a psychophysical chain greatly contributed to the conceptual foundations of classical theories of perception and was instrumental to the development of *psychophysics,* the corpus of behavioural methods for studying quantitative relations between percepts and stimuli. Initiated by Gustav Theodor Fechner around the mid-nineteenth century, psychophysical methods remain one of the key sources of data about perception along with modern techniques for recording or visualizing neural activity. The conceptual model, however, has proved less useful in the long run. Consider the way the boxes and the arrows are displayed in Figure 1.1, and note that the whole process is summarized by two arrows only. This reflects the idea that for each of the senses there is one psychophysical chain. The senses are separate and independent. Interactions between them can occur, but they take place *after* the primary processing within each sense has been carried out. In addition, note that the arrows point in one direction, and in one direction only. The flow of information proceeds from input to output. Provide initial conditions, and after some processing this will result in a final state. The processing can be very complex, no doubt. But the notion captured by the model is that of a passive response to incoming stimulation. In short, the model described by the psychophysical chain has two key features: it applies to separate and independent senses, and it conceives each of these as passive receptors of the incoming sense data.

For many researchers in perception science today, both these features are fundamentally wrong. The senses are not separate. In fact, even providing a scientifically satisfactory definition of what a 'sense' might be proves much harder than our naïve psychology suggests (see Box 1.1). Moreover, perception is not a set of passive channels for inputting data. Perceptual mechanisms work as active seekers of stimulus information. Perception is not just a sequential chain of events, but a cyclical process, because we are mobile organisms and through our movements we continuously obtain new sensory signals from the environment. For this reason, contemporary theories model perception not as a psychophysical chain, but as a perception-action cycle (Jeannerod, 2006; Jacob & Jeannerod, 2003; Nöe, 2004; Milner & Goodale, 1995; for the earlier work that introduced the term, see Neisser, 1976)—in fact, a *multisensory* perception-action cycle. This is also the model adopted in this book. In the next sections, we provide further arguments for this choice.

Box 1.1 The five senses reconsidered

The idea that humans have five senses is so deeply rooted in our culture that one could justly consider it as a key component of the way we think about ourselves (Figure 1.2). But are the senses really five? Ask anybody and you will get a puzzled look: of course they are. Yet a quick tour to the libraries, real and virtual, brings about quite a few surprises. Aristotle, and after him all philosophers in the Aristotelian tradition, maintained that we have six senses, not five. In addition to sight, hearing, smell, taste, and touch, he believed that humans have a *common sense* (see Gregoric, 2007). We return to this intriguing idea in the final part of this book. According to the witty *Book of General Ignorance* (Lloyd & Mitchinson, 2006), the senses are nine. In addition to the usual five, humans have senses for temperature, balance, pain, and bodily awareness. If instead we chose to lend credence to the 'sense' entry on *Wikipedia* (last checked on May 1, 2017; interestingly, this one keeps changing), the senses are ten. To the usual five, we must add other five 'non-traditional' senses for pain, balance, body position and movement, temperature, and other internal senses. Who is right?

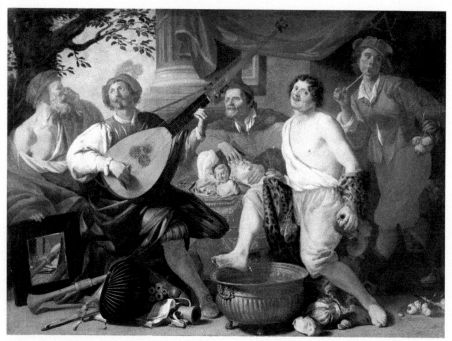

Figure 1.2 Allegory of the five senses. In this painting by Theodoor Rombouts (1597–1637), sight is represented by the man holding a pair of spectacles; hearing by the man playing a theorbo; touch by the blind man touching a statue; taste by the man holding a glass of wine; smell by the man smoking a pipe. The history of art is rich in paintings and, to a lesser extent, statues celebrating the 'five' senses. But are there really five senses?
Museum voor Schone Kunsten, Ghent, Belgium/Bridgeman Images

Box 1.1 Continued

Let's take a look at a handbook of neural science (Kandel & Schwartz, 1985). We learn that sensory channels are defined in relation to the concept of a *receptor*. A receptor is a cell in the nervous system whose job is to transform external energy into a neural sign, a function that is called *transduction*. This is not a book about human physiology, but we can try to apply this criterion. First of all, there are only two known mechanisms of transduction in vertebrates: those based on ion channels, which in humans code mechanical and thermal stimuli as well as acid and salty tastants, and those based on G-protein coupling, which code light patterns, odorants, and sweet, bitter, and umami tastants (see Chapter 5). However, a complete list of receptors includes five types in the retina, the light-sensitive layer of tissue lining the inner surface of the eye (the three cone types for day vision, the rods for night vision, and the less-known light-sensitive ganglion cells for the regulation of night/day cycles), two types of receptor in the organ of Corti within the inner ear (the outer hair cells for pre-amplification and the inner hair cells for converting sound to a neural signal); at least nine different types in the skin (Pacinian corpuscles, Ruffini's organs, Meisnsner's corpuscles, and Merkel's disks for pressure and vibration, thermal receptors for cold and warm, receptors for pain, plus specialized mechanoreceptors for itch and affective touch); two types in the muscles and joints (muscle spindles for changes in muscle length and the Golgi tendon organs for muscle tension); additional balance mechanoreceptors in the semi-circular canals and in the otolithic organs also within the inner ear (hair cells respectively sensing head rotation and linear acceleration); additional internal mechano-receptors and nociceptors within internal organs; and a large number of chemoreceptors in the tongue, palate, cheek, epiglottis, and upper oesophagus (for gustation) and in the olfactory bulb in the nasal cavity (for detecting odorants). In short, if we were to use the receptor criterion, we would have to conclude that the number of human senses is either two or well above 20, depending on which criterion we choose for classifying.

But reading on through the handbook of neural science, we would also learn that sensory systems can be studied at the organ level. We certainly have sophisticated organs that play a fundamental role in perception. The eye, the ear, the tongue, and the nose immediately come to mind, as they are well localized and identifiable, and obviously re-latable to four of the 'senses'. But what about touch? That the skin can be considered the organ for touch is less obvious. The skin covers the whole body and coincides with it. It certainly is not as localized and identifiable as the previous four, and there are also sen-sory signals from the interior of the body, where there is no skin. If these are not part of touch, what sense should they be grouped with? But let us concede for the moment that we can consider the skin an organ. Do we now have a criterion for stating that there are five senses? Not really. There is at least another obvious organ that has a well-defined sen-sory function: it is the organ of balance within the inner ear. Do we have six senses then?

In response, a psychophysicist might argue that human senses respond to informa-tion carried only by three forms of physical energy: electromagnetic (light), mechanical

Box 1.1 Continued

(pressure, stretch, vibration including sound), and chemical (tastants and odorants). Therefore, sensory receptors could also be grouped into three categories only: photoreceptors, mechanoreceptors, and chemoreceptors, suggesting that in reality humans have only three senses. An evolutionary biologist might, however, respond that humans senses evolved to serve only two basic functions: obtaining information about the external world, and knowing about the internal state of one's body. Perhaps we have only two senses after all? Perhaps. But we might then stumble into the work of English neurophysiologist Charles Scott Sherrington (1906), who argued that we should distinguish between two types of internal sense, proprioception that codes the position and movement of our body in space, and interoception that codes internal signals related to states such as hunger, drowsiness, or the need to go to the toilet. Maybe three is a more correct count of the number of senses?

If all this sounds confusing, perhaps we should change the angle of attack completely. Let us try a philosopher. An old and respected philosophical approach is that of *phenomenology*, the study of the qualitative character of percepts (phenomena are, indeed, things as they appear to us in our perceptual conscious experience). Incidentally, phenomenology also plays an important role in perception science, as mentioned in Tutorial 1.1, so the idea that we might find there useful criteria for 'sensehood' is not so far fetched. We could therefore ask our philosopher if all phenomena are of the same kind, or if there are distinguishable perceptual *modes* that have unique, specific phenomenal characters that belong to each mode and to no others. Presumably, he will respond that percepts are certainly not all of the same kind. For instance, there is something about the character of visual phenomena that is intrinsically different from that of auditory phenomena. These two kinds of perceptions have different *qualia,* the term invented by philosopher of mind Lewis (1929) to define 'what it is like' to experience a given percept (Nagel, 1974). Our analysis might eventually lead to the conclusion that there are at least seven different such modes of human perception: the visual, auditory, tactile, gustatory, olfactory, noxious, and thermal. In addition, and importantly, there is an eighth mode that is different from the previous seven because it is defined not by the presence of a certain perceptual character, but by its absence. In this mode, something is actually perceived, not merely imagined or thought-of, but the way the percept is given to our consciousness does not have a modality, i.e. it is *a-modal.* The notion of amodal perception is somewhat counterintuitive, and may seem puzzling. But consider Figure 1.3. It is quite clear here that recognizable grey letter figures are perceived as if they were behind the grey occluding blobs. Yet about 50 percent of those figures are not given in the visual modality, because the black occluders prevent you from actually seeing the corresponding parts. We return to the issue of amodal perception in section 1.6, and elsewhere, for it has several important implications. For the purpose of the present box, however, it will suffice to stress that phenomenological analysis also fails to provide a clear justification for the notion that we have five senses.

Box 1.1 Continued

So how many senses do humans have? Having tried different angles of attack, we can appreciate that providing a scientifically accurate answer is far from trivial. Paradoxically, the only firm conclusion that seems to emerge from our list of potential answers is that by no criterion the senses are five. This leads to a different, and at least as interesting question: why then are the five senses such a deeply ingrained idea in our language and in our naïve psychology? The answer lies, in our opinion, in the tight coupling between perceiving and acting that characterizes the human mind (and, we suspect, the minds of most non-human animals). Perception is a complicated business that must be studied at several different levels of analysis. Our criteria for sensehood focused either on the initial levels (the 'input' to the mind, so to speak), or on the final product (the 'output'). Thus we discussed external stimuli, receptors, and consciously perceived qualities of objects in the world. However, the path from external stimuli to percepts is not a linear one. Sensory channels do not act as passive sensors recording levels of external energy, but are part of systems that actively seek information in flows of ever-changing energy patterns. Perception is a form of exploratory activity, and there are exactly five ways that humans can actively and consciously explore the environment: by looking, listening, feeling, tasting, and sniffing. Presumably, it is this fundamental feature of the way we relate to our environment that forms the basis for our impression that there are five senses.

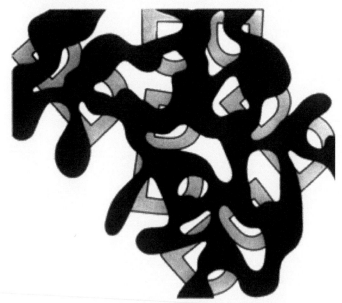

Figure 1.3 Amodal completion. You perceive capital Bs, but only about 50 percent of your experience of the Bs is in the visual modality, such that you actually have a visual percept. A large part of the Bs is perceived amodally. Yet, the experience that these are complete Bs is compelling and quite different from imagining the Bs or consciously reconstructing them by a reasoning process.

1.2 **Is perception modular?**

Component parts that function independently as units but can be used within a larger, more complex structure are called *modules*. The idea that the mind consists of a collection of modular input systems is deeply ingrained in the way we think of cognition. For instance, apart from a handful of academic reference books, written for specialists and highly technical (Calvert, Spence & Stein, 2004; Murray & Wallace, 2012; Spence & Driver, 2004; Stein, 2012), college textbooks on perception are books about visual, auditory, tactile, and chemical input systems, each discussed separately and on their own terms. There are of course some good reasons for adopting this view, at least in certain contexts.

First of all, the initial step of perception is always a neural response at the level of receptors, the cells in the nervous system that convert physical stimuli into neural impulses. This process is called *transduction* by sensory physiologists, and if you are one it makes perfect sense for you to focus on the behaviour of a single receptor type. For instance, we now have a very good understanding of the physical and biochemical mechanisms that underlie the ability of retinal photoreceptors in the eye to transduce electromagnetic energy. At this level of analysis, reference to multisensory processes is of course of no use.

In addition, ample evidence suggests that there are sensory channels in the nervous systems. Within these channels, information is initially processed in parallel by neurons specialized to code it most efficiently and then relayed to unique sensory areas in the cortex. This is especially clear for the large majority of visual signals, which after an intermediate stage of processing in a structure located deep in the brain (the so-called lateral geniculate nucleus of the thalamus) reach their cortical target in the occipital lobe (the so-called area V1, the primary visual cortex). Similarly, somatosensory signals reach cortical area S1, the primary somatosensory cortex, in the parietal lobe, and auditory signals reach area A1 in the temporal lobe (Figure 1.4). The existence of a unique primary sensory area is somewhat less clear for olfactory and gustatory signals.

Finally, we know that each cortical region that seems to serve the function of primary sensory area is organized in a distinct way (that is, has a specific *functional architecture*). For instance, it is well established that at the level of the primary somatosensory cortex there is a precise mapping of somatosensory signals from specific body parts to specific parts of S1. This suggests that S1 contains a spatial representation of the body which is based on a *somatotopic* frame of reference, that is, on coordinates that are measured in relation to the body. We discuss this mapping in greater detail in Chapter 2 of this book. Similarly, at the level of V1 there is a precise mapping of signals from the retinas which is based on a *retinotopic* frame of reference, and at the level of A1 there is a mapping based on the frequency of incoming sound—a *tonotopic* frame. This is illustrated in Figure 1.5 for S1 and A1. For an illustration of the functional architecture of V1, which requires consideration of binocular and colour processing, we recommend consulting any standard perception textbook (e.g. Wolfe at al., 2012). Although olfactory and gustatory areas are not

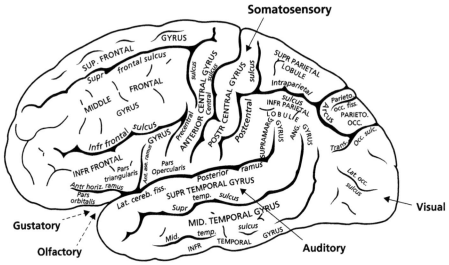

Figure 1.4 Approximate locations of the so-called primary sensory areas. We reproduce Figure 726 from Henry Gray's classic human anatomy textbook (Gray, 1918). Primary visual area V1 is located in the striate cortex of the occipital lobe; primary auditory area A1 is located in the superior gyrus of the temporal lobe; primary somatosensory area S1 in the postcentral gyrus of the parietal lobe. The primary gustatory cortex AI/FO is generally believed to be located in two structures called the insula and frontal operculum within the inferior frontal gyrus of the frontal lobe, although its precise location in humans has not been determined conclusively. Primary olfactory cortex has been related to several structures that are located deep within the medial temporal lobe. Due to their location, the latter two cortical regions are not directly visible in the figure. To expose them, you would need to separate the frontal from the temporal lobe at the lateral fissure using surgical instruments such as retractors.

Reproduced from Henry Gray, FRS, *Anatomy of the Human Body, 20e*, ed. Warren H. Lews, BS, MD, Lea and Febiger, New York, 1918.

so easily understood in terms of spatial encoding, the presence of neurons responding to specific taste or olfactory qualities is also consistent with specific functional architectures.

Specificities in the functional characteristics of receptors, primary sensory areas, and cortical mappings are consistent with an account of perception as a collection of independent, domain-specific mechanisms. The broad psychological theory underlying this account is that of the *modularity of mind* (Fodor, 1983). In a classic monograph, American philosopher Jerry Fodor proposed that the functional architecture of the human mind is best captured by a distinction between *horizontal* and *vertical* faculties. Horizontal faculties subserve 'the fixation of belief' whereas vertical faculties are for 'input analysis' (p. 120). The former include general purpose cognitive processes, such as memory, attention, and reasoning. The latter are mechanisms that transform sensory information into abstract representations for later processing by 'higher-level' mental processes. Fodor called these mechanisms *input systems,* and argued that the fundamental difference between input systems and horizontal faculties is that input systems are modular. Modular

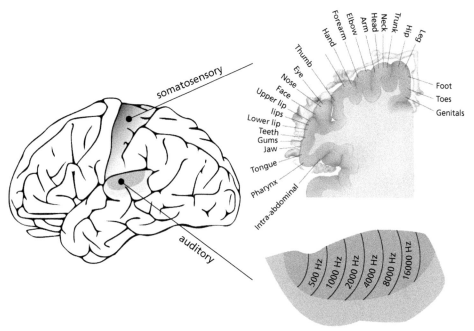

Figure 1.5 Maps in primary sensory areas. A schematic illustration of somatotopic (top) and tonotopic (bottom) maps in the primary somatosensory and auditory cortices.

input systems are characterized, according to Fodor, by several distinguishing properties, the most important here being *domain specificity, fixed neural architecture,* and *information encapsulation.* The first, domain specificity, refers to the fact that individual input systems are tuned to special classes of stimulus properties: for instance colour, shapes, or spatial relations between objects for vision; melodic structure, rhythm, or the human voice for hearing. The second, fixed, neural architecture refers to the fact that neural substrates of input systems are largely hardwired in specific neural architectures that do not change over development. The third property of modular systems, information encapsulation, refers to the fact that any input system processes information only within its own domain and is not affected by processing done within other domains. For instance, processing of spatial relations within vision proceeds independently of spatial processing within hearing.

Fodor's conception of perceptual mechanisms as independent modules has been greatly influential in cognitive neuroscience, and still lurks in the theoretical background of a lot of research papers. One of the reasons, presumably, is that several perceptual phenomena appear quite consistent with Fodor's criteria for modularity. Consider, for instance, phenomena like the so-called optical-geometrical illusions. In Müller-Lyer's illusion, for instance, two segments are physically the same length, but perceptually they seem to have different lengths due to the effect of inward- and outward-pointing fins. This illusion occurs automatically, and is not affected by knowing that the segments are, in fact, the same. Most important, for a long time it has been generally believed that these effects are strongly visual, and are not altered by concomitant input from other (modular) sensory channels. For instance, in a much-cited study, Rock and Victor (1964) had participants wear prismatic goggles that optically shrunk the retinal projection of a test square. While they looked at the shrunken square, participants could feel it with their hand (a clever arrangement prevented them from seeing the hand itself). Thus, participants received veridical haptic information about the square's size along with the distorted visual information. Yet, Rock and Victor reported that vision dominated perceived size: when asked to pick, on a graded scale, a square that had the same size as the one they were currently seeing and feeling, they picked a size consistent with the optical distortion.

In the last two decades, however, the theoretical and empirical bases of Fodor's conception of input systems have been questioned. Evidence from animal models demonstrates that sensory channels interact at intermediate stations in the neural path from receptors to cortex; for instance, in the superior colliculus (Wallace, Meredith, & Stein, 1998), amygdala (Nishjo, Ono, & Nishino, 1988), and thalamus (Cappe, Morel, Barone, & Rouiller, 2009; Komura et al., 2005). For higher level neural processes, there is even stronger evidence that most of them are in some form multisensory (Alais, Newell, & Mamassian, 2010; Ghazanfar & Schroder, 2006; Klemen & Chambers, 2012). These studies cast doubt on the validity of Fodor's characterization of input systems. Parts of the primary auditory cortex have been shown to respond to visual signals during lip reading (Calvert et al., 1997), the primary visual cortex has been shown to respond to somatosensory signals in tactile tasks (Sathian & Zangaladze, 2002), and the putative primary gustatory and olfactory areas receive abundant input from other channels, in particular visual and somatosensory ones (we discuss this in greater detail in Chapter 5). It has been argued (Driver & Noesselt, 2008) that these observations are very difficult to reconcile with the view that the cortical centres of input systems are strictly specific for certain classes of stimuli. To some extent, Fodor himself was aware of this issue, as he conceded (in a footnote) that, in some limited cases, domains for modular inputs systems could be defined across sensory channels (see note 13 in part III; the example given being language perception by ear and eye, a problem that had been extensively studied at the time of publication of Fodor's book). Similarly, several studies have demonstrated that primary sensory areas that are deprived of their normal sensory input can be recruited for processing of other kinds of input. This has been documented, for instance, in early blind individuals where primary visual areas can become responsive to non-visual input (Collignon et al., 2013). These results argue against a fixed neural architecture for input systems.

Finally, and most importantly for the purposes of this book, behavioural studies suggests that in many perceptual tasks multisensory interactions are much more important than was originally believed (Driver & Spence, 2000). For instance, rub the back of your left hand with your right hand. How does the skin feel? Dry or well hydrated? Smooth or wrinkled? Whatever you have answered, note that your perception has a specific tactile character, is localized on the skin, the 'feeling' comes from the skin. Yet, it can be demonstrated that your percept does not depend merely on the tactile signal, but is also modulated by hearing. If the sound produced by the rubbing is experimentally modified, for instance, by emphasizing higher frequencies, the hand will feel smoother and drier (the *parchment-skin illusion,* Jousmäki & Hari, 1998). Or recall the last time you saw a movie. Where did the voice of the actors on screen come from? Naturally, it seemed to come from the lips of the actors. Yet, the sound did not come from the lips on screen, but from loudspeakers variously positioned in the theatre. What you experienced is a form of visual capture of hearing, often called the *ventriloquist illusion* (Figure 1.6). Effects such as these are far from rare, and provide strong evidence that input systems do not function as encapsulated modules. In perception, multisensory interactions are the norm rather than the exception (Shimojo & Shams, 2001).

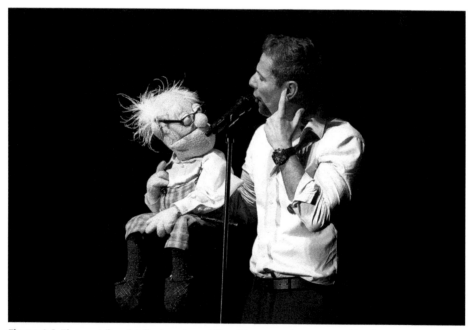

Figure 1.6 The ventriloquist illusion. A ventriloquist can produce acceptable, funny-sounding speech without moving the lips or while masking minimal lip movements. If this is done while moving the puppet mouth, the illusion arises that the sound comes from the puppet, not the ventriloquist. The effect is an instance of visual capture of sound; the reverse effect (auditory capture of vision) can also happen in certain conditions. Ventriloquist Paul Zerdin performs onstage at the Paramount on March 25, 2016 in Huntington, New York.
© Debby Wong/Shutterstock.com

1.3 **Is perception passive?**

We now address the second implication of the classic psychophysical chain. Is perception passive? To answer this question, we draw on the work of James J. Gibson, one of the most influential perception scientists of the past century. A little more than 50 years ago, Gibson published a pioneering study entitled 'Observations on active touch' (Gibson, 1962). In this paper, now considered a classic of the field, Gibson did two things.

The first thing that Gibson did in his study was to collect a rich set of observations using a deceptively simple task: a participant described various properties of an object that was felt with the hand, when both hand and object were hidden behind a cloth curtain. The set-up allowed Gibson to witness the participant's hand movements while recording his or her verbal reports, and to compile a list of perceptual features that can be perceived by touch alone. This list included the object's unity, stability, rigidity, three-dimensional shape, and motion relative to the skin surface, as well as the texture, substance, curvature, slant relative to gravity, and slant of the object's surface, as well as its distance relative to another surface. Gibson observed that all these are readily perceived when freely exploring with the hand, whereas they often lead to misperception and difficulty if the hand was stimulated passively by pressing objects on the skin.

The second thing Gibson did was to perform an experiment. He went to his kitchen at home and grabbed six small cookie cutters from a drawer. These were nothing but metal strips bent to the forms shown in Figure 1.7. He showed the set to participants and told them that each corresponded to a number: the triangle was number 1, the star was number 2, and so on. After participants had learned this, he tested them for tactile recognition with no vision. Each cookie cutter was placed behind a curtain, participants felt them and had to call out the right number. Chance performance in this task is about 17 percent. Gibson found that the average accuracy of participants was 95 percent with active touching, but dropped to 29 percent if the cutters were passively pressed on the palm by a mechanical lever system. Thus, participants could recognize the shapes better than chance in both conditions, but there was a dramatic difference between active and passive touch. With active touch, performance was practically perfect. With passive touch, it dropped to just slightly better than chance.

That objects should be perceived best by way of active exploration makes good intuitive sense. Gibson, however, was able to see beyond what seems obvious. He recognized that the advantage of active touch cannot be easily reconciled with a model like the standard psychophysical chain. If perception is merely interpretation of proximal stimuli, then

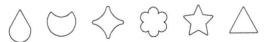

Figure 1.7 Gibson's cookie cutters. The six shapes employed in Gibson's seminal study on active touch.

Adapted from James J. Gibson, Observations on active touch, *Psychological Review*, 69 (6), pp. 477–491, doi: 10.1037/h0046962 © 1962, American Psychological Association.

conditions that enhance the precision and accuracy of responses to these stimuli should result in more precise and accurate percepts. Passively pressing a shape on the palm of the hand should provide exactly this type of enhancement, because the stimulus is stable and unvarying. Gibson's findings, however, went exactly in the opposite direction. The hand exploratory movements that he witnessed produced a continuously changing, seemingly chaotic constellation of mechanical events. Localized pressure on the finger-tips, mechanical deformations of the hand palm, and stretching of the skin in various lo-cations followed each other in a complex sequence. Passive stimulation instead produced a spatiotemporally well-defined pattern of proximal stimulation. Yet, the former seemed far superior in promoting accurate perception.

By adding a third condition, Gibson was also able to show that this superiority is not just due to the fact that in active touch the proximal stimulation changes over time. In this third condition, the cookie cutters were passively rotated on the palm of the hand by the experimenter. The location of the stimulation therefore was the same as the passive touch condition, but the stimulation changed continuously rather than re-maining stable. In this condition, recognition accuracy was 72 percent, much better than passive but still much worse than active touch. Near perfect performance, he concluded, requires a spatiotemporally varying stimulus but this must result from de-liberate exploration, not from passive motion. As Gibson himself stated: 'The living animal is stimulated not only from sources in the environment but also by itself. Its in-ternal organs provide stimulation, and so do the movements of its extremities and sense organs or feelers, and the locomotor movements of its whole body through space. [...] Action-produced stimulation is *obtained,* not *imposed* [...]. It is intrinsic to the flow of activity, not extrinsic to it [...]. The input is not merely afferent, in the terminology of the neurologist, but *reafferent*—that is, contingent upon efferent output.' (Gibson, 1966; p. 31; our italics).

Gibson's classic cookie cutter study is widely recognized as a theoretical turning point for perception science. So important has been its long term impact, that at least in the opinion of philosopher of science Rom Harré the cookie cutters belong to the 'twenty ex-periments that changed our view of the world' (Harré, 1981). One of the reasons for this is historical. In the early sixties and throughout the seventies and eighties, psychology was dominated by cognitivism. Researchers conceived of input systems pretty much in the way that Fodor described, and studied them as passive channels for inputting data into higher-level cognitive processes. To this aim, the instrument of choice was the tach-istoscope, an instrument that permits precise control of stimulus durations. Typical tach-istoscopic experiments involved extremely brief stimuli, very often lasting just a small fraction of a second. This permitted to determine exactly what input was provided to the system, but prevented participants from engaging in any form of exploratory activity. Gibson developed this point in his most famous last book, *The ecological approach to visual perception* (Gibson, 1979), which contains among many other things a forceful plea for active perception not only in exploratory touch, but also in vision and in all forms of perception.

For the purposes of this book, however, there is at least another feature that is worth examining. This is the often-neglected point that the cookie cutter experiment was a *multisensory* study. Specifically, it was a study of crossmodal recognition (see Chapter 4) requiring participants to match current tactile percepts to previously experienced visual percepts. We believe that this was not just a convenient methodological choice, but a direct consequence of Gibson's interest in studying active, exploratory perception. Perceptual exploration implies that the perceiver's body becomes, in a very concrete sense, a sort of organ for obtaining information from the environment—it becomes part of one's perceptual mechanisms rather than a mere actuator of motor behaviours. This in turn has two interesting implications. The first concerns the role of the body in all this. Perceptual exploration entails that sensory signals about the body, such as, for instance, signals about the hand in space or about the movements of the eye, need to be taken into account even in tasks involving the perception of external objects. The second concerns the role of movement in multisensory processes. If perceptual stimuli are obtained contingent on exploratory movement, then movement itself can become a common frame of reference for binding sensory signals from different channels (Fogassi & Gallese, 2004). Both implications play a key role in contemporary theories of 'embodied' cognition (see Wilson, 2002). In Gibson's work, they became the building blocks for his seminal notion of *perceptual systems*.

1.4 Perceptual systems

A 'system' may be defined as a set of interconnected elements forming a complex whole. The word is used in many contexts. In particular, it can be used in biology to refer to a set of organs having a common function (i.e. the digestive system, the respiratory system, and so on). In general systems theory (von Bertalannfy, 1968) a system is a model for a set of phenomena whose behaviour is critically dependent on structure and hierarchical organization. Crucially, a system exhibits *emergent properties,* that is, properties that result from the interaction between the components but cannot be reduced to the components alone. In natural phenomena, two examples are found in weather patterns, which develop at a global level from local interactions involving factors such as temperature or atmospheric pressure, and in the growth of crystals, which is driven by local interactions within the random motion of water molecules. The idea that perception includes processes of organization according to specific hierarchies, and that this can result in emergent properties, was a key idea of the Gestalt movement in psychology. We will return to some of the contributions of the Gestaltist to perception theory in Chapter 4. That Gestalt ideas had an influence on Gibson's theorizing was not coincidental. In the early years of Gibson's career, the German psychologist Kurt Koffka fled from Nazi Germany and landed a job at Smith College in Massachusetts, where Gibson held his first teaching position. Koffka was one of the founders of the Gestalt movement, the author of a vast monograph on the subject (Koffka, 1935), and an intellectual of great culture and scientific creativity. Meeting and discussing with Koffka did not make Gibson a Gestaltist, but it was certainly one of the spurs for his adoption of a systemic approach.

Gibson embraced systems in his second book, published four years after the famous cookie cutter study (Gibson, 1966). The book was entitled *The Senses Considered as Perceptual Systems*, as motivated in this famous passage: 'We shall have to conceive the external senses [...] as active rather than passive, as systems rather than channels, and as interrelated rather than mutually exclusive [...] they [...] should be denoted by a different term. They will here be called *perceptual systems*.' (Gibson, 1966; p. 47; italics are ours). In the book, Gibson argued two key points. First, he rejected the classic notion of the 'senses' as a collection of passive, unidirectional psychophysical channels. The functional units of perception are for actively sampling the available stimulation within perception-action cycles, not for passively inputting data. Second, he suggested that these units are fundamentally multisensory. Perceptual systems are interrrelated, not independent and modular. To fully understand Gibson's notion of a perceptual system, however, it is instructive to examine the actual list of systems that Gibson discussed in separate chapters of the book.

Gibson proposed that human minds have five perceptual systems (Gibson, 1966; table 1, p. 50), for basic orientation (balance, posture, velocity, and acceleration of the body), hearing (nature and location of vibratory events), haptics (mechanical and thermal properties of objects), smelling and tasting (volatile substances, nutrients), and vision (anything specifiable by patterns of light to the eye). He maintained that these are inherently multisensory. Consider perceiving one's posture. Postural information is provided by signals from the vestibular organs, but also from stretch receptors in the joints and in the muscles, from mechanical events on the skin, from sound localization, and from visual information about posture and movement of the body. Gibson argued that sensory signals in many instances provide equivalent information to the perceiver. For instance, he maintained that a fire is a source of four kinds of stimulation: sound, odor, heat, and light. The information to any of the corresponding perceptual systems may be considered equivalent to the extent that each specifies the same event. In addition, Gibson argued that the five perceptual systems have complex relations with motor systems, which he tentatively classified into seven categories: postural (compensatory movements for balance), orienting-investigating (any movement by head, eye, mouth, and hand to obtain external information), locomotor (any movement to change position relative to the environment), appetitive (any movement to take from, or give to, the environment, such as eating, breathing, or evacuating), performatory (any movement to alter the environment, such as displacing things or using tools), expressive (facial, postural, and vocal movements to specify emotions and the identity of the actor), and semantic (signalling movements including speech).

Gibson's systemic approach entailed a radical restructuring of the way scientists think about sensory processing and perception. Many features of his theorizing have been controversial, but the emphasis on multisensory processing and on active perception has gradually become a staple of the way most researchers think about perception. After almost fifty years, unsurprisingly, there are also parts that appear outdated. For instance, Gibson's notion of a unitary visual system is difficult to reconcile with evidence suggesting at least partly separate visual functions for spatial processing in near and far space, whereas Gibson's clear distinction between the visual and auditory systems contrast with the well-documented fact that audiovisual interactions are important in the perception of far space. In general, Gibson's categories of perceptual systems appear somewhat arbitrary. Why he chose to limit them to five remains poorly justified, and how these are interconnected is unclear. Gibson's notion of equivalent information oversimplifies the complexity of multisensory interactions within different contexts. On the motor side, Gibson was almost certainly right in postulating complex relations between perceptual and motor functions, a suggestion that was indeed revolutionary at the time. However, his treatment of motor systems as separate from perceptual systems now appears too drastic. As we have seen, perception is an activity in itself and exploratory activities are what we do when we perceive. Thus, many contemporary models of perception do not to make a sharp distinction between perceptual and motor functions, but think of functional units of analysis that have both perceptual and motor properties (e.g. Fogassi & Gallese, 2004).

1.5 **This book**

In planning the structure of this book, we have also adopted a systemic approach. But instead of starting from a list of senses, or of perceptual systems, however defined, we have chosen to organize our material around subsets of what is to be perceived. This has lead us to identify a set of functions that are typical of what perception does for all us throughout our lives: perceiving our own body and ourselves as its owners and controllers; perceiving other objects beyond our bodies; perceiving those special objects that provide nourishment; perceiving spatial and temporal relations between objects. To complement our discussion of these domains of human perception, we have also included chapters on the intriguing phenomenon known as synaesthesia, which may be regarded as an anomaly in the multisensory processes involved in object perception; and on multisensory attention and learning. In addition, in most chapters we have tried to include examples of the many applications of multisensory perception science. We treat our topic as inherently multisensory from the start, asking what different sensory channels are typically involved in providing information relevant to each function, how they interact, and how this is relevant to our ability to perceive those specific features of the world. In addition, our discussion of each of these topics strongly emphasizes the active and exploratory nature of perceptual processes, and therefore the strong links between perception and action. When compared to other monographs about perception, the resulting organization is unusual but, we hope, engaging and accessible even to readers who are not specialists. In fact, it seems to us that our choice of topics and our approach follows quite naturally from adopting a multisensory perspective. Most of naturally occurring perception and sensorimotor control is multisensory, as both exploratory and performatory movements require combining external information with information about the state of our own body. And on the other side of the perception-action coin, internal models of actions turn out to be important for understanding a host of other perceptual phenomena even when these do not require overt movement.

Thus, this book retains many of Gibson's early ideas, but does not make an attempt to carve perception into specific subsystems a priori. In principle, it should be possible to identify a set of processing mechanisms for specific functions, to describe their functional and underlying neural structure, and perhaps even to evaluate to what degree they can function in a modular fashion. We believe, however, that Gibson's list of perceptual and motor systems eventually turns out to be not particularly useful. The study of the multisensory and active processes involved in perceiving objects such as our own body or the food we eat instead seem to suggest that these complex functions are subserved by several highly adaptive multisensory and sensorimotor mechanisms. These involve rather complex neural circuits, implementing sophisticated neural computations. We are just beginning to understand some of these, and a fuller specification of these presumed functional components of perception has yet to be achieved (although, of course, some interesting attempts in this direction have been made; see, for instance, Previc, 1998).

In contrast with Gibson's approach, who was little interested in the neural bases of perception, this book also takes a more eclectic stance on the issue of levels of explanation. This is a key issue in the study of the mind (Marr, 1982), and a serious analysis would require discussing the deep problem of what constitutes a causal explanation in biology and in the cognitive neurosciences in particular (Hogan, 1994). For the purposes of this book, it will suffice to draw a clear distinction between two levels: neural substrate and adaptive function. We adopt the first when we discuss perception in terms of receptors, organs, or brain circuits; we adopt the second when we discuss the potential added value of multisensory over unisensory processing or inquire about formal models of multisensory integration. For many years, cognitive psychology stressed the functional level. For functionalists such as Fodor himself (1968) or Putnam (1975), minds can be studied by asking *how* and *for what* purpose we process information, and this can be done independently from *what* implements these functions, that is, the neural substrate. Mind states can be understood as a set of abstract logical relations (as in a computer program), and the concrete mechanisms that implement them (be they neural networks or silicon chips) are less important. In the contemporary cognitive neurosciences, however, a different approach has proved more fruitful. Rather than choosing a single level of analysis, many scholars seek to bridge across different levels (see for instance Teller, 1984). In this perspective, what implements a function also provides constraints on how it can be implemented. This is very much the principle that has inspired us in choosing our material for the different chapters of this book, which draws on findings from studies at several different levels and employing a variety of different methods (see Tutorial 1.1).

Tutorial 1.1 Methods in multisensory perception

To study multisensory interactions, psychologists and cognitive neuroscientists use a variety of methods and approaches. For the purposes of this tutorial, we will divide them into behavioural methods, neurophysiological and brain imaging methods, and patient studies. All three categories largely coincide with standard methodologies in perception science, but often take a new twist when applied to multisensory problems. This tutorial aims at providing a brief introduction to the research methods that will be cited in the chapters. Further details will be provided when necessary.

Perhaps the simplest research method, and a most useful one for the purposes of scientific communication, is phenomenological analysis and demonstration. Phenomenology is the study and description of one's perceptual experience, and it often leads to identification of the best conditions for experiencing a certain perceptual effect. These can then be exploited for demonstrating the effect itself to an audience, even in poorly controlled conditions, or even on the internet, as the identified conditions are cogent. One of our favourite such demonstrations is the illusion that one has two nosetips (a variant of the so-called Aristotle's illusion, discussed in Chapter 7), which is readily obtained in a large classroom by almost all students, and with entertaining but also pedagogically useful consequences. Very often, phenomenological demonstrations are based on creating conditions of multisensory conflict; that is, by pitting different sensory signals one against the other. This is a common strategy in perceptual psychology (see for instance Gregory, 1986) and an excellent way to discover conditions leading to dominance of one channel over others, as in the examples of visual capture that we introduced in the relation to the ventriloquist's illusion; or to reveal conditions where the conflicting signals result in percepts that cannot be reduced to either of the unisensory signals, as in some examples that we discuss on the next page. Information about participant's phenomenal experience can sometimes be gathered by appropriately constructed questionnaires. This is especially useful for higher-level perceptual contents, such as, for instance, the perception of a seen limb as belonging to one's own body, or the unusual associations between perceptual modalities that are experienced by synaesthetes.

Behavioural methods also continue to play an important role to collect quantitative data about perceptual tasks. Such data can be collected by psychophysical procedures to measure sensory thresholds or, more generally, the sensitivity of a perceptual mechanism in coding certain stimulus characteristics. Thresholds are derived, statistically, from estimates of accuracy and precision in discrimination tasks. For readers less versed in statistics and measurement theory, think of accuracy as one's ability to perceive an environmental feature correctly, and of precision as a measure of one's consistency in responding. Data about accuracy and precision provide key information for modelling multisensory interactions. For instance, some such interactions are well modelled by a weighted sum of the component sensory signals, where the more precise components are weighted more than the less precise. Additional useful information about perceptual efficiency lies in processing speed, which is estimated by measuring response times as a function of various multisensory manipulations. By comparing these manipulations, it is possible, for instance, to determine if the presence of redundant signals from different sensory channels improves efficiency, or if conflicting signals reduce it, putting different models of multisensory integration to test. Finally, another important source of behavioural data is the measurement of movement kinematics in response to unisensory or multisensory signals. This data allows us to understand how multisensory perception is used to guide actions and to test models of multisensory action control.

Over the last decades, the scientific study of perception has greatly benefited from technologies that let us visualize or modulate brain activity during specific tasks. Two widely used such techniques are *functional magnetic resonance* (fMRI) and *positron-emission tomography* (PET). These measure the metabolic consumption of substances such as oxygen and glucose in different brain areas. By comparing measures during task execution with appropriate baselines, it is possible to infer which areas are selectively active during the task under study. In addition to providing information on neural circuits involved in perception, the data are often useful to test models of multisensory interactions. Another often-used technique is the analysis of *event-related potentials* (ERP). This technique uses non-invasive electroencephalographic technology to measure weak electrical signals at different locations on the scalp while participants perform experimental tasks. ERP and fMRI data are often combined as the former have good temporal resolution but provide only very approximate information on the brain location of origin, where the latter fares much worse in timing activations but is more precise in localizing them. Theoretical predictions about the involvement of certain brain structures can also be tested using *transcranial magnetic stimulation* (TMS). This technique induces transient and well-localized electromagnetic fields to target brain areas, testing whether the magnetic interference modulates performance in tasks that are hypothesized to be subserved by those areas. Finally, important data about perceptual processing at the single neuron level have come from microelectrode recordings in animal models. For instance, key information about the rules of low-level multisensory integration has come from studies of single neurons in the superior culliculus (SC) of the cat (for a review, see Stein & Stanford, 2008).

Behavioural and physiological data can be collected from healthy participants but also from populations with atypical or clinical conditions. Synesthetes are examples that we already mentioned. Individuals suffering from sensory deprivation of some kind, such as blind or deaf people, are another example. Yet another example is found in patients who suffered brain damage due to stroke or other neurological conditions. These populations offer unique opportunities to test wide-ranging questions. For instance, comparing early and late-acquired forms of sensory deprivation can be informative about the role of innate mechanisms vs learning in multisensory interactions. Investigating how special populations learn to compensate for deficits can provide useful guidelines in the development of sensory prostheses, such as for instance cochlear implants. Recent developments in limb transplantation have begun to raise similar problems even for somatoperception. Patients suffering from sensory deafferentation often also provide opportunities to evaluate perceptual performance in the absence of one of its normal components. For instance, studying patients who have been deprived of sensory signals coming from the body (somatosensory *deafferentation)* has allowed researchers to test models of motor control in ways that would have been very difficult to achieve in humans with different methodologies.

Independent of the technology and the research method of choice, multisensory studies can also be grouped based on the general nature of the question of interest. It seems to us that in general terms questions motivating multisensory research can be grouped into three general categories. We will call them *what for* questions, *how* questions, and *whether* questions. Studies asking 'what for' questions are typically interested in understanding what added value multisensory perception brings, in comparison to unisensory conditions. Studies asking how questions are instead interested in determining the algorithms, or natural computations, that actually join different sensory signals into a unified percept, as well as their neural correlates. Studies asking whether questions, finally, are typically interested in what turns multisensory perception on or off, that is, on what makes the brain decide that multiple sensory signals must be unified rather than kept separate. We conclude this tutorial by providing examples of each kind of question.

Studies asking 'what for' questions typically compare performance under multisensory conditions and performance with the component unisensory signals only. These comparisons often document that performance becomes faster, more accurate, or more precise in multisensory conditions, in comparison to the unisensory component signals. An interesting party game that exemplifies this point is asking friends to identify food items with the nose and eyes closed. Many foods become hard to identify on the basis of taste signals alone, and surprisingly so in comparison with performance after adding smell or of course vision. In some cases, multisensory conditions even result in perceptual experiences that do not resemble any of the percepts experienced in unisensory conditions. An example is the McGurk effect (McGurk & McDonald, 1976; you can easily find an example by searching 'McGurk demo' on the net). Imagine a video showing a young woman pronouncing the syllable 'ga' while the soundtrack plays the syllable 'ba'. In these conditions, one hears 'ga', a syllable that was neither seen nor heard! Thus not only the perception of spoken speech, experienced as auditory, is in fact heavily influenced by vision of the articulatory movements; but also what is heard is a bit like an emergent property of the multisensory interaction, not reducible to any of the components. That visual signals are exploited to understand heard language makes good sense when you consider the adaptive value of perception. We often must strive to understand fellow humans that are talking to us in noisy environments (student parties, crowded trains, and narrow-band video conferences being the first examples that come to mind). Lip reading provides additional information that can help disentangle the speech signal from the noise.

Studies asking 'how' questions typically compare multisensory and unisensory signals with the goal of obtaining quantitative data on unisensory and multisensory responses that can then be modelled statistically. This can be done at the cell level, recording from multisensory neurons to determine how the cell codes simultaneous input from two or more converging sensory signals. It can also be done at a more global system level, for instance, by studying activity in brain areas of interest during multisensory stimulation. In most studies, however, how questions are addressed by psychophysical studies collecting various indices of perceptual efficiency in unisensory and multisensory conditions, and comparing them with modelling predictions. Over the last decade or so, many of these models have embraced conceptual tools derived from statistical sampling theory (see Chapter 4), although this is not the only possible approach and is probably not applicable to all forms of multisensory interaction. In sampling theory, the best (or 'optimal') way to combine statistics from separate samples into a single estimate of a population parameter is to weight each statistic by its precision. When applied to multisensory integration, this idea provides an ideal optimal integrator against which multisensory performance can be evaluated. An excellent example of this is the study of the ventriloquist effect performed in his Pisa laboratory by the Australian-born perception scientist David Burr (Alais & Burr, 2004). Alais & Burr manipulated the reliability of vision by blurring their visual stimuli to various degrees, and paired them with auditory stimuli at different locations. Using this paradigm, they were able to show that visual signals capture the location of auditory signals when vision is reliable (i.e. unblurred and therefore well-localized stimuli), whereas auditory signals capture the location of the visual ones when vision is unreliable (i.e. blurred and therefore less well-localized stimuli). This suggests that the integration of visual and auditory signals in the multisensory perception of location is approximately optimal (in the statistical sense). Thus, the classic ventriloquist effect turns out to be a special case of a more general principle of audio-visual interactions.

Studies asking 'whether' questions, finally, aim at identifying rules or constraints that the brain could exploit to correctly decide when to join multisensory signals together and when to keep them separate. This is a key issue which is still not well understood. When multiple sensory signals are present, they may or may not originate from the same object or event. If they do, then binding them might be advantageous, but if they do not keeping them separate would be more appropriate. Let us consider the so called *mirror illusion*, another well-known effect that can be reproduced easily at one's home. Sit down in front of a table and have a friend hold a mirror in the direction of your body's midline, such that you can place one hand behind the mirror and the other in front of it. Now look diagonally into the mirror. You will see a reflection of the hand in front, but most likely you will have the impression that you are actually looking at the hand behind, as if you were seeing through the mirror. We return to various implications of this set up in Box 2.2 in the next chapter. For now, it will suffice to say that in this case there is a very strong tendency to bind the visual and somatosensory signals, and the perceived location of the (unseen) hand behind the mirror depends as much on the visual signal (actually from the reflection of the other hand) as on the somatosensory signal. It is generally very difficult to keep the two signals separate, even though one knows very well that this would be the correct interpretation of what is going on. The tendency to bind, however, becomes increasingly weaker as the spatial separation between the seen and the felt position is increased, or if one of the signals is delayed. In general, therefore, for the multisensory perception of location a spatial rule and a temporal rule appear to determine whether binding takes place or not. When the conflict between the two signals is large enough, binding seems to be prevented. This of course begs the question, how does the brain determine whether the two signals originate from the same location in space, or moment in time. We will address these issues in later chapters of the book.

1.6 **A note on terminology**

Before we begin our discussion, a final note on terminology is in order. In writing this book, we have had a chance to survey a large part of the literature on multisensory perception over several decades and have been forced to think about connections with more traditional perception research. This has led us to notice some terms that are now commonly used in multisensory work but have, traditionally, different meanings and refer to different levels of analysis in perception science. Although this often has no serious consequences, in some cases it can create ambiguity, terminological confusion, and even potential misunderstanding. This section is somewhat technical, as we added it for readers that are familiar with the multisensory literature (if you do not belong to this category, you might consider skipping it or perhaps reading it after you have finished the book), but we believe it is important to clarify how we will use some key terms and how our usage might differ from those of others at least in certain contexts. The main issue regards the notion of *sensory modality* as it is often used in multisensory research either in this form or in related expressions that use the adjectives *modal, amodal, crossmodal, polymodal,* and *supramodal.*

The expression *sensory modality* is commonly used in the multisensory literature to refer to 'the senses'. It has been used, to mention only a few examples, to argue that 'sensory modalities are not separate modalities' (Shimojo & Shams, 2001); that 'inputs to different sensory modalities can bring information about the same event' (De Gelder & Bertelson, 2003); that the brain 'binds together signals from multiple sensory modalities' (Bushara, Hanakawa, Immisch, & Toma, 2003); that the perception of flavour 'arises from the combination of inputs from several sensory modalities' (Marks, Elgart, Burger, & Chakwin, 2007); that there are 'brain areas tuned to a modality' (Klemen & Chambers, 2012). It is clear from these representative examples that the term *sensory modality* is used to refer to neural or functional mechanisms, or to sensory information coded by those mechanisms. This poses at least two problems.

First, what such mechanisms are may be obvious from the standpoint of naïve psychology. In the everyday use of language, talk of the five senses is commonplace. However, from a scientific standpoint defining the senses proves quite hard. As we have seen, there is no obvious way to answer even the simple question how many senses there are (Keeley, 2013; see also Box 1.1). Second, usage of the terms *modal* and *modalities* have a long tradition in perception science, but with a completely different meaning. This use can be traced back to Helmholtz (1867), who proposed that contents of experience belong to different modalities when they are so different that no transition or comparison is possible between them, i.e. they have distinct phenomenal characters that can only be defined in terms of first-person experience. In this notion, modalities refer to qualitatively different modes of perceptual experience, such as the visual or the olfactory mode, not to sensory mechanisms. They are a property of percepts, not of their neural or functional counterparts. The notion of *perceptual* modalities and the associated concept of *amodal* perception have later been central to the work of Michotte (Michotte, Thinès, & Crabbé, 1964). The Kanizsa triangle (Kanizsa, 1955) is a good example of how these terms are traditionally used. When we see the triangle (Figure 1.8) we are experiencing *modal completion*, that is, we are perceiving the edges of a foreground (illusory) surface in the visual modality; at the same time, we are experiencing *amodal completion* of the inducing structures

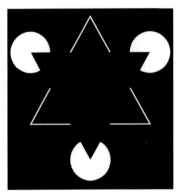

Figure 1.8 The Kanizsa illusory triangle.
Drawing from Kanizsa, G, 'Margini quasi-percettivi in campi con stimolazione omogenea', *Rivista di Psicologia*, 49 (1), pp. 7–30, 1955.

behind the illusory triangle, that is, we have a perceptual experience of those structures as continuing and forming complete shapes behind an occluder.

The vagueness of the notion of sensory modalities and the terminological inconsistency with earlier perception science are undesirable. However, the issue becomes even more problematic when considering several composite locutions that use the adjective *modal*. These are often used with meanings that are inconsistent with the earlier usage, sometimes also carrying parasite theoretical implications. Perhaps the most salient case in point is the use of *amodal* in the notion of *amodal features*. These have been defined as features that can be used to identify an object or event in more than one sensory modality (see, for instance, Spence, 2011). This definition is ambiguous: it can be understood to allude to *stimulus* features that can be coded by more than one neural sensory mechanism (e.g. spatial extent); or to *perceived* features that are somewhat the same or similar across different perceptual modes (e.g. perceived intensity). In either interpretation, moreover, the definition is self-contradictory. The privative alpha means 'absence of', whereas the definition implies 'presence of several'. In the traditional sense, amodal percepts are experiences that lack (privative alpha) the characteristics of a perceptual mode, experiences 'between perceiving and thinking' (Kanizsa, 1979). In the current multisensory usage, amodal features have become features that are not associated with a specific perceptual mode or neural sensory mechanism, and can thus appear in, or be coded by, many.

In this book, we have adopted a slightly modified terminology which, in our opinion, avoids these problems. We will use the term *perceptual modality* to refer to the quality, or mode, of perceptual experience. In Box 1.1 we have argued that seven such modes can be identified—visual, auditory, olfactory, gustatory, tactile, thermal, and noxious. Each of these has a distinct phenomenology, that is, a distinct quality which can only be defined in terms of first-person experience (see Box 1.1). Accordingly, we will use the adjective *amodal* to refer to phenomenal experience that lacks a perceptual modality, as in the experience of amodal completion. In contrast, we will refer to object features that can be experienced in more than one perceptual modality (such as, for instance, the object's size) as *modality aspecific,* while we will refer to features that can be experience only in one modality (such as colour) as *modality specific.* Finally, we will reserve the adjective *multimodal* for all those events or conditions whereby multisensory perception produces conscious content in more than one perceptual modality. This happens in many contemporary man-machine interfaces, such as, for instance, your smartphone or your laptop. But multimodal experience is also typical of more basic phenomena which are also discussed in this book, such as, for instance, *crossmodal recognition* (see Chapter 4: you experience X1 in modality A, say vision, then you experience X2 in modality B, say touch; you recognize X2 as the same as X1), and *crossmodal correspondence* (see Chapter 5: you experience X in modality A, say vision, then you experience Y in modality B, say hearing; although there is no obvious connection between X and Y, you spontaneously experience a natural connection, a sense that X and Y 'go together').

Our proposed usage of *modality* pertains to the phenomenology of perception, not to underlying neural mechanisms nor to their function. When referring to mechanisms, we will use instead the adjective *sensory.* Thus, psychophysical mechanisms coding a specific type of stimulus will be called *sensory channels,* in accord with well-established usage in psychophysics and physiology (e.g. Livingstone & Hubel, 1987). Sensory channels will be described as mechanisms that code specific *sensory signals,* and perceptual mechanisms that process signals from different channels will be called *multisensory.* To fully appreciate the distinction, consider how multisensory stimuli and multimodal experiences relate to one another. Multisensory stimulation does not necessarily lead to multimodal experience. In fact, in many cases, stimulation from multiple sensory channels results in a unified percept in a *single* modality. A striking example of this is how we perceive the flavour of food (see Chapter 5), which is entirely experienced in the taste modality, whereas it depends crucially also on signals that come from olfactory, somatosensory, and even visual and auditory channels. Conversely, unisensory stimulation does not necessarily lead to unimodal experience. In the peculiar condition known as synaesthesia (see Chapter 6), a single stimulus causes the synaesthete to have a percept in the modality usually associated with that stimulus (say, a sound is perceived as a musical tone), but also a concurrent percept in another, seemingly unrelated modality (say, a coloured flash). For consistency, we will also talk about *multisensory brain areas, multisensory neurons,* and about processes of *multisensory binding, combination,* or *integration,* even though the adjective 'multimodal' is sometimes used in the literature to refer to these things.

Chapter 2

Perceiving Your Own Body

2.1 The homuncular enigma

Have you ever visited the neuroscience section of a museum or science fair? If you are reading this book most likely you have, and you have probably encountered the concept of the somatosensory *homunculus*. Next to illustrations of the strips of brain cortex receiving signals from the body, termed primary somatosensory cortex or S1 (Figure 2.1a), museums often display the somatosensory homunculus in two ways: as a series of body parts draped along S1, from the fissure between the brain hemispheres to the most lateral part of the cortex (Figure 2.1b), and as a grotesque 'small man' with dwarfish trunk and limbs but oversized hands, ears, lips, tongue, feet, and genitalia (Figure 2.1c). Both these visual representations of the body in the brain have become icons of psychology and neuroscience (Schott, 1993), and they are meant to represent two key notions about the brain basis of body perception. We start by considering each in turn.

The first notion is the existence of some sort of map of the body in the somatosensory cortex, i.e. an ordered topography of the peripheral somatosensory signals in S1. Consider Figure 2.1b. As we travel through S1 starting from the fissure between the hemispheres, we first encounter cortical territories receiving afferents from the genitalia, toes, foot, leg, and trunk. Next, we find territories that receive inputs from the shoulder, arm, hand, and fingers. Adjacent to the region dedicated to the thumb, we find territories receiving sensations from the eyes, nose, and face. Finally, in the most lateral part of the hemisphere, we find territories receiving afferents from the oral cavity, tongue, pharynx, and abdomen. The second important notion illustrated by the somatosensory homunculus is the remarkably different amount of cortical territory devoted to the somatosensory signals originating from different body parts. As can be seen from Figure 2.1b, the regions of S1 dedicated to certain body regions are disproportionately large in comparison to those of other body parts. For instance, compare the amount of cortical area devoted to the hand with that dedicated to the arm.

Despite its approximations, the somatosensory homunculus effectively conveys the message that the brain holds a representation of the body, but also that the representation is markedly dissimilar from the actual body. One important discrepancy concerns the relative size of body parts in our actual body and in the body represented in the brain. Another discrepancy pertains to topology rather than size. If one considers the relative location of the different body part representations, it becomes apparent that cortical relative locations do not always respect those of the actual body. For instance, the face is immediately adjacent to the hand, whereas it is distant from the neck and nape. Yet, we do

(a) (b) (c)

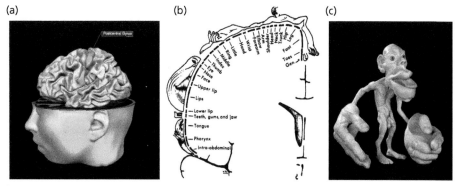

Figure 2.1 Is this the body you know? (a) The location of the primary somatosensory cortex
(or S1) in the human brain (drawn with BrainVoyager Brain Tutor). (b) The approximate
correspondence between cortical territory within S1 and peripheral somatosensory signals.
(c) One three-dimensional rendering of the somatosensory homunculus, in which relative size of
body parts is approximately proportional to the extent of dedicated somatosensory cortex.

Figure 2.1b) Reproduced from Wilder Penfield and Theodore Rasmussen, *The Cerebral Cortex of Man: A Clinical
Study of Localization of Function*, Copyright © 1950, Gale, a part of Cengage, Inc. Reproduced by permission. www.
cengage.com/permissions.

Figure 2.1c) Mary Evans/Natural History Museum.

not perceive contiguity between the face and the hand, nor do we experience detachment
between the face and the neck. On top of having swollen hands and face, the homunculus
should look a bit like a cubist painting, with body parts in unrealistic positions relative to
each other!

The existence of a somatotopic map in the brain was predicted by English neurologist
John Hughlings-Jackson in 1863 (see Jackson, 1931). While working with patients with
epilepsy, Hughlings-Jackson noted regularities in the sequence of tactile percepts evoked
during seizures. He, therefore, hypothesized that seizures propagate across a cortical territory containing an orderly representation of body parts. This was later confirmed using
direct electrical stimulation of S1 by Canadian neurosurgeon Wilder Penfield and his
collaborators (Penfield & Boldrey, 1937), who had also the insight of introducing the pictorial representations of the homunculus shown in Figure 2.1. Today, the organization of
SI can be shown in healthy humans with neuroimaging techniques such as fMRI (Hlustík
et al., 2001).

The homuncular representation is there to remind us that the perception of our own
body begins with brain representations that are remarkably distorted. Yet, of course, how
we perceive our bodies does not resemble the homunculus in Figure 2.1. If the brain
representation of the body is nothing more than the somatotopic map in S1, how we
perceive our own bodies indeed becomes an enigma. Given the perspective of this book,
our readers will not be surprised that there is, however, a solution to the enigma: when
perceiving the body, we do not rely only on somatosensory afferents; instead, we use also
information from other sensory channels and from the motor system. Presumably, these

multisensory and motor contributions lead to representations that resemble more closely the actual metrics and topology of our body. But which sensory channels are employed to perceive our body accurately? And how does this happen in the brain?

2.2 Sensory signals from the body are not just touch

Although the perspective of the five senses that we learned in school treats touch as a single channel for sensations coming from the skin, somatosensation actually relies on a much richer repertoire of sensory signals. Let's begin by focusing on the skin surface. The skin is the largest layer of tissue endowed with sensory properties in the whole body—up to 1–2 square meters. On this vast *sensory epithelium* we can distinguish between receptors that convey mechanical displacement of body tissue, leading to touch and vibration percepts; receptors sensitive to thermal changes, leading to percepts of heat and cold; and receptors that are sensitive to different energies (mechanical, thermal, chemical) and respond whenever there is a damage to the skin or even just the possibility of damage. The latter class of receptors are termed nociceptors and are associated with the percept of pain. Furthermore, since the end of the last century, scientists have discovered a sub-group of nerve fibres (termed C-fibres) that are preferentially activated by pruritic stimuli (Schmelz et al., 1997) or by slow and gentle stroking by soft objects on the hairy skin (Nordin, 1990). The former lead to the perception of itch; the latter, to a pleasant experience that is generally categorized as *affective touch* (Olausson et al., 2010).

This compound of receptors on the skin reveals the remarkable and often underestimated richness of the information that we constantly receive from our own body. If we now turn to the inside of the body, another set of fundamental inputs is revealed. Muscle and joints, as well as the internal organs of the body, are rich in receptors that capture mechanical, thermal, and chemosensory forms of energy. Receptors contained in muscles and joints, in particular, provide essential information for own-body perception and body movement: *proprioception*. We owe the term to the Nobel-laureate Charles Sherrington, a pioneer in the study of somatosensation (Sherrington, 1906). Proprioception is something of a secret sense, because it remains undetected to most people until they are explicitly informed about it, but plays a fundamental role in recording changes of posture and muscle tone that are necessary for controlling our body in space. It is also the fastest of the sensory channels that convey inputs from the body: its signals travel to the central nervous system at a whopping 80-120 metres per second (roughly 360 km/hour), through large fibres called A-alpha that are also naturally shielded against electrical dispersion by a layer of specialized cells that wrap around the length of the nerve. For comparison, consider that pain travels through thin and poorly shielded fibres called A-delta, at 5–30 metres per second, or even through completely unshielded C fibres, at 0.5–2 metres per second.

Another concept originally introduced by Charles Sherrington is that of *interoception*. Sherrington originally used it to refer to the visceral sensation that we derive from internal organs (heart, lungs, intestines). He distinguished these bodily signals from exteroception (in which he included touch, temperature, and pain) and proprioception (Sherrington, 1948). However, this conceptualization of interoception has recently undergone a substantial change. It has been proposed that all the information that represents the physiological condition of the body, whether on its surface or inside, contributes to a dedicated pathway, clearly distinct from touch and proprioception (Craig, 2002). According to this view, visceral feelings (such as vaso-motor activity, hunger, and thirst), but also non-visceral inputs (such as pain, temperature, itch, and affective touch) would all be processed within a specialized system. Put it more simply, the brain treats together all the signals that can provide useful information about the on-going physiological condition of the body. This specialized afferent would be critical to the rapid functioning of a continuous regulatory activity aimed at maintaining the body's physiological equilibrium (homeostasis). This re-definition of the concept of interoception as 'the sense of the physiological condition of the entire body, not just the viscera' (Craig, 2002, p. 655) has been motivated by the observation of a distinct neural pathway for all small-diameter fibres (A-delta and C) that convey inputs from temperature, pain, and affective touch and innervate virtually all tissues of the body. This pathway has a common hub in a region of the spinal cord and brain stem (Lamina I of the dorsal horns) and terminates in a portion of the brain cortex different from the primary somatosensory cortex: the right insular cortex. This notion is in agreement with the evidence that lesions of the primary somatosensory cortex affecting somatosensory touch leave temperature or pain sensations unimpaired. Moreover, it captures the important observation that—unlike somatosensory touch—temperature, pain, and affective touch convey emotional qualities as well as automatic regulatory responses in the autonomic system.

Vestibular sensations are another fundamental source of information about our bodies. Whenever our body changes from an upright to a horizontal position, when our head tilts back and forward, or whenever our head moves in space, a group of organs in the inner ear can be activated and signal these changes to the brain. Two of these vestibular organs (the otoliths) detect linear motion of the head in three-dimensional space, such as the motion imposed on our head when we start walking or when the train leaves the station. The remaining vestibular organs (three semicircular canals) detect angular motion, such as head turning movements. Importantly, all these vestibular sensors are sensitive to changes of our body with respect to the Earth's gravitational pull and therefore are crucial for our equilibrium (Day & Fitzpatrick, 2005). They signal if the body changes its vertical orientation in the physical world. Furthermore, the vestibular systems also contribute to the distinction between self-motion and non-self-motion (Dichgans & Brandt, 1978).

2.3 Seeing the body

There is little doubt that the abundant and diverse somatosensory signals play quite an important role in how we *feel* our own body. However, the body can also be *seen*, that is, perceived through a set of sensory channels that are most typically associated with the perception of things outside the body. Although perception of own-body can develop in the total absence of visual information (consider for instance the case of individuals who are congenitally blind), throughout life vision provides us with continuous valuable information about the shape, size, and position of our body. Importantly, vision provides information that has a degree of spatial precision that is typically higher with respect to the one that can be achieved through somatosensation. As such, it is a valuable concurrent source of input for perceptual estimates of the body.

As a first step into the interactions between vision and somatosensation in body perception, consider the following experiments. Imagine you are asked to respond as quickly as possible to a tactile stimulus delivered to your right hand. In some conditions, you can see the hand through a video monitor, but in other conditions you have to perform the task without seeing your hand. Importantly, in either case vision will be entirely irrelevant to the task, because the monitor will show the hand, but not the stimulator touching it. Would you nonetheless predict a difference between the two conditions? Or imagine another experimental setting. You are asked to make a tactile spatial judgment on touches applied to your forearm. In some of the trials you are touched in two distinct locations, in other trials, at a single location. Do you think it would be easier for you to make this spatial discrimination of touch if your arm were seen through a magnifying lens?

As you may have imagined, the experiments we just described have been actually performed (Tipper et al., 1998 and Kennett, Taylor-Clarke, & Haggard, 2001, respectively). They illustrate a phenomenon first documented at the end of the twentieth century and known as Visual Enhancement of Touch (VET). VET is defined as improved tactile detection and discrimination at a specific body part (typically a hand), when the body part is either seen directly (Kennett, Taylor-Clarke, & Haggard, 2001; Press, Taylor-Clarke, Kennett, & Haggard, 2004; Taylor-Clarke, Kennet, & Haggard, 2002; Whiteley, Kennett, Taylor-Clarke, & Haggard, 2004) or indirectly (for instance in a video or photograph; Tipper et al., 1998, 2001). Critically, VET emerges despite the fact that vision of the body part is completely task-irrelevant and uninformative about somatosensation. Furthermore, although this multisensory effect has been mainly reported in neurologically healthy participants, there is evidence that vision of body parts can also temporarily ameliorate the somatosensory deficits in patients who suffered from stroke (Serino et al., 2007a; see also Rorden, Heutink, Greenfield, & Robertson, 1999 for related findings with vision of a rubber hand).

Studies using electroencephalography (EEG, see Tutorial 1.1) have started to reveal the brain basis of VET (Taylor-Clarke, Kennet, & Haggard, 2002; Sambo, Gillmeister, & Forster, 2009; Longo, Pernigo, & Haggard, 2011). In particular, Longo and colleagues (2011) examined the electrical potentials evoked by stimuli delivered directly to hand nerves, comparing conditions when participants looked directly at the stimulated hand to when they looked a small wooden block which was approximately hand-size. Results showed that vision of the hand, compared to vision of the object, modulated a very early somatosensory response in the brain, occurring approximately 30 ms after stimulation to the nerve was delivered. What is most relevant is the fact that this early response occurs in S1, the primary somatosensory cortex. Recall that this is the brain region that we described at the beginning of the chapter and that has typically been conceived as selectively dedicated to somatosensation. Yet, vision influences S1, suggesting that multisensory interactions can modulate processing of body related information from very early on.

While the VET phenomenon is already evidence that multisensory interactions can change somatosensory inputs, it does not clarify to what extent own-body perception can be affected by vision. To illustrate this specific aspect, let us examine how vision contributes to the perception of *body metrics,* the extension and size of body parts. One of the first systematic observations on our ability to estimate body metrics was conducted more than 150 years ago, by German physiologist and anatomist Ernst Heinrich Weber. In 1834, he discovered a tactile illusion that occurs when comparing the distance between pairs of tactile stimuli applied to the skin. Curiously, the same distance seems larger when the stimulation is applied to the index finger, compared to when it is applied to the forearm. This is now called Weber's Illusion. You are encouraged to try it yourself: get an ordinary caliper, set the opening to about two cm, and apply the two points to a blindfolded friend's finger or forearm. Intriguingly, Weber's illusion reveals that the distorted body representation in S1 *can* influence behaviour to some extent, leading to misjudgements of the size of objects that touch the skin. As you might recall, the cortical territories devoted to the index finger are considerably larger compared to ones devoted to the forearm (Figure 2.1). However, as we have stressed before, our perception of body metrics is usually accurate, and quantitative assessments of Weber's illusion on different body parts have conclusively shown that the size illusion is, in fact, considerably less than one would expect based on differences in the proportion of cortical areas in S1 (Green, 1982). Even in the conditions that produce Weber's illusion, therefore, we see the signature of processes that go beyond the representation of the body coded in S1.

If the representation of the body is not limited to the S1 homunculus, what happens afterwards? An intriguing study published in 2004 by Patrick Haggard and colleagues (Taylor-Clarke, Jacobsen, & Haggard, 2004) has suggested that part of what happens after S1 is due to the brain taking into account other sources of information about the body, and, in particular, using visual signals to rescale somatosensory inputs relative to an internal model. The experiment worked as follows. Participants were asked to report the longer of two tactile distances delivered to the index finger or the forearm. At the beginning of the study, and in agreement with Weber's illusion, distances on the index finger were perceived as longer. But this was just the beginning. After the initial measurements, participants were subjected to a very special training session. For a full hour, they saw a computer screen showing their hand optically reduced to half its size, their forearm magnified to double its size, and repeated presentations of markers on the hand or arm. In addition, for the whole hour, they had to judge the distance between the markers. Once they had completed this somewhat tedious learning phase, they were tested again for Weber's illusion. Remarkably, in this post-test phase the bias to perceive distances on the finger as larger than those on the forearm reduced by 9 percent relative to pre-test. Thus, visual information about body metrics seems to affect the way the brain interprets tactile information about external objects. This underscores a key principle of multisensory perception: under multisensory conditions, signals from one sensory channel can be used to recalibrate or rescale signals from another channel, and this can then carry over to unisensory conditions.

The intriguing results reported by Haggard and collaborators are consistent with a sort of recalibration of somatosensation based on visual inputs. Other phenomena indicate that visual modulations of somatosensation can take place even in more complex contexts. In these contexts, perceived features of body parts such as their location or size appear to result from a sort of 'intelligent' solution to the problem posed by concomitant sensory afferents from vision, touch, and proprioception. One such phenomenon is the multisensory Ames window described by Bruno, Dell'Anna, & Jacomuzzi (2006). The Ames window is a classic visual demonstration originally conceived to study motion and depth perception in vision. It was created by Adalbert Ames, one of the most creative developers of spectacular perceptual effects in the history of perception science. We encourage our readers to search the internet to see it live. As you will see, the window is simply a trapezoid, which tends to appear as a slanted rectangle—i.e. as an open window. Ames used this to create an interesting motion illusion, whereas what Bruno and collaborators did was to build a small-scale model of the window, and then ask participants to hold this model in their hands while keeping an eye closed. Monocular viewing is needed here to remove binocular cues to depth and help the brain process the perspective cues that make the trapezoid appear as a slanted rectangle. The interesting thing about the demonstration is that, when holding the window as illustrated in Figure 2.2, one 'feels' as

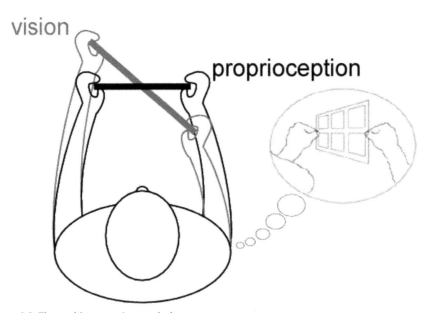

Figure 2.2 The multisensory Ames window.

if one hand is closer that it is, while the other is farther away. This is a proprioceptive il-lusion, as the hands are actually equidistant from the body. Some participant also experi-ences a sort of paradoxical stretching of one arm and shrinking of the other. They feel a bit like the famous Marvel comics character, Mr Fantastic of the Fantastic Four (a superhero who has the power to elastically stretch his limbs).

The Mr Fantastic illusion is indeed a weird phenomenon. But, if you think about it, that one would perceive a stretching of the arms is a rather reasonable conclusion, given the sensory premises. Consider the sensory signals that are simultaneously presented to the brain mechanisms responsible for representing the body. Somatosensory signals veridically inform the brain of the actual hand position relative to the trunk (equidistant) and of the shaping of the arms (fully extended). Visual signals, in contrast, are consistent with an ob-ject that is slanted in depth: one side is closer to your trunk than the other. But there is a third element, and this does the trick. There is also a tactile signal from your fingers, which is telling your brain that the hands are making contact with the object (one could argue that the felt weight of the object is doing the same). So, the brain has this problem: how can the hands be equidistant from the trunk, if they contact an object on locations that visually appear at different distances from the trunk? The arms should be of different lengths, and the hands should be at the visual, not felt locations! This may sound somewhat too far away from rigorous, quantitative science, but in our opinion effects such as these do highlight a more complex, higher-level form of visual influence on somatosensation. There are, in fact, several other intriguing multisensory illusions that are based on the exactly the same ingre-dients: visual and proprioceptive signals about the body, and something else that forces the brain to reach surprising perceptual solutions. We discuss some of these illusions in Box 2.1.

Box 2.1 Ping-pong half balls, Pinocchio, and fMRI

Visual sensory signals can have surprising effects on how we perceive our body parts. In the main text of the chapter we introduced the multisensory Ames window. A re-lated illusion that is very easy to reproduce at home has been described recently by Ekroll, Sayim, Van der Hallen, & Wagemans (2016). Try it: all you need is a ping pong ball. Use a cutter or sharp scissors to cut the ball in half. Next, turn your hand to point your index finger straight up toward the ceiling, and cup the fingertip with one half ball. The half ping pong ball should rest on your fingertip like a small hat. Keep the hand near your belly, and look down towards the finger. You will see the half ball, of course, and the hand underneath. You will notice that, because of the position of the finger and the balancing of the half ball on top, the half ball actually looks like a regular (complete) ping pong ball, a little sphere somehow balanced over the tip of your finger. This is an instance of amodal completion (similar to the one created by the well-known Kanizsa triangle; see Chapter 1): your visual system had direct infor-mation about the visible half, and tends to use that to infer, incorrectly in this case, that the ball continues on the other side. We do this all the time with all objects, if you

Box 2.1 Continued

think about it. We see the parts facing us, but we are also aware that there are other parts in the back. And now for the fun part. You may have noticed at this point that your finger feels shorter. To quantify this feeling, Ekroll and collaborators performed a very simple test. They asked participants to point, with the index finger of the other hand, the vertical position of the fingertip with the half ball. Try it on yourself, almost certainly, you will find that you point a good 2–3 cm below the real position of the tip of your finger. Why? The explanation is the same as that for the multisensory Ames window. There is a touch signal that tells your brain that the tip of the finger is contacting an object. Visually, this object is a full sphere. In reality, of course, you finger is at the same level as the visible tip of the half sphere (only inside it) but knowing this does not help—perceptual illusions are typically impenetrable to rational knowledge. So the location of the finger contacting the object must be where the (illusory) sphere ends, which is much lower than the true position of the finger.

Interested? It turns out that such visual modulations of the felt body parts are not entirely new. They are in fact all offsprings of another classic illusion: the Pinocchio illusion (Lackner, 1988). This is a multisensory set-up that causes participants to experience that parts of the body stretch or shrink. For instance, one can induce the illusion that one's nose gets longer—hence the reference to the famous child-marionette of Collodi's book. To get this to work is a bit harder that the ping pong ball demonstration, but the general idea is similar. You need to apply a vibration to the tendon of the bicep of your experimental participant while she holds the tip of her nose with a pincer grip. Usually, equipment used by physiotherapists or masseuses provides the right kind of vibratory stimulus. The vibration stimulates your stretch receptors, specialized cells that signal stretching of muscles and tendons, and this results in a sensory signal that is equivalent to what would be sent to the brain if you were extending your arm. This is so because to extend the arm you need to flex your triceps muscle (in the back of the arm) and this results in stretching of the opponent muscle biceps. The situation, from the standpoint of the brain mechanism representing the body, is as follows. Proprioceptive signals indicate that the arm is flexed and that the hand is near the nose. Kinaesthetic signals due to the vibration, however, indicate that the arm is being extended, which should cause the hand to move away from the nose. At the same time, however, there is a touch signal that continuously informs the brain that there is physical contact between the fingers and the nose. You continue to hold your nose, but your hand is moving away from it. How could that be? You get the idea: the nose must be getting longer, Pinocchio-like. In reality, more rigorous tests of what happens in these conditions have revealed that things are more complicated. For instance, many participants do not report that the nose is getting longer, but that the fingers are. Some feel that both the nose and the fingers get longer, both by a smaller amount. In addition, the opposite effect can also be elicited. All you need to do is vibrate the tendon of the triceps instead of that of the biceps. The kinaesthetic signal will now be that the arm is flexing and the hand is getting closer to

Box 2.1 Continued

the nose. Under these conditions—you guessed it—one does not feel that the nose gets longer, but that it shrinks. One can even feel that the finger penetrates inside the nose towards the skull, a somewhat unpleasant sensation. The explanation, however, is still the same: the brain needs to resolve the conflict between proprioception, kinaesthesia, and touch. And is happy to do so by updating the representation of the body part, even if consciously one knows very well that the feeling is illusory.

If you get the general idea, you have perhaps thought that in principle one could induce 'Pinocchio' illusions over different body parts. This is quite true, and has been put to good scientific use by Henrik Ehrsson, one of the leading investigators in current multisensory studies of body representations. Ehrsson et al. (2005) exploited a variant of the Pinocchio illusion which requires participants to place the palm of their hands on the sides of the body, approximately at the level of the navel. If one then administers vibratory stimulation on the tendons of the wrists, this results in the feeling that the wrist is flexing, as if the hand were moving closer to the centre of the body. In other words, this feels as if you are suddenly getting thinner in your midsection, an effect that could be termed the 'wasp waist' illusion. This is cool, but not particularly new—the explanation is the same as that of the classic Pinocchio or the visually induced variants discussed earlier. The advantage of the wasp waist variation, however, is that it can be applied to a participant who is lying flat inside an fMRI scanner. This allowed Ehrsson and collaborators to actually record neural activations, and to perform comparisons between the conditions that cause the illusion and several control conditions. At the end of a somewhat complex analysis, Ehrsson and collaborators were able to identify brain areas that were selectively activated by the change in body representation. One such area, for instance, was a small region in the left superior parietal lobe. Ehrsson observed that the intensity of the differential activation of this area, in comparison with the controls, was statistically associated with the reported intensity of the wasp waist illusion, assessed by a questionnaire administered to the participants after the scanning. Thus, it is tempting to speculate that this region forms part of a brain network for body representation. Tutorial 2.2 in this chapter presents on overview of our current understanding of this network. We are now beginning to have at least a general idea of the main cortical nodes of this network. In contrast, it remains a major challenge to understand the dynamics of the network, that is, how the nodes talk to each other to achieve a representation of the body. One interesting approach to this issue has been recently described by Kanayama, Morandi, Hiraki, & Pavani (2017).

2.4 Embodying visible body parts

The importance of vision for the perception of one's body goes beyond the rescaling effects that we have described in the previous section. In certain conditions, vision can even trick your brain into mistaking a fake limb for your own body part. Something of this sort was reported for the first time by French researcher J. Tastevin (1937). He noted that if he arranged a cloth such that a fake finger was poking out of it, and if he had a person place a hand hidden not too far away from the cloth, the observer would sometimes misjudge the finger as belonging to their real hand. This peculiar phenomenon described by Tastevin has been rediscovered and greatly extended in more recent years. This trend began in 1998, when psychologists Matthew Botvinick and Jonathan Cohen published a brief but very influential paper in the journal *Nature*. Botvinick and Cohen asked participants to place their left hand behind a vertical screen on a table. The screen hid the hand and the arm so that participants could not see them. Well visible in front of the participants, they instead placed a fake rubber replica of a left hand and forearm. Participants were instructed to gaze at this fake hand and do nothing else. In the meanwhile, an experimenter gently touched the hidden real left hand and the visible fake hand using two paintbrushes, taking care to touch the same fingers on the real and fake hands at the same times. After 10 minutes of this synchronous stroking, participants started to report three surprising percepts concerning their hand. First, when asked *where* they felt that they were being touched, they typically responded that they felt light touches *in the locations where they saw that the brush was touching the rubber hand*. This was remarkable because the felt touch was located outside of their body and seemed to be caused by the paintbrush touching the rubber hand. Second, when Botvinick and Cohen asked their participants to close their eyes and to point to the perceived location of their left hand, they observed that they pointed to a location closer to the rubber hand, in comparison with a control group in which a small asynchrony was introduce between touching of the two hands. Third, those participants in which multisensory stimulation was synchronous were more incline to describe the rubber hand as their own. In short, it was almost as if the fake hand had paradoxically become their true hand. This was a paradox, for participants knew that the rubber hand was not part of their body, yet they seemed to truly experienced ownership of the rubber hand.

This revamped version of Tastevin's observation quickly became known as the 'rubber hand illusion' (Botvinick & Cohen, 1998; but a better name is probably 'fake hand illusion', as the hand certainly does not need to be made of rubber), and has been employed in many other studies afterwards, according to our estimate, over 250 in almost 20 years and we are still counting (for review see Makin et al., 2008). Thus, it is clear that the fake hand illusion is much more than an enjoyable party trick. It is a powerful experimental tool for studying multisensory interactions in the perception of one's body, in particular with respect to the perception of body ownership. This is important, because studying bodily ownership in healthy humans is far from trivial. Consider researchers interested in the perception of faces. If you have such an interest, it is easy to present face stimuli, and compare these with control non-face stimuli, such as, for instance, a scrambled mix of eyes, nose, and mouth that no longer retain the global configuration of a face (Johnson, Dziurawiec, Ellis, & Morton et al., 1991). In contrast, experimental manipulations of ownership are not easy to achieve. The fake hand illusion provides an elegant way to do just that, defining conditions of ownership for the fake arm that can be contrasted with conditions in which the fake arm is perceived as extraneous. Using this approach, researchers have been able to investigate the factors that are critical for perceiving owner-ship, as well as the functional and neural underlying mechanisms.

Given the potential of the fake hand illusion as a tool for studying ownership, it is not surprising that several studies have focused on identifying what factors are critical for experiencing it. For instance, we now know that the illusion depends on the relative pos-ture and relative distance of the fake and the real hands. If the fake hand is aligned with the real hand and it is relatively close to it, the illusion is readily obtained. This is the case illustrated in Figure 2.3. However, if the fake hand is rotated by more than 90 degrees relative to the real hand (Pavani, Spence, & Driver, 2000; Tsakiris & Haggard, 2005), or if it is placed more than 30 cm away from it (Lloyd, 2007; Preston, 2013; see also Kalckert & Ehrsson, 2014), the illusion does not work as well. When postural and spatial con-straints are satisfied, another manipulation that promotes the illusion is the synchronous stimulation of the fake and real hand. As in the original Botvinick and Cohen study, even small asynchronies between multisensory stimulations can hinder this bodily illusion. The explanation of this repeatedly documented difference between synchronous and asynchronous stimulation in inducing the illusion (for a review see Makin, Holmes, & Ehrsson, 2008) is likely related to the tendency of our mind to bind together sensory

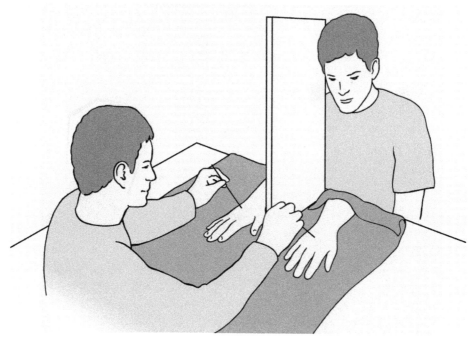

Figure 2.3 Typical set-up for the fake hand illusion. The participant looks at the rubber hand while his real hands are hidden from view. The experimenter touches the rubber hand and the corresponding left hand of the participant with two paintbrushes. When the stimulation is synchronous on the two hands, the illusion emerges.

signals that co-occur in time, i.e. are simultaneous or within relatively short temporal windows. Instead, it treats signals that do not co-occur in time as separate. This is a fundamental principle of multisensory integration, the so-termed *unity assumption* (Welch & Warren, 1980), and we will return to this notion in various chapters of this book. Interestingly, it has even been argued that visuo-tactile simultaneity could promote somatosensory illusions also when no fake body part is shown. Armel and Ramachandran (2003) devised an experiment in which several synchronous conditions were possible. In some blocks, they synchronously stroked the participant's hand and a rubber hand (the standard illusion setting). In other blocks, they synchronously stroked the participant's hand and the bare surface of the table. They reported that participants could perceive touch on the rubber hand, but also on locations on the table.

These observations reported by Armel and Ramachandran suggest that synchronous multisensory stimulation can affect processes related to body perception even in very peculiar conditions. However, even in their experiment, the condition that elicited the strongest illusion was when a plausible fake hand was visible. This reveals an important principle of the multisensory perception of our own body: when the brain must decide whether a visible body part is ours or not, it compares incoming multisensory signals with representations of the body that are available in long-term memory. In other words, it searches for potential correspondences between the on-going flow of sensory signals and some existing internal model of what our body must be like. These long-term representations need not be conscious or directly accessible for scrutiny, yet they clearly affect the multisensory interactions that involve the perception of the body or of objects near the body (To learn more the long-term body-representations stored in our mind read Box 2.2). The fake hand illusion has the potentials to shed light also on the nature of these internal representations of the body.

Consider, for instance, the following surprising finding: the similarity between the fake and the real hands is largely unimportant for the emergence of the illusion. What this means is that the fake hand illusion is not undermined by differences in form or luminance (one of the psychophysical dimensions of colour) between the participant's own hand the fake hand (Longo et al., 2009), nor by the use of unrealistic colours (Pavani, Spence, & Driver, 2000), or by the evidence that the fake hand belongs to a different racial group than that of the participant (i.e. a black hand in a group of white participants; Farmer, Tajadura-Jiménez, & Tsakiris, 2012). Correspondence in size also appears to be largely irrelevant (Bruno & Bertamini, 2010; Haggard & Jundi, 2009; but see Pavani & Zampini, 2007). Finally, studies that extended the fake hand illusion paradigm to the whole body (see next paragraph) revealed that even gender differences between the participant and the observed body are insufficient to block the illusion (Slater, Spanlang, Sanchez-Vives, & Blanke, 2010)! What this means is that as long as the seen object is interpreted as a body part, the brain can be deceived into thinking that it is part of the own body. What this also suggests is that the internal representations of the body that are consulted when deciding whether to embody a fake hand or not specify certain information but not others. In particular, they seem to include the current spatial arrangement of the

Box 2.2 Multiple internal models of the body

The notion that the brain may contain at least two distinct representations of the body is quite old. It was first proposed by the British neurologists Henry Head and Gordon Morgan Holmes (1910/1911), and it has been reiterated many times. In a nutshell, the idea is the following. One representation is largely unconscious; it is primarily based on proprioceptive and motor signals and used for the control of action and posture. Another representation is considerably more accessible to conscious scrutiny, is primarily based on visual signals, and contributes to our awareness of how our body is and looks to others. Head and Holmes originally named the first representation 'postural schema', although several authors adopted later the term 'body schema' (Berlucchi & Aglioti, 1997; Gallagher, 1986; Paillard, 1999), which in fact was first introduced by Bonnier in 1905. The second representation has been referred to as 'body image' (Head & Holmes, 1910/1911; Lhermitte & Tchehrazi, 1937), a term that has become even more widespread even in everyday language.

Head and Holmes' distinction fits some neuropsychological observations. Some patients seem to be impaired in their body schema, but not in their body image. For instance, patient G.L., who suffered peripheral deafferentation caused by permanent damage of the nervous fibres from the skin and muscles receptors and the spinal cord, was perfectly capable of reporting verbally which body part was touched. She was also capable of indicate that location on a schematic body silhouette. At the same time, she was unable to point directly to the stimulated body part. Thus, G.L. was aware of the presence of the tactile event on the body, was capable of attaching a verbal label to its location, and was able to localize it with respect to a generic visual body description (the silhouette). Yet, she was incapable of using the same information for sensorimotor planning (Paillard, 1999). Other patients show the opposite pattern, with poor body image processing but preserved body schema functionalities. For instance, patient R.S., who suffered central deafferentation following a lesion in the left parietal lobe, was unaware of static tactile stimulations applied to her right hand and forearm. Nonetheless, she was remarkably capable of correctly pointing to the touched location on the right hand with her left index finger (Paillard, 1991). Based on these observations, the distinction is frequently adopted in may textbooks and scientific papers.

However, and despite its heuristic value especially for studying patients, in the last decades the distinction between body schema and body image has often been challenged. Some authors have proposed that both these body representations should be unified within a unique and genetically determined representation (the so-called 'neuromatrix' proposed by Melzack, 1990). Others (Schwoebel & Coslett, 2005; Sirigu, Grafman, Bressler, & Sunderland, 1991) have instead proposed a further subdivision within the concept of body image between the aspects which are more strictly visual ('structural body description') and those who are related to more verbal knowledge ('body semantics'). This distinction was again motivated by the behaviour of

Box 2.2 Continued

brain-damaged patients. Specifically, there have been reports of patients who are incapable of planning and executing actions in the absence of motor deficits (*apraxia*, considered evidence for a deficit in the body schema), patients who are incapable of localizing body parts on the own body, on the body of the examiner or on a mannequin (*autotopoagnosia*, considered evidence for a deficit in the structural body description), and of patients who are selectively impaired in naming specific body parts (*selective aphasia for body parts*, considered evidence for a deficit in body semantics).

The interested reader can find more extensive discussions of these multiple representation of a single body elsewhere (de Vignemont, 2007; Dijkerman & De Haan, 2007). What is important to emphasize here, however, is that these multiple representations are surely not based on somatosensation alone. The representations of the body are derived from processes of multisensory perception. As we have sought to show in this chapter, although research is only beginning to understand these processes in detail and to see their clinical implications, the evidence supporting this fundamental conclusion is overwhelming and will inform all future studies of the brain representation of the body.

body (as evidenced by the sensitivity of the fake hand illusion to changes of this sort), but they do not seem to specify the shape, colour, size, race, and gender of the body (as shown by the irrelevance of this information for the illusion).

2.4 From fake hands to fake whole bodies

That a fake hand can be perceived as part of our own body is certainly striking: it documents the important role of visual inputs in body perception and it offers a useful tool for experimenting with complex mental processes, such as body ownership. But can the illusion be extended to a whole fake body? In the early days of experimental psychology, George Malcom Stratton (1899) had already noted that certain multiple mirror images of the body could induce some sort of disembodiment. He tried the experience of walking for hours with special goggles that projected his body ahead of him, floating in the air, and reported a sort of out-of-body experience (see Figure 2.4; Stratton experiments with prism are discussed in greater detail in Chapter 3). In the current era of virtual reality, ways of experimenting with the visible body have expanded substantially. Faster and more realistic computer graphics, goggles that allow three-dimensional immersive contexts, and sensors capable of detecting body movements in real-time are making the experience of visual duplicates (avatars) of ourselves increasingly common.

In 2007, using virtual reality, two studies successfully expanded the rubber hand illusion to the whole body (Ehrsson, 2007; Lenggenhager, Tadi, Metzinger, & Blanke, 2007), taking this multisensory body illusion a step forward. The set-up used in the two studies was largely similar and is illustrated in Figure 2.5. In both studies,

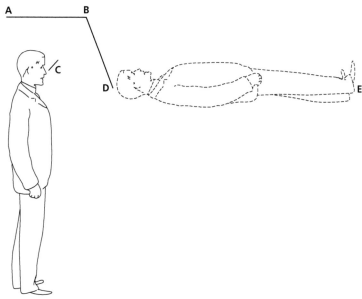

Figure 2.4 Altering the seen body with mirrors. This set-up was used by George Stratton (1899) to visually project his body in the air, ahead of him.

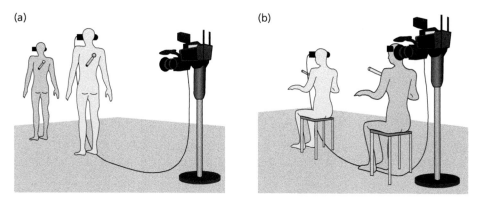

Figure 2.5 Experimenting with virtual bodies. (a) The virtual reality set-up adopted by Lenggenhager et al., 2007. Participant are stimulated on the back and perceive an illusory self in front of them. (b) The virtual reality set-up adopted by Ehrsson, 2007. Participants are stimulated on the chest and perceive an illusory self behind their physical body, in the location where they see the fake touch.

Reprinted by permission from Macmillan Publishers Ltd: *Nature Reviews Neuroscience*, 13 (8), Olaf Blanke, Multisensory brain mechanisms of bodily self-consciousness, pp. 556-571, doi:10.1038/nrn3292. Copyright © 2012, Nature Publishing Group.

participants observed an image of their own body captured by a video-camera located several metres behind them, and delivered to them through head-mounted displays: special goggles that allow for a three dimensional immersive experience in virtual reality. In essence, they saw their own body filmed from behind. As in the fake hand illusion, the experience was amplified by stroking the participant's body in synchrony with a visual stroking on the body's seen image. Lenggenhager and colleagues (2007) touched participants on the back while they saw the virtual body also touched on the back about 2 metres in front of them (Figure 2.5a). Instead, Ehrsson (2007) touched participants on the chest and at the same time, extending his other arm towards the video-camera, mimicked touching an illusory body placed 2 metres behind the participant (see Figure 2.5b). In both cases, participants experienced illusory self-locations for their real body: either forward, towards the virtual body seen in front of them (Lenggenhager, Tadi, Metzinger, & Blanke, 2007), or backward, towards the illusory body placed behind them (Ehrsson, 2007). Moreover, just as in the fake hand illusion, participants reported that they experienced the touch on the virtual visible body, and provided various reports that suggested some degree of disembodiment. Their skin conductance documented a fear reaction when the experimenter 'hit' the virtual body with a hammer (Ehrsson, 2007; see also Guterstam & Ehrsson, 2012). Thus, both set-ups produced some sort of disembodiment, with a substantial change in perspective: because of the visual illusion participants experienced the bizarre experience of a third person view on their own body.

Another set-up capable of triggering whole body illusions, this time retaining a first-person perspective, was developed by Petkova and Ehrsson (2008). In this set-up, two video-cameras were positioned on the head of a male mannequin, such that each camera captured the view from the position of one of the mannequin's eye (see Figure 2.6a). The cameras showed the abdomen of the mannequin and the surrounding body parts. Meanwhile, the participant wore a head-mounted display and received the

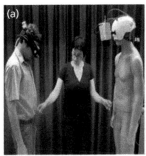 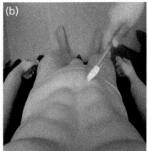 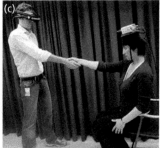

Figure 2.6 Body-swapping. (a) The set-up for the body-swapping paradigm (see text for details). The experimenter touches the participant's body and the mannequin in synchrony (to induce the illusion) or out of synchrony (to prevent the illusion) (b) The participants sees the body of the mannequin in first-person perspective. (c) The set-up for body-swapping with the experimenter; participant see themselves from the first-person perspective of the experimenter.
© Courtesy of BeAnotherLab, beanotherlab.org

visual inputs captured by the video-cameras. This produced in the participant the three-dimensional impression of looking down on the mannequin's body (see Figure 2.6b). As in other body illusion settings, a visuo-tactile stimulation was added to promote or to contrast the illusion: in half of the blocks the experimenter touched the abdomen of the participant and the mannequin in synchrony, and in the remaining half touches on the real and fake body were delivered out of synchrony. The results documented again the robustness of these visual illusions. After synchronous stimulation, participants reported the impression that the mannequin's body was their own and that they could sense touches delivered on the mannequin's abdomen! Moreover, if the experimenter threatened the mannequin with a knife, the participant exhibited an increased physiological response (as measured by skin-conductance) that was largest after synchronous compared to asynchronous stimulation. In a follow-up experiment, Petkova and Ehrsson (2009) also showed this 'body swapping' illusion holds also when the experimenter takes the position of the mannequin and shakes hands with the participant. In this alternative set-up for the illusion (Figure 2.6c), the video-cameras were mounted on a helmet, which was then placed on the head of the experimenter. This gave the participant the first-person view of the experimenter and the remarkable experience of swapping body with the experimenter. As noted by one participant 'I was shaking hands with myself' (Petkova & Ehrsson, 2008, p. 5). This remarkable body swapping experience is now making possible embodiments that novelist conceived since the end of the nineteenth century, and until recently appeared only as something that could occur by mysterious magic acts (see Box 2.3).

Box 2.3 Body-swapping art

In 1882, Thomas Anstey Guthrie, a young Cambridge-educated lawyer, published a comic novel under the pseudonym F. Anstey. The novel, titled *Vice Versa* (the Latin words for 'the other way round'), tells the story of a business man named Dr Grimson, who swaps his body with that of his son Dick. The body swapping is unintentional—it is made possible by the powers of a magic stone brought from India. However, it leads Dr Grimson to experience his son's life at boarding school, and permits Dick to live the challenges of running his father's business in the City of London. Although at the end of the novel father and son return in their original bodies and lives, for both of them the experience brings a better understanding of each other's perspectives. Guthrie's narrative idea has been so tantalizing that several other novelists proposed body swapping in their works. For instance, body swapping has been the core idea of a later children's novel, *Freaky Friday* (1972) by Mary Rodgers, and it was proposed also in Ian McEwan's *Daydreamer* (1992). Furthermore, it has been presented in several movies and television series, which reiterated both the original scenario of a body swapping between father and son (or mother and daughter in the case of *Freaky Friday*, first produced as a movie in 1976), or expanded into the scenario of gender swapping (as in the case of Blake Edward's *Switch*, 1991).

Box 2.3 Continued

As we have described in this chapter, some degree of body swapping is now becoming a reality. Instead of relying on magic stones brought from India, as in *Vice Versa*, affordable virtual reality technology allows taking the visual perspective of a different person, and sharing of experiences between individuals. This possibility has now been explored

(a)

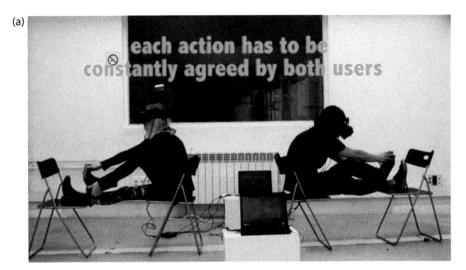

(b)

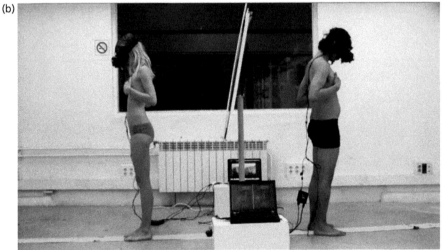

Figure 2.7 Swapping gender. Still frames from the video describing *Gender Swap—investigation on Gender Identity, Queer Theory and Mutual Respect,* performance presented at the Mu Art Space in Eindhoven (Netherlands) in 2014. See www.themachinetobeanother.org for the video and further details.
Courtesy of BeAnotherLab, beanotherlab.org

Box 2.3 Continued

by various research group throughout Europe (Henrik Ehrrson's lab in Sweden; Olaf Blanke and Andrea Serino's labs in Switzerland; Mel Slater's lab in Spain; Alessandro Farnè's lab in France), but notably also made it into less scientific contexts, at the boundaries between art and design. One of these examples is the insightful project called 'The machine to be another' (www.themachinetobeanother.org), a web-based platform that shares ideas on the potential of a low-cost and low-tech version of the paradigms developed in the research laboratories. The procedure they propose is simple and yet effective, based on a combination of telepresence achieved through head-mounted displays and headphones, and active performance (Figure 2.7). The couple involved in the body swapping makes an active effort to act in synchrony, touching identical objects available to both, while each of them sees in real-time the perspective recorded from a camera placed on the head of the body-swapping partner. Additionally, any spoken utterance made by the one member of the couple is presented through headphones and heard intracranially by the other member of the couple. With this simple set-up the BeAnotherLab has already explored the impact of sharing personal stories through the other's perspective, to 'embody the narratives' when heard and seen through narrators voice and eyes. In addition, they have tested the experience of swapping gender, or the experience of being in the body of a physically disabled person. The potentials of these approaches are just in their infancy, but it is already apparent from these explorations in science and art that body swapping could prove a useful tool for promoting empathic experiences or—at the very least—prompt perspective changes on fundamental topics such as gender, ethnicity, or social stereotypes.

Since these early observations, several other studies have now documented whole-body illusions (for review see Kilteni, Maselli, Kording, & Slater, 2015). What is becoming increasingly clear is that, unlike multisensory illusions for single body parts, whole-body misperception can allow researcher to manipulate some of the fundamental aspects of body perception, including the ones that potentially ground self-consciousness and self-awareness. Several authors (Gallagher, 2005; Blanke & Metzinger, 2009) have proposed that the experience of owning a body is the most basic kind of self-consciousness, a form of *minimal phenomenal selfhood*. According to Blanke and Metzinger (2009) the three main aspects that characterize minimal phenomenal selfhood are (1) the identification with the body as a whole (full-body ownership), (2) the experience of looking at the world from within our body (first-person perspective), and (3) the feeling that the body occupies a specific volume of space at any given time (self-location). As we have briefly seen in this section, each of these aspects can be altered using whole-body illusion paradigms, opening the possibility of experimentally manipulating these parameters of body perception and self-recognition. Studies on the brain correlates of body perception are starting to reveal partially distinct brain networks subtending some of these cognitive mechanisms (see Tutorial 2.1).

Tutorial 2.1 The multisensory body in the brain

Own body perception is functionally complex and a variety of distinct sensory channels—for touch, proprioception, vision, interoception, and vestibular signals—concur to the rich phenomenal experience that we have about our own body. In addition, own body perception entails sensorimotor processes, spatial transformations, and multisensory binding. Although the neural correlates of such a complex cognitive machinery involve an articulated network of brain regions, partial solutions to the puzzle of the brain basis of own-body perceptions are beginning to emerge (see Figure 2.8).

The first piece of the puzzle concerns the systematic involvement of the premotor cortex (PMC) and the superior portions of the posterior parietal cortex (particularly a sulcus termed the intra-parietal sulcus, IPS) in tasks that challenge body ownership. In fake hand illusion paradigms, these brain regions are active in both hemispheres in association with changes in perceived hand ownership and perceived hand position (Ehrsson et al., 2005; Tsakiris et al., 2007). Likewise, in whole-body illusions paradigms, they are involved during illusory self-identification with the visible body duplicate (Petkova et al., 2011; Lenggenhager, Halje, & Blanke, 2011; Guterstam, Björnsdotter, Gentile, & Ehrsson, 2015).

The second piece of the puzzle concerns the role of sensory cortices in body perception. In agreement with the multisensory perspective that we have adopted in this book, the sensory cortices involved in body perception include those dedicated to processing of somatosensory stimuli (S1; Ehrrson et al., 2007; Petkova et al., 2011), as well as those dedicated to processing visible instances of the body (particularly a region called the extrastriate body area, EBA; Ionta et al., 2011). Although the contribution of these brain areas to own-body perception has emerged using modern brain imaging techniques (e.g. fMRI, PET, electro-encephalography) in healthy people, concurrent evidence comes from the study of people with brain damage who show body disturbances (see Tutorial 2.2). In disorders

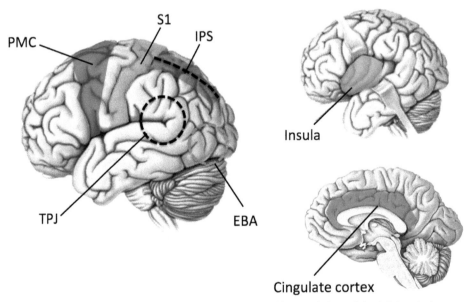

Figure 2.8 Brain areas involved in own body perception. (a) Lateral view of the left hemisphere. PMC: premotor cortex; S1: somatosensory cortex; IPS: intraparietal sulcus; TPJ: temporo-parietal junction; EBA: extra-striate body area. (b) View of the insula, once the lateral sulcus of the hemisphere is spread. (c) view of the cingulate cortex of the right hemisphere, once the left hemisphere is removed.

like asomatoagnosia or somatoparaphrenia, structural and functional changes have been documented in the cortical territories dedicated to somatosensation (primary and secondary somatosensory areas) and action planning (premotor brain regions). In addition, subcortical lesions involving the brain structure or fibres conveying somatosensory, vestibular, and visual signals from the receptors to the cortex have also been observed. Crucially, posterior brain areas such as the superior and inferior parietal lobule have also been associated with body disturbances (Vallar & Ronchi, 2009). The parietal lobes can accomplish the integration of multisensory and motor signals in space. Damage or deprivation of critical body afferents could contribute to the abnormal disintegration of the multisensory representation of the body (Wolpert, Goodbody, & Husain, 1998).

A third fundamental piece of the puzzle concerns the brain regions primarily supporting perception of self-location. As we highlighted in this chapter, self-location perception is essential for binding together multisensory and motor information about our own body and maintaining a coherent unity of the body and the self. The key region for this process seems to lay at the intersection of temporal and parietal lobes, and involve also the insular cortex (which is not visible on the side of the brain, but it can be exposed by spreading apart the cortices along the lateral sulcus of the hemisphere). The name of this region is the temporo-parietal junction (TPJ). When eliciting whole-body illusions in fMRI, this brain area was active during illusory self-location as well as during changes in first-person perspective. Interestingly, this area of the brain corresponds well also with the key region for cortical processing of vestibular information, an area called the parieto-insular vestibular cortex (PIVC). It is important to note here that the PIVC is a highly interconnected brain region, receiving multisensory and motor inputs from several of the brain areas already mentioned (the somatosensory cortex, the premotor cortex, the posterior parietal cortex). Furthermore, out-of-body experiences have been linked to disturbances in the TPJ (Blanke, Ortigue, Landis, & Seeck, 2002; Ionta et al., 2011).

Two final pieces of the puzzle are also noteworthy. One is the insular cortex, which we mentioned above. This hidden region of the brain is a multisensory hub for somatosensory, motor, visual, auditory, and vestibular inputs. In addition, it plays a role in the integration of interoceptive signals (Craig, 2002; Critchley et al., 2004) and is modulated by limbic signals (from the amygdala, the perirhinal cortex, and the cingulate cortex) that can contribute affective and emotional components to the multimodal body experience (e.g. Ebisch et al., 2011). The other is the cingulate cortex, which is also a brain region invisible on the lateral view of the brain, because it is hidden in the depths of the fissure that divides one brain hemisphere from the other. The more anterior portion of the cingulate cortex has been studied in studies adopting the fake hand illusion, and it has been linked with the involvement of an interoceptive neural circuitry (Ehrsson et al., 2007). In contrast, the role of the posterior portion of the cingulate cortex has only been recently revealed in a study inducing the whole-body illusion and triggering self-location changes in the participants (Guterstam, Björnsdotter, Gentile, Ehrsson, 2015). This brain activation has been linked to the spatial transformations linked to self-location processing.

As a final remark on the neural correlates of body perception, it is interesting to note that while the brain networks described in healthy people using brain imaging typically involve both brain hemispheres (for a review see Blanke, 2012), studies in patients who suffer body disturbances often document a more prevalent role for the right hemisphere. Disturbances such as asomatoagnosia and somatoparaphrenia are most often associated with lesions occurring in the right hemisphere of the brain. For this reason, they are most typically observed for left body parts (Vallar & Ronchi, 2009). Interestingly, the same happens also in behavioural pathologies that are not associated with brain lesions. For instance, xenomelia (see Tutorial 2.2) is considerably more common for left compared to right limbs (at least in men), suggesting a prominent role of the right hemisphere in this body disownership syndrome (e.g. see McGeoch et al., 2011 for evidence suggesting a key role of the right superior parietal lobule in processing touch from the non-accepted body part in xenomelia).

2.5 **The role of interoception in body perception**

Having made the case for multisensory body perception with examples from the inter-actions involving vision, it is time to return to the sensations originating from within the body and, in particular, to explore the contribution of interoception and vestibular signals. Interoceptive and vestibular signals are central to body perception, but they have remained surprisingly marginal until recent years. However, new lines of investigation are starting to show that the degree to which individuals are capable of processing their interoceptive signals could influence their overall susceptibility towards body illusions, i.e. the 'malleability of their body representation' (Tsakiris et al., 2011). We will start by considering the role of interoception and move to vestibular contributions in the next section.

The first study to experimentally address the link between interoception and body perception was conducted by Manos Tsakiris and collaborators (Tsakiris, Tajadura-Jiménez, & Costantini, 2011). Taking advantage of the fake hand illusion, they examined whether different degrees of interoceptive awareness could modulate the likelihood of incorporating the fake arm into body representations. Manipulating interoceptive sen-sations experimentally is rather difficult and potentially invasive. In extreme cases, it may entail introducing sterile water into the stomach through a naso-gastric tube and measuring the subject's ability to detect the induced stomach contractions (Whitehead & Drescher, 1980). However, Tsakiris and colleagues took a much less invasive ap-proach: they measured the ability of participants to track and count their heartbeats over a short time interval. This ability is variable in the population and correlates with other indices of interoceptive awareness (Herbert, Muth, Pollatos, & Herbert, 2012). You can try this task yourself, just relax and pay attention to your heartbeats without attempting to sense them through touch which would be far easier. Tsakiris and colleagues found that participants who were less able to monitor their heartbeat, that is, were less aware of their interoceptive states, were also more sensitive to the rubber hand illusion (see also Tajadura-Jimenez & Tsakiris, 2014).

Interestingly, this inverse relationship between interoceptive awareness and the fake hand illusion seems to hold also in clinical populations. For instance, people with eating disorders typically report altered interoceptive awareness. In one study (Eshkevari et al., 2012) it was shown that women suffering from eating disorders are also more sensi-tive to the fake hand illusion. Interestingly, their interoceptive deficits were among the variables that predicted the degree of body illusion (together with the tendency for self-objectification; see also Mussap & Salton, 2006). Another study (Schauder, Nash, Bryant, & Cascio, 2015) tested a group of children with autism spectrum disorder in the heartbeat monitoring task and in the fake hand illusion. They found that children with autism spec-trum disorder showed better interoceptive awareness in the heartbeat task compared to a group of children with typical development, particularly as the task became more com-plex. Interestingly, this group of children also showed the inverse relationship between interoceptive awareness and the fake hand illusion.

The current interpretation of the intriguing link between interoceptive awareness and body perception is that any *exteroceptive evidence* concerning seen body parts is constantly weighted against the *interoceptive predictions* of how the body feels (Critchley & Seth, 2012; Tajadura-Jimenez & Tsakiris, 2014). Put it more simply, whenever a visible fake hand is touched in synchrony with your real hand, your mind starts wondering whether it could be part of your body or not—a process of self/other distinction triggered by the available exteroceptive evidence. If you are highly sensitive to internal states of your body (you have good interoceptive models of how your body should feel) you may be more prone to reject the perceptual hypothesis that the fake hand is yours. This because none of your interoceptive sensations are a plausible match to the fake-arm you see. In contrast, if your monitoring of interoceptive sensations is poor, your ability to notice that your internal bodily sensations do not match the seen arm will also be less efficient. As a consequence, your body representation would be more malleable and more affected by body illusions.

Although this interpretation awaits systematic experimental testing, it makes an interesting prediction: if we incorporate interoceptive signals into the fake hand or fake body illusion, we should make the discrimination between self and other harder. In support of this prediction, two studies have recently developed interoceptive versions of the fake hand illusion (Suzuki, Garfinkel, Critchley, & Seth, 2013) and of the whole-body illusion (Aspell et al. 2013). In both cases, the experimenters introduced into the visible body a visual cue (a pulsating red light or a visible beating heart) which was synchronous or asynchronous with the participant's own heartbeat. As predicted, this visual-interoceptive synchrony increased the body illusion.

2.6 Vestibular signals and body perception

Somewhat similar to interoception, vestibular signals have also remained rather marginal in many multisensory accounts of body perception. Vestibular signals are critical for the interactions between the body and the environment, as evidenced by the hugely disabling consequences of vestibular dysfunctions such as vertigo. These sensations originate from sensory organs on each side of the head, located within the inner ear and next to the structure that hosts the mechanisms for the sound transduction (i.e. the cochlea). These vestibular organs comprise the semicircular canals and the otolith organs, which together form the vestibular labyrinth. Each semicircular canal appears as a circular tube, filled with fluid and mounted on an ampulla bearing hair cells that detect fluid movements. Because each vestibular labyrinth comprises three semicircular canals oriented in the x, y, and z planes, it can signal changes in head orientation with respect to gravity. The otolith organs, the utricle and saccule, are made of hair cells embedded in a gelatinous medium surmounted by stone-like elements (the otolith, literally the 'stones of the ear', from the Greek words for 'ear' and 'stone'). They detect linear acceleration and rotation of the head, and are the sensory organs that signal to your brain when the train actually starts to move.

Although vestibular contributions to body representation have been hypothesized by several authors (Lopez, 2013), systematic studies of this relationship started only in the last decade (for an insightful review, see Lenggenhager & Lopez, 2015). This is most surprising if one considers that gravitational forces have been present throughout human evolution and may have thus imposed substantial constraints on our body representation. Furthermore, it is rather striking if one considers that the vestibular system provides unambiguous sensory signals about body movements in space (Lenggenhager & Lopez, 2015). For vision, hearing, or touch, changes in the sensory input are potentially ambiguous in relation to body movements, because these sensory channels code body motion relative to an external reference (e.g. changes on the retina can result from the movements of the distal object or of the eyes; changes in time of arrival of a sound to the two ears (an auditory cue that can be used for localization, see Chapter 7) can arise from movement of the sound source or of the observer; changes on the skin can result from movements of the object or of the object). By contrast, vestibular sensations code head motion relative to a fixed, common reference: gravity.

Evidence that vestibular changes can impact on body representation comes from the neuropsychological literature. Body disturbances such as perceived changes in body-part size or experiences of body-part disownership (see Tutorial 2.2) have been reported

---

Tutorial 2.2 Disorders of multisensory body perception

In this chapter, we argue that the body as we know it is the result of representations created through multisensory processes. What can happen if these multisensory processes fail temporarily or permanently? Disorders of body perception have been known for a long time and several authors hint that at least for some pathological misperceptions of the body the problem is precisely a malfunction of multisensory processes (Brugger & Lenggenhager, 2014; de Vignemont, 2010; Haggard & Wolpert, 2005; Semenza, 2001). Here we provide brief descriptions of five misperceptions involving the body and likely attributable to multisensory malfunctions: misperceptions of limb size, paradoxical disappearances of a limb, limb disownership, autoscopic hallucinations, and 'phantom' limbs.

The perceptual magnification or minification of one's limb have been called *macro-* and *microsomatognosia*. Since the original observations of Bonnier (1905) who documented several patients reporting that their body or body parts felt larger or smaller, this body disturbance has been seldom reported. Increase in the perceived size of the face and hands is also known to occur during migraine auras (Robinson & Podoll, 2000). Interestingly, anaesthetized body parts are usually perceived as larger than they are (Gandevia & Phegan, 1999), and Fisher (1976) reported that upon awakening some people feel their body size to be reduced. As discussed at the beginning of this chapter, the representation of the body in primary and secondary somatosensory areas devotes a disproportionally large amount of cortex to the hands and face, in comparison to other body parts (see Figure 2.1). The brain exploits information provided by visual and kinaesthetic sensory signals to rescale these distorted somatotopic maps and generate higher level representations of body structure. It has been suggested that macrosomatoagnosia may be caused by a malfunction of the multisensory processes that contribute to these higher-level body representations (Haggard & Wolpert, 2005), resulting in perceptually enlarged hands or faces. Although the same logic would predict perceptual minification for cortically underrepresented parts, microsomatoagnosia seems to be less frequent than macrosomatoagnosia. One possible explanation for this finding is that somatotopic distortions in the homunculus are in the direction of an enlargement of body parts (such as the face, hands, and oral cavity), whereas the body is relatively undistorted (including the head, trunk, arms, and legs). This may make minification less likely.

The tendency of limbs to disappear has been termed *feeling of absence*. Most patients are aware that the fading of limbs is illusory, although they don't have an explanation for the illusion. The disappearance has therefore a paradoxical character. Wolpert, Goodbody, and Husain (1998) described a patient with lesions in the left parietal lobe who experienced fading of right limbs when she could not see them and did not move them. Haggard & Wolpert (2005) suggested that these symptoms may be related to a problem in the interaction of kinaesthetic and somatosensory signals, causing an inability to maintain a representation of limb position in the absence of changing proprioceptive signals from muscles and joints, or signals from vision. Arzy, Overney, Landis, and Blanke (2006) described a patient with lesions in the right premotor area who experienced visual fading of her left forearm and hand. These authors interpreted this dramatic experience as due to a disturbance of multisensory interactions between visual and somatosensory signals at the level of the premotor cortex, which is known to receive visual and somatosensory input from parietal regions and to contain neurons with visual–somatosensory receptive fields. Although we don't know how these interactions may account for visual disappearance, the case suggests that the premotor cortex collaborates with the parietal cortex in multisensory body perception and representation.

In brain-damaged patients the loss of body parts can also emerge in combination with productive symptoms, whereby the body part becomes the object of delusions. These misperceptions were first described by Gerstman (1942), who termed them *somatoparaphrenias*. They typically involve somatosensory hallucinations, such as the feeling that the limb is separated from the body or the delusional attribution of one's limb to others ('This is my niece's hand. She works here (i.e. in the hospital). I do not know why her hand is here, she should be around.'; Romano, Gandola, Bottini, & Maravita, 2014). Patients with somatoparaphrenia often also have difficulties in attending the body side opposite the brain lesion and can have visual or somatosensory deficits. In particular, a loss of position sense for the body (proprioception) is quite characteristic. However, somatoparaphrenia can also occur in the absence of these deficits, suggesting that they are not sufficient causes (Vallar & Ronchi, 2009). Presumably, instead, what goes wrong in these patients are multisensory processes for representing the space surrounding one's own body. Key to these processes is solving a binding problem: somatosensory signals and visual information about the body need to be integrated when they both originate from ourselves, but kept separate otherwise (Vallar & Ronchi, 2009). When such integration fails, seen limbs can feel extraneous to one's body. In the words of one patient: 'My eyes and my feelings don't agree, and I must believe my feelings. I know they look like mine, but I can feel they are not, and I can't believe my eyes' (quoted by Nielsen, 1938, p. 555). A puzzling manifestation of body disownership is called *xenomelia* (also termed apothemnophilia or body integrity disorder). Patients with xenomelia perceive their body veridically and verbally acknowledge ownership of each body part. At the same time, however, they experience such a deep detachment from certain body parts as to actively seek their surgical removal (Blom, Hennekam, & Denys, 2012; First, 2005). Patients with xenomelia do not have brain lesions, and this seems to set them apart from somatoparaphrenics. As for somatoparaphrenia, however, it has been suggested that xenomelia may be caused by a dysfunction of parietal-lobe multisensory processes that represent the body (Brang, McGeoch, & Ramachandran, 2008). Supporting this conjecture, a recent MRI study by Hilti et al. (2013) revealed brain structural changes in the right parietal lobe of patients with xenomelia, relative to controls.

One further example of body disorder attributable to a breakdown of multisensory processes are autoscopic phenomena. Autoscopy literally means self-seeing, from the Greek *autos* (self) and *skopein* (looking at), and consists of vivid illusions of seeing one's own body from outside, as if the self had somehow abandoned the physical body. Note that this implies a change of the perceived location of the 'centre of conscious experience', that is, of the self (Blanke & Mohr, 2005). These illusions come into three kinds: *out-of-body experiences, autoscopic hallucinations,* and *heautoscopy* (Brugger, Zosh, & Warren, 1997). During an out-of-body experience, people report floating outside their physical body and looking down on it from an elevated perspective. This is a combination of disembodiment (the self outside the physical body), change in perspective (a third-person view on one's own body), and autoscopy proper. It is important to remark here the sensations of floating, of being elevated, and without weight, that frequently accompany out-of-body experiences. These sensations are compatible with transient alterations of the vestibular function and testify the importance of this sensory system for body perception (see section 2.7). During autoscopic hallucinations, people instead see a duplicate of themselves, but this is a bit like looking at oneself into a mirror, there is no perception that the self is outside the physical body (no disembodiment). Finally, during heautoscopy, one can have a somewhat intermediate experience. Similar to autoscopic hallucinations, patients who experience heautoscopy report seeing a copy of themselves, right in front of them. However, it is difficult for them to establish whether their self is anchored within their physical body or it is projected into their double. This produces the very unsettling feeling of occupying *both* locations at the same time: the real one and the extra-personal one. Heautoscopy differs from the other autoscopic phenomena also for the great unpleasantness of the experience. People suffering this condition report the terrifying feeling of being split into two parts or two selves; in other words, the feeling of being two people at the same time.

The last form of body misperceptions in our list is probably the best known. *Phantom limb* experiences consist in vivid percepts originating from a limb that no longer exists due to amputation or is deafferented (Mitchell, 1871). These percepts can include feelings of limb position in space, limb movement, light touch, or hitching. About 50–80 percent of amputees also report pain (Jensen & Nikolajesen, 1999). The condition can last for many years and even for one's whole life, although many patients report that over the years the phantoms disappear in part or completely, often undergoing a perceivable gradual retraction towards the stump (a phenomenon known as telescoping, which could be also classified as a special case of microsomatoagnosia). Phantom limb is independent of general intelligence, age, degree of awareness of the mutilation, or acceptance of the mutilation. Most importantly, there is no relation between the emotional significance of the amputated part and the prevalence of phantoms (Weinstein, 1969), a fact that argues against psychodynamic accounts. As an alternative, it has been proposed that the neural representation of the missing limb remains active, and that the brain interprets this activity as originating from the body part that was originally represented there. Studies of non-human primates (Merzenich et al., 1984) and human amputees (Ramachandran, Rogers-Ramachandran, & Cobb, S., 1995; Aglioti, Bonazzi, & Cortese, 1994) have documented substantial reorganization of primary and secondary somatosensory cortices following amputation. Cortical regions that represent the missing hand can be invaded by afferents from cortical neighbouring regions, such as that of the face or the upper arm. Supporting this proposal, it has been observed that arm amputees often report feeling phantom tactile percepts on the missing limb when they are touched on the cheek (Ramachandran & Altschuler, 2009). This is indeed what one would expect if, after cortical reorganization, regions representing the hand were stimulated by face afferents, but continued to refer these signals to the hand. Although we believe that phantom limb phenomena should not be considered pathological breakdowns of multisensory processes—unlike the other disturbances described above—they clearly speak of the possibility of dissociation between sensory information from the body and awareness of body parts. In our view, they offer strong arguments for the proposal that high level representations of the body originate from multisensory and motor signals, not just from somatosensation. This proposal may also have useful implications for the treatment of phantom limb pain (see BOX 2.4).

in association with alterations of the vestibular system. The Austrian psychologist and psychoanalyst Paul Ferdinand Schilder (the father of the term 'body image') noted that vestibular patients make claims that extremities became larger or elongates during dizziness (Schilder, 1935; cited in Lopez et al., 2012). The Italian neuropsychologist Edoardo Bisiach and colleagues studied a right-brain-damaged patient with pathological delusions of disownership for the left arm. They observed that pouring cold water in the left ear induced activation of the vestibular system, eventually alleviating symptoms related to

Box 2.4 Shooing phantoms with mirrors

In the fourth episode of its sixth series, the celebrated TV show *Dr House* featured the protagonist treating a war veteran who has phantom limb pain in his amputated arm (see Tutorial 2.2). House shows up with a strange box holding a mirror in the middle, and literally forces the amputated veteran to undergo 'a little bit of neurological trickery'. The patient has to sit in front of the box, with the mirror parallel to the sagittal body plane and facing the healthy arm (Figure 2.9), and is asked to clench his fist in the healthy arm while he imagines clenching the fist of the phantom hand. As he moves the good arm, he sees its reflection, located exactly where his amputated arm would have been behind the mirror. After this, House says: 'now let go'. The patient stretches the hand (or hands, if you include the phantom) … and breaks into tears of joy. After more than 30 years, his phantom limb pain has gone away.

House's procedure is, of course, a piece of medical science fiction ('If only it was that easy!' complained a neuropsychologist friend). Behind the dramatization, however, are some intriguing observations and an experimental rehabilitation procedure: *mirror box therapy*. A mirror box (Ramachandran & Ramachandran, 1996) is essentially a poor man's virtual reality. By exploiting mirror reflection and body symmetry, it affords a simple way of creating a virtual image of a hand and arm, independently of its actual

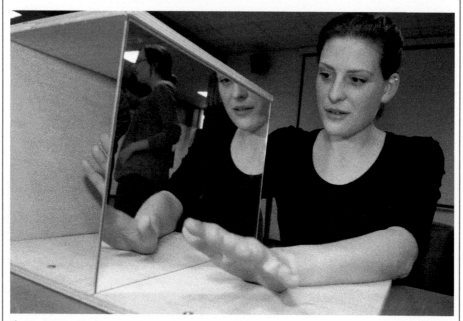

Figure 2.9 A simple mirror box. The left arm of the participant is in front of the mirror; the right arm is hidden behind the mirror. The participant looks at her left arm while she also sees the reflection of the left arm in the mirror, looking just as a right arm.
Paul Avis/Alamy Stock Photo

Box 2.4 Continued

position. You can easily try it yourself. Get a mirror, place it sagitally in front of your body midline with the reflecting side facing left, and put your hands symmetrically on both sides. Now look rightwards into the mirror. You will see your left hand, of course, but because of the mirror it will look just like your right hand. And quite convincingly so: if, unknown to you, your right hand is displaced so that its true position is no longer symmetrical to that of the left hand, you will still feel it in a position consistent with what you see in the mirror (Holmes, Crozier, & Spence, 2004). Even more surprisingly, if you try moving the right hand, you will have the most alarming paradoxical experience of paralysis. You willed your hand to move, but you did not see it move—because you were seeing the reflection from the left hand, and this hand you did not move. Now suppose that you suffered amputation of your right hand. Using the mirror box, you can generate a visual signal that will tell your brain that your hand is there again. And if you were experiencing a phantom limb, this will remove the conflict between the felt phantom and the unseen hand. The idea behind mirror box therapy is, in a nutshell, simply this. The pain arises somehow because of the conflict between the visual and the somatosensory signals. Remove the conflict, and the pain will go away.

In real life, real mirror box therapy is a little different from House's version. First of all, it usually consists of relatively long sessions spread out over several days—no sudden healings in real life. Second, it is now often performed using virtual reality rather than an actual mirror box (Cole, Crowler, Austwick, & Slater, 2009; Murray, et al., 2006). The way this works is the following. Using motion capture apparatus, the motion of the stump in three dimensions is used in real time to render a computer-generated arm that is seen to move on a VR display in the appropriate position relative to the stump. This frees the patient from the need to perform movements with the healthy arm, allowing a greater variety of movements over longer periods and extending the approach to bilateral amputees. Third, there is evidence that mirror box therapy can reduce phantom limb pain in comparison to control conditions (Chan et al., 2007; Lamont, Chin, & Kogan, 2011), but not for all patients (Cole, Crowle, Austwick, & Slater, 2009; Brodie, Whyte, & Nive, 2007) and not without minor but noticeable side effects (Casale, Damiani, & Rosati, 2009). The technique, therefore, remains somewhat controversial. Interestingly, however, recent evidence also suggests that mirror box therapy can help with other forms of chronic pain (Karmarkar & Lieberman, 2006) and in rehabilitating hemiparetic patients (Dohle, et al., 2009; Samuelkamaleshkumar et al., 2014; Wu et al., 2013). Thus, mirror therapy is no miracle cure, but can be justly considered an interesting, and potentially useful, clinical application of basic findings in multisensory research.

body disownership (Bisiach, Rusconi, & Vallar, 1991; see also Rode et al., 1992). More recently, it has been shown that similar procedures affecting the vestibular system can also alter body perceptions in healthy participants (Lopez, Schreyer, Preuss, & Mast, 2010).

Lopez and collaborators applied electrical stimulation behind the ears to induce predictable changes in the vestibular sensory organs (galvanic vestibular stimulation) while participants were tested in the fake hand illusion set-up. When the electrical stimulation increased vestibular functions on the right side, the feeling of ownership for the fake hand as well as the tactile mislocalization towards it increased. In another study, Lopez and colleagues (2012) induced vestibular stimulation by pumping a constant air flow of warm air in the right ear canal and concurrently a flow of cold air in the left ear canal. Participants were asked to compare tactile distances applied to the palm of their left hand with those applied to the forehead (note that this is the same procedure used by Taylor-Clarke, Jacobsen, & Haggard, 2004, which we described in section 2.3 to document the effects of visual arm elongation on body size perception). Remarkably, distances on the hand were judged longer during caloric vestibular stimulation, indicating that the temporary changes in the vestibular signals modified the internal representation of hand-size.

One recent study has shown that galvanic vestibular stimulation can also affect the extent to which participants hold first-person vs third-person perspectives on their body (Ferrè, Lopez, & Haggard, 2014). To assess the preferred adopted perspective, they used the so-called graphesthesia task (Natsoulas & Dubanoski, 1964). Imagine an experimenter in front of you draws the letter 'b' on your forehead while you are blindfolded: do you think you would see it from the same perspective as the experimenter (third-person view) and read it also as 'b', or instead you would see it from your perspective (first-person view) and read it as 'd'? Although both perspectives are possible, by studying which one prevails over the other it possible to infer which perspective (first- vs third-perspective) was preferentially chosen by the participant. Interestingly, Ferrè and colleagues (2014) found that low-intensity galvanic vestibular stimulation causes first-person perspectives to become more frequent and suggested that this could reflect augmented vestibular contributions to embodiment.

These findings on vestibular contributions to body representation highlight the importance of adding this sensory system to the multisensory accounts of body perception. Several authors have hypothesized that vestibular sensations could play a key role in the process of binding multiple sensory signals. Such binding is necessary to produce the coherent and embodied first-person perspective experience that characterizes own-body perception (Blanke, 2012; Lenggenhager & Lopez, 2015).

2.7 The multisensory body and the social self

A rubber hand, a mannequin, or a virtual reality avatar are not experienced as truly animate entities. They are not conspecifics that have 'another mind'. But what would happen if we could elicit a multisensory illusion with a whole-body or a body-part that recognizably belongs to another person? Can the multisensory illusion create some form of binding between the self of a participant and the self of someone else? This question bridges multisensory perception body perception with social cognition (for a recent review see Maister, Slater, Sanchez-Vives, & Tsakiris, 2015), and allow us to conclude by showing some broader and rather unexpected implications of the multisensory phenomena we describe in the chapter.

One important starting point for this research line was when investigators realized that the fake hand paradigm could be adapted to accommodate a situation in which the stimulated body part clearly belongs to another person. This occurs if the experimenter simultaneously touches the face of a participant while she watches the face of another person being similarly touched in a video feed (Tsakiris, 2008; Sforza, Bufalari, Haggard, & Aglioti, 2010). When the stimulation is applied to both faces synchronously, some components of the perceptual experience are similar to those of the classic fake hand illusion. For instance, participants may report feeling the light touches where they see the other person being touched. Another component of the illusion, however, is more surprising. After synchronous stimulation, participants often perceive the face of the other person as looking more like their own—hence the description of this effect as 'enfacement' (Tsakiris, 2008; Sforza, Bufalari, Haggard, & Aglioti, 2010). If participants are exposed to a graded series of morphs between their own face and the face of the other person, they identify as their own face morphs having a larger proportion of facial features coming from the other person (Tajadura-Jiménez, Grehl, & Tsakiris, 2012). In Figure 2.10 we present an example of what gradual facial morphing can look like, using two well-known faces instead of the stimuli adopted in the real enfacement studies. These results therefore seem to suggest a certain degree of bodily merging between the participant and the stranger stimulated in synchrony.

Even more strikingly, multisensory stimulation can trigger a perceived similarity between self and other that expands beyond physical appearance to encompass personality traits. Recent research has shown that participants are more inclined to attribute personality traits that belong to themselves to the stranger in the video feed after synchronous multisensory stimulation with the stranger, but not after asynchronous stimulation (Paladino, Mazzurega, Pavani, & Schubert, 2010; Mazzurega, Pavani, Paladino, & Schubert, 2011). Remarkably, participants in the synchronous conditions are also readier to conform to a judgement expressed by the stranger. This behaviour is typically observed when strangers are considered as in-group members (Castelli, Vanzetto, Sherman, & Arcuri, 2001). Thus, these studies reveal that multisensory perception can cause a

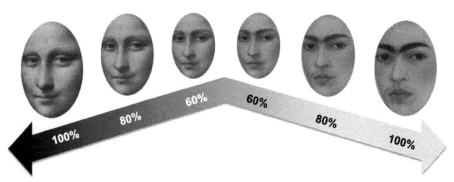

Figure 2.10 Morphing from Mona Lisa to Frida Kahlo. In white the percentage of Mona Lisa's facial features in each oval; in black the percentage of Frida Kahlo's facial features in each oval.

merging between self and others along conceptual and social dimensions, extending the impact of multisensory body illusions to the domain of social cognition.

Researchers are taking the link between multisensory body perception and social cognition even further, exploring to what extent sharing a body through multisensory illusions could promote empathy and perspective taking. For instance, Maister, Tsiakkas, and Tsakiris (2013) tested emotion recognition before and after the induction of the enfacement illusion. Emotion recognition improved for the synchronous other, selectively for the fearful facial expressions, compared to control conditions using asynchronous stimulation or no-stimulation. Even more strikingly, in a study using immersive virtual reality to embody adults in a 4-year old child, it was observed that participants classify themselves using child-like more than adult-like attributes to a greater extent after they experienced the bodily illusion (Banakou, Groten, & Slater, 2013).

Another line of research has explored to what extent the conceptual consequences of multisensory body illusions could change social attitudes towards groups: in other words, the possibility that blurring self–other boundaries at the perceptual level could also change long-term categorization that people apply to social groups (i.e. stereotypes). Two studies so far have attempted to change attitudes towards social groups using multisensory body illusions. Maister, Sebanz, Knoblich, and Tsakiris (2013) induced the rubber hand illusion in a group of Caucasian participants using a dark-skinned fake hand. Before and after the illusion, they measured the racial bias of each participant against people with dark skin using a well-known implicit test based on speeded responses to verbal and pictorial stimuli (the Implicit Association Test; Greenwald, McGhee, & Schwartz, 1998). Results showed that the more participants experienced the illusion of ownership for the dark-skinned hand, the more positive their implicit attitudes towards the dark-skin outgroup became. Convergent findings were documented in the same year by a different research group, using a whole-body illusion in a virtual reality set-up (Peck, Seinfeld, Aglioti, & Slater, 2013). In this study, light-skinned participants were embodied either in an avatar with a similar skin tone, or in an avatar with a dark skin tone or alien-like avatar with bright purple skin. Similar to Maister, Tsiakkas, and Tsakiris (2013), embodiment in a dark-skin avatar (but not in an alien-like avatar, which is obviously also an outgroup member) reduced implicit racial biases.

What these recent lines of investigation show is that a multisensory perspective to body perception, as well as the multisensory paradigms used to elicit bodily illusions, can have an impact that reaches well beyond body perception alone. Conceptual representation of the self, including social constructs such as interpersonal bonding or stereotypes, appear to be influenced by these seemingly simple manipulations. When looking at social behaviours common to all cultures, it is actually quite striking how multisensory and motor synchronizations across individuals have been used throughout human history to promote social bonding (Durkheim, 1915; Fiske, 2004). Consider, for instance, the strong interpersonal impact of social behaviours like ritual dancing, choir singing, or marching, which rely all on acting in synchrony in response to visual, auditory, and somatosensory stimulations. Although the complexity of these behaviours surely entails more than multisensory integration alone, we believe that the conceptual tools that we outlined in the present chapter could prove when attempting a cognitive explanation of their origins.

Chapter 3

Perception for Action

3.1 **Motor behaviours**

Multisensory interactions play a fundamental role in the multifaceted representations subserving how we perceive our bodies. Our bodies, however, are not static, and sensory signals are constantly being processed by the brain also to guide actions and control body posture. Given this plain fact, it will come as no surprise that multisensory interactions are also fundamental in motor control. In this chapter, we will discuss some examples of such interactions, with special attention to reaching and grasping with the hand, to locomotion, and to the control of one's posture. In addition, we will discuss the intricate problems that arise when tackling the perception of *agency,* arguably one of the most important features of selfhood—on the motor side of body ownership. Motor control is a complex field of study with a large literature (for comprehensive treatments, see Rosenbaum, 1991; Schmidt & Lee, 1999). As this is mainly a book about perception, we will not attempt to review this literature in full. Rather, we will concentrate on few selected examples to elucidate how multisensory perception impacts on how we understand motor behaviours. An advantage of studying simple tasks involving multisensory motor control is that these are more easily reproduced in well-controlled laboratory settings. In these settings, an investigator can use state-of-the-art equipment for recording the trajectory of the movements in space, and eventually extract key kinematic signatures of the processes that take sensory signals as input and produce organized motor commands as output.

Our choice to focus on grasping, locomotion, and agency does not mean of course that perception scientists are not interested in other, more naturalistic situations. For instance, Gray (2008) reviewed a series of empirical results concerning the role of multisensory signals in sports and in driving automobiles and aeroplanes. One of these concerns how pilots control flying direction in conditions that involve a sudden forward acceleration of the aeroplane. As illustrated in Figure 3.1, three sources of sensory information are available to the pilot about the forward movement of his or her body in these conditions. The first is the focus of expansion (FOE) of the optic flow, recorded through the visual channel, and potentially specifying the flying direction relative, for instance, to the underlying terrain. The second is a constellation of pressure signals, caused by gravity (g), on the portions of the skin that contact the pilot seat, coded through somatosensory channels. The third is the vestibular signal caused by the inertial force (I) which results from forward acceleration. Note that, as shown in the figure, the resultant of the g and I forces can be a vector that points downward. This means that the combination of the sensory signals caused by

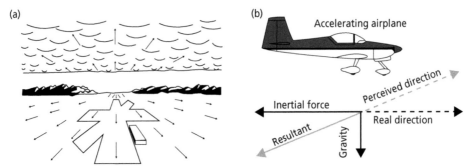

Figure 3.1 The *heads-up* illusion. A pilot can experience the heads-up illusion when conditions degrade visual information and the plane is subjected to a sudden acceleration, such that the resultant of the gravitational and inertial forces is a vector pointing downward. (a) schematics of the focus of expansion (FOE) of optic flow, providing visual information about flight direction. (b) Schematics of the proprioceptive information from inertial and gravitational forces during forward acceleration.

g and I could, in principle, inform the brain that the body is moving upward (opposite to the inertial plus gravitational pull) even if the plane is in reality flying level. Often this will not be a serious problem because pilots can rely on visual signals for controlling flying direction. But now suppose that, for whatever reason (clouds? nightime flying?), visual signals became less reliable or absent altogether. Inexperienced pilots could be tricked by some combination of gravitational and inertial forces into perceiving an upward movement of their body. They might then erroneously attempt to correct the flying direction by pushing the joystick forward, and by this action cause the plane to nose-dive with potentially dangerous consequences. This situation is known in aviation parlance as the *heads-up illusion,* and it is an excellent example of the many practical implications of multisensory research in real-world conditions.

The skill of an expert pilot is a fine example of the process that takes sensory signals as input and produces organized motor commands as outputs. An organized sequence of goal-directed motor behaviours is often termed an *action,* and because actions are the focus of this chapter, we begin with a discussion of four conceptual distinctions that are useful for defining them: The distinctions between discrete, continuous, and serial motor behaviours; between open and closed motor behaviours; between a preparatory and an online phase; and between closed-loop and open-loop control. A brief discussion of each will reveal (although by no means exhaust) the complexity of the mental functions involved in guiding actions, and the sheer number of brain mechanisms potentially involved. Given this complexity, one might very reasonably expect that multisensory interactions are heavily involved in how we guide actions. Examples of how researchers are accumulating evidence for this prediction will be introduced after this introductory section, starting with reaching and grasping.

Organized goal-directed movements come in many kinds, and the motor control literature offers several useful classifications. An important distinction is that between discrete, continuous, and serial motor behaviours. *Discrete* motor behaviours have a well-defined beginning and end. Throwing a ball or striking a match are good examples. *Continuous* motor behaviours, in contrast, do not. Swimming laps or steering a car, for instance, are continuous motor behaviours. *Serial* motor behaviours, finally, are sequences of discrete behaviours performed one after the other. This happens, for instance, when one prepares a cup of coffee or completes an assembly line task. In addition, and irrespective of whether the action is discrete or continuous, another important issue is whether the environment where the action takes place is predictable or not. Here, motor control scientist often think of a continuous dimension with *open* and *closed* behaviours as defining opposite polarities. Suppose, for instance, that you are playing a football game, and that you are pushing the ball towards the goal to score. There are many environmental features that are continuously changing and that you should take into account in guiding your action, including the actions of your teammates, of the opposing team players, and especially of the goalkeeper, and your own internal state. All these features are largely unpredictable, and a skilled player needs to adjust to them flexibly as the action progresses. This is therefore a prime example of an open motor behaviour. In contrast, consider the conditions of a bowling contest. Here the conditions are relatively stable and predictable, as each throw is done in the same conditions, your lane in the bowling alley. This would therefore be a good example of a closed skill. Most natural motor behaviours fall somewhere in between the extremes of a fully unpredictable or completely predictable environment. When steering a car on the highway, for instance, the behaviour of other drivers and the features of the road will be to some extent always the same, but there can be unexpected happenings or unusual road conditions that violate your expectations.

The distinctions outlined in the previous paragraph have implications for the sensori-motor processes that one would expect to be most relevant. Note that the tripartite distinction between serial, continuous, and discrete motor behaviours pertains mainly to the actual movements that are part of an action and to their temporal unfolding. The polarity between open and closed actions, in contrast, pertains mainly to the nature of the typical environment of a given action. When combined together, these two classifications suggest that some kinds of motor behaviours can be executed using mostly sensory signals that were collected before initiating any actual movement. A closed discrete action, for instance, is a sequence of well-defined movements to be executed in relatively fixed conditions. To a large extent, therefore, it should be possible to pre-programme the sequence and then execute it rapidly, paying relatively little attention to the sensory input during the actual movement. Other actions should instead require constant monitoring of external conditions. An open serial action, for instance, implies a sequence of discrete movements in relatively unpredictable conditions. Successful performance of this type of task therefore requires processing sensory signals that become available during the execution. This analysis implies that the sensory guidance of actions can, in principle, take place in two different ways, namely, exploiting mostly sensory signals that are collected before movement onset (preparatory phase), or mostly signals that become available during movement (online control phase). These two strategies, in turn, imply different effects of movement velocity, as has been known for more than a century. The next paragraph introduces this idea.

The distinction between a preparatory and an online phase is, perhaps, one of the most fundamental conceptual tools in the psychology of action. Its roots can be traced at least as far as the PhD thesis written by the influential early experimental psychologist Robert S. Woodworth at Columbia University. A Harvard undergraduate, Woodworth studied under William James and was later admitted to the Columbia Graduate School to work with James McKeen Cattell, the first professor of experimental psychology in the USA. In his doctoral thesis, Woodworth used a somewhat rudimentary, but effective method for recording multiple hand movements. A continuous roll of paper was mounted on a device called a kymograph, which moved the paper while a participant traced a set of successive straight lines with a pencil. In the simplest, and most used, task participants were required to make each line equal to the immediately preceding line. In this way, each trial effectively created the target for the following trial, ensuring that participants planned each movement afresh instead of repeating them mechanically. The method, however, had another important advantage: it allowed Woodworth to test participants in two conditions, with eyes open but also with eyes closed. Finally, Woodworth employed a mechanical metronome to pace participants in the task, thus varying the speed of execution of each trial. In each trial, Woodworth measured the error in reproducing the length of the preceding line.

The results reported by Woodworth are reproduced in Figure 3.2. In the 'eyes open' condition, participants looked at each line while they tried to reproduce it. In the 'eyes closed' condition, instead, they kept the eyes closed and had to resort to the immediate memory of the previous movement. In the 'automatic' condition, finally, participants kept the eyes open but did not look at the lines—they were left free to move their eyes around the room without any specific constraint. Two features are apparent in the data. First, average error grows with speed in the 'eyes open' condition, but not in the other two conditions.

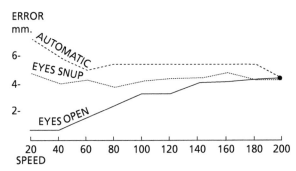

Figure 3.2 Woodworth's results. Average error is plotted as a function of tracing speed in the three conditions of Woodworth's line-tracing task. Reproduced from the original graph in the dissertation (Figure 3 in Woodworth, 1899). Author of the pencil marks unknown.

Reproduced from Woodworth, R.S., 'The accuracy of voluntary movement', figure 3, PhD thesis, University of Columbia, 1899.

Second, average error remains mostly constant in these other two conditions, but not perfectly—it tends to be slightly larger at very low metronome settings in the 'automatic' and to some extent also in the 'eyes closed' conditions. Woodworth interpreted these results as evidence that sensory guidance of movement involves two phases. He called them *initial adjustment* and *current control*. The initial adjustment of the target length is performed before starting the movement, on the basis of the available sensory signals, whereas the current control is performed *during* the movement, and consists in a series of 'later and finer adjustments by means of which a movement is enabled to approximate more and more closely to its goal.' (Woodworth, 1899, p. 42). Note that the longer the time of the movement, the larger the opportunity to perform these online finer adjustments. Thus, one would expect that errors increase as velocity increases (and movement time accordingly decreases), as observed. But these finer adjustments are mostly based on visual signals about hand position, relative to the goal of the movement. When these visual signals are not available, therefore, one would not expect to see this effect of velocity, and this is also observed. In addition, Woodworth noted that his use of a metronome caused the interval between successive responses to co-vary with speed. At slower metronome settings, movements were slower but there was also a longer interval between the presentation of the target (the preceding response) and the onset of the response. Woodworth suggested that the initial adjustment 'becomes less certain as the interval that has elapsed increases' (Woodworth, 1899, p. 42), causing the small increment in average error at the lower metronome settings.

Woodworth's two-phase model provided a tremendously influential framework for understanding sensorimotor transformations in simple movements, and it remains an important foundation of much work in this area (Elliott, Helsen, & Chua, 2001). It is now generally agreed that both aiming and reach-to-grasp movements involve two phases, and that the relative importance of these phases depends on specific compromises between speed and accuracy that seek to achieve fluidity of movement within the constraints of a specific task.

3.2 Multisensory interactions in aiming

Although he manipulated only visual signals, Woodworth was well aware that the aiming movements he studied were guided by a multisensory process. He wrote: ' [...] any sense whatever may conceivably serve as the sensory basis for controlling the extent of movement. Those which actually do so serve are the 'muscular,' tactile, visual and auditory, and probably in some cases the sense of smell.' (p. 72). In his opinion, two empirical questions stemmed from this realization: to determine if aiming with eyes open relied only on vision or also relied on other channels; and to determine what sensory channels are used to guide the movement when eyes are closed and vision is excluded. These remain key questions in the study of multisensory perception for action. Regarding the first question, Woodworth believed that in his experiment only vision was used: '...the movement entirely disregarded the muscle sense and relied solely on the eye.' Regarding the second, he argued that aiming was guided using an internal, abstract motor representation. He called this 'a sense of the extent of movement', not reducible to the perception of either its force, duration, or its starting and ending positions. This representation was, in his conclusion, '…the real basis on which control is based' (p. 80). We now know that the first of Woodworth's intuitions is not true in general, whereas the second is largely correct. Key data supporting these conclusions comes from studies employing a technique known as prismatic adaptation.

Prismatic adaptation involves exposing participants to a systematic disturbance of the optical input and observing how performance adapts (see Tutorial 3.1). It is most easily

---

Tutorial 3.1 The intriguing world of prismatic adaptation

One of the most deeply ingrained naïve assumptions about vision is that vision begins with a retinal 'image.' Many of us have been taught in school that the eye works like a camera, focusing light rays on the receptive surface in its back. The image thus formed on the photoreceptor mosaic is then processed and passed on to the higher visual centres where it is interpreted. This eye-as-a-camera analogy is no doubt useful to understand focusing defects such as myopia or hyperopia, that cause the rays to be focused before (near-sightedness) or after (far-sightedness) the retina, and to prescribe glasses that can correct these defects. When we try to understand the whole process of visual perception, however, the analogy immediately becomes the source of a theoretical puzzle. The optics of the eye, just like those of a camera, invert the putative image such that objects on the left (or right) visual field are projected on the right (left) parts of the retina, and likewise objects on the upper (lower) field are projected on its lower (upper) parts. How come then that we see the world right-side up and with left and right in the correct environmental positions? Clearly, the brain must be doing something much more complicated than merely 'looking' at the putative retinal image to determine where things are out there.

Important insights on how the brain does this have come from experiments with head-mounted devices that alter the input available to the eye. This has been done most often with wedge prisms that deflect the light rays by a certain amount (usually 10 to 20 degrees) laterally, and that are relatively easy to obtain. In more extreme cases, special devices have been used to completely invert the direction of the rays vertically (such that the 'image' is no longer upside-down) or horizontally (re-inverting left and right), or both. The results of these experiments have been tremendously instructive, and here we will try to give you a brief introduction to these intriguing observations. To this end, we will begin by travelling back in time to George Stratton's laboratory at Berkeley and then to Ivo Kohler's psychology department in Innsbruck.

George Malcolm Stratton (1865–1957) was one of the pioneer experimentalists in perceptual psychology. Trained as a philosopher, after a period in Wilhelm Wundt's Institute for Experimental Psychology in Leipzig, Germany, in 1896 Stratton came back to his Alma Mater, the University of California at Berkeley. In the same year, he published the first of two studies on vision 'without inversion of the retinal image.' During his long and productive career, Stratton devoted himself to the study of many other topics in psychology, but his early inversion studies are his most enduring contribution. Stratton started his research programme with a simple, well-defined empirical question: Is an inverted image on the retina necessary for vision? To answer this question, he built a head-mounted display with two convex lenses arranged in such a way that, when wearing the device, the 'image' cast on the retina corresponded to the field of view after a rotation around the line of sight of 180 degrees. In other words, he re-inverted his retinal 'image' both vertically and horizontally. Stratton wore these peculiar glasses for about three days in a preliminary study, and for eight straight days in a later investigation (Stratton, 1896; 1897). He reported that, at the beginning of each period, the environment appeared upside-down and that movements were awkward and uncertain. For instance, if he aimed his arms forward they seemed to enter his visual field from above, and reaching for an object required painstaking trial-and-error. As the experiments progressed, however, controlling movements became easier and visual appearances changed. Although 'the feeling that the field was upside down remained in general throughout the experiment,' the nature of this feeling changed depending on how he looked at scenes. He reported that if his attention was directly 'inward,' then the scene seemed clearly inverted. However, if he attended to outer objects, then 'these frequently seemed to be in normal position, and whatever there was of abnormality seemed to lie in myself, as if head and shoulders were inverted.' Stratton had discovered what is now called prismatic adaptation (although he did not use prisms). An inverted retinal image is not necessary, for the brain can adapt to alterations of the optical input to the eyes. This process has a motor side, in that after adaptation one is again capable of fluid movements, and a perceptual side, in that visual experience feels more and more 'normal' despite the optical inversion.

Stratton's experiments had limitations. With his lens system convergence of the eyes was very hard to achieve. Thus, Stratton was forced to experiment with monocular viewing only. Adaptation to the distortion occurred only for one eye and one brain hemisphere. Most likely, this is the reason why he did not notice after-effects upon removing the lenses after the first three days. On that occasion he reported that 'On removing the glasses ... normal vision was restored instantaneously and without any disturbance in the natural position of objects' (Stratton, 1896). After the second session, he instead took care to ask an assistant to remove the lenses from the glasses, but kept the glasses on—preserving a monocular field of view. He then experienced that 'the scene had a surprising, bewildering air which lasted for several hours' but that 'it was hardly the feeling that things were upside down.' This report seems to suggest that he did not experience obvious perceptual consequences. He found, however, that he had definite difficulties in guiding his own movements. For instance, in walking around he 'frequently ran into things in the very effort to go around them,' and he often found himself 'at a loss which hand to use to grasp' (Stratton, 1897). This was, to the best of our knowledge, the first report of motor after-effects due to adaptation. After the brain has adapted to an optical distortion, when the normal input is restored there are, for a certain period of time, some consequences. Stratton did not seem to fully understand what these are. However, later studies filled this gap.

After the publication of Stratton's papers, there were some attempts to extend his observations in the 1920s, but these were limited in scope. In 1946 and 1947, however, Ivo Kohler at the Institute of Experimental Psychology of the University of Innsbruck, Austria, started an extensive research programme on the effect of long-term adaptation to optical disturbances of the visual input. The optical alterations he studied included up–down reversals, achieved by a head-mounted mirror device, left–right reversals using a prism device, deflections with distortions, using wedge prisms, and many others. He even studied the effect of altering the spectral composition of the input light in various ways. Most of his results are described in English in a monograph published in the journal *Psychological Issues* more than 50 years ago (Kohler, 1962; a wonderful movie, with no less that James J. Gibson providing the narrating voice, can be seen on You Tube at https://www.youtube.com/watch?v=C-Opnrb6l9A). Kohler showed that motor adaptation could go well beyond what had been observed before. In one study, after a few days wearing the up-down reversing device one participant was able to ride a bicycle, and even to ski. Kohler also confirmed that the perceptual appearance of objects was often normal despite the reversal, and that both motor and perceptual after-effects followed removal of the device. Experiments using wedge prisms included in-depth studies of these after-effects, sometimes in studies lasting for impressively long times. In one study, Kohler himself wore prisms deflecting light rays by 15 degrees and then by 20 degrees for 124 days. These studies revealed that after-effects could be long-lasting and, most important, that they were independent of the adapted retinal region. This conclusion stemmed from the nature of the optical disturbances produced by wedge prisms. Deflection of light rays is at the minimum when one looks through the centre of the prism, and increases whenever one deviates from this line of sight either horizontally or vertically. As a consequence, in the proximal 'image' angles are distorted, and horizontal or vertical lines are displaced, depending on the line of sight. For instance, the projection of the same object is shrunk when viewed through one side of the prism, and broadened when viewed through the other side. Thus, prismatic adaptation occurred for qualitatively different displacements despite the fact that they were always presented on the centre of the retina which 'fixated' objects in different viewing directions. Even more interestingly, after removing the prisms the observed after-effects depended on viewing direction. For instance, objects were now broadened when viewing form the side of the prism that during adaptation had shrunk them. Kohler called this feature of the after-effects 'situational,' that is, contingent on the situation in which the displacements occurred originally.

After-effects contingent on viewing direction suggest a role of body representations and motor processes in realigning visual and proprioceptive spatial maps during perceptual adaptation. This has been largely confirmed by later studies, which have identified two distinct phases of the adaptation process, called *error correction* and *spatial realignment* (see Redding, Rossetti, & Wallace, 2005). The error correction phase is thought to reflect a form of strategic control. The participant realizes that she is making a systematic error, and deliberately plans a correction. As a consequence, in a simple aiming movement accuracy can be greatly improved already after two or three failed attempts. However, strategic error correction is short lived and does not cause the after-effects that are the signature of a more permanent change in the system. Spatial realignment is instead a slower process that requires several repetitions of the movement. Spatial realignment, which manifests itself in an additional improvement in accuracy, is essential for after-effects to develop fully after removal of the disturbance. The neural and psychological mechanisms underlying this key spatial realignment process have been studied extensively in more recent years. In particular, monkey lesion (Kurata & Hoshi, 1999; Baizer, Kralj-Hnas, & Glickstein, 1999), patient (Martin et al., 1996; Newport et al., 2006), and fMRI (Chapman et al., 2010) studies suggest that spatial realignment is implemented by a network including posterior cerebellar, ventral parietal, and ventral premotor areas. Appropriately, these areas have been also shown to have multisensory and motor functions. In addition, several behavioural studies have confirmed that spatial realignment can be specific for the conditions of adaptation. For instance, it has been reported that after-effects are stronger when tested from the same starting position employed during adaptation (Baraduc & Wolpert, 2002) or with movements having approximately the same duration as those performed during adaptation (Kitazawa, Kimura, & Uka, 1997). These results are very much reminiscent of Kohler's 'situational' after-effects.

At this point, you may be wondering what is it like to experience prisms. The effect of prisms causing lateral deflections can be experienced easily in most science museums, which often host a prismatic adaptation demo in the section on the sensory sciences. Our hope is that you will feel encouraged to try these. If you can get a hold of prismatic goggles, a simple experiment can be performed using a plastic bag filled with dry beans (a beanbag will not roll away from the place where it lands). Make a mark on the floor with tape to serve as the target and ask a friend to stand four metres away from it. Give her the bag and ask her to under-hand throw the bag aiming to the basket. Repeat for, say, five attempts. She will be more or less accurate (give or take random aiming errors). This is called the *pre-adaptation* phase, and it will serve you to establish a baseline for your friend's accuracy and precision in throwing the bag. Now ask her to put on the goggles and throw again. Suppose the goggles displace the optical input by, say, 15 degrees to the right. Her first throws should be clearly off to the right. Repeat for, say, 20 throws. This is called the *peri-adaptation* phase, and after a few attempts you should already notice that the tendency to throw to the right of the target decreases. Most likely, after the 20 attempts the aiming will be again accurate. Now remove the goggles and throw again five times. This is the *post-adaptation* phase, and the first throw will most likely be to the left of the target. This is the motor after-effect, and it is evidence for a modification of the sensorimotor process using the visual and proprioceptive input to programme the throw.

Under these conditions, this modification is short-lived and at the end of post-adaptation the tendency to throw to the left should be already gone or greatly reduced. Now note that beanbag-throwing is a ballistic movement—once you release the bag, you cannot use visual information to modify its trajectory. Therefore, adaptation is based on registering the terminal error and re-adjusting the throwing movement accordingly. If the task had been aiming with your hand towards a nearer target, the situation would have been more complex. In this case, you will have visual and proprioceptive information about the position of the hand relative to the target before but also during the movement. Unless the aiming is very fast, your brain will have opportunities to monitor the movement and to perform corrections based on the online sensory feed-back. As a consequence, you will eventually land on target, but its trajectory will not be a straight line from the hand's initial position to the target as it would be normally. Instead, the hand's path will initially curve to the right (if the goggles are right-deflecting) and then curve back towards the target. Adaptation will then manifest itself as a gradual reduction of this curvature, but measuring it will be trickier. You will need appar-atus to record the hand's trajectory in space, and statistical tools to extract kinematic parameters, including the duration of the preparatory phase (from presentation of the target to the onset of movement), the move-ment time (from onset to the moment you touch the target), the actual trajectory, and its velocity and ac-celeration profiles. Several experiments measuring some of these parameters are described in this chapter.

done using wedge prisms that deflect light rays by a certain amount in a given direc-tion (most typically, along the horizontal) and that can be worn like ordinary spectacles (Figure 3.3a). Technically, adaptation experiments can be, and have been, done also using mirror devices, lenses, or computer-controlled visual displays. For simplicity, here we will group all of these manipulations under the rubric of prismatic adaptation. This is not completely correct as these techniques sometimes use optical disturbances that are not exactly equivalent to those of wedge prisms (again, more details on this in Tutorial 3.1). But these differences are not important for the purposes of this section of the chapter. It is well known that adaptation to optical disturbances involves a realignment of visual and proprioceptive maps within sensorimotor mechanisms. This multisensory process can be quantified elegantly by measuring adaptation after-effects, that is, motor errors observed when the participant removes the spectacles after wearing them for a given amount of time. Consider the following experimental set-up. Your hand is at a starting position near your body and there is a target dot at about arm's length. However, you see both your hand and the target through a combination mirror plus lenses device. The effect of this device is that you see the target at its true position, whereas the hand is displaced—the displace-ment is equivalent to having your hand 4 cm to the right of where it actually is. Suppose now that you have to point with your index finger to the target, but as soon as you start the movement you no longer see your hand. Where will you land? Will the optical dis-turbance affect your aiming, and how?

The above situation was designed by Rossetti, Desmurget, and Prablanc (1995) specific-ally to study multisensory interactions between vision and proprioception in aiming. They framed the problem in this way. The aiming response is programmed while viewing the hand and the target, but then executed while viewing the target but no longer viewing the hand. The motor programme is therefore akin to pre-computing a vectorial displacement in space, from the initial position of the hand to the position of the target. (And yes, this is essentially Woodworth's 'initial impulse' concept.) If the computation of this vectorial dis-placement were based entirely on visual signals, one would expect that the participant fin-gers would land about 4 cm to the left of the target, that is, there should be a pointing bias equal to the optical shift caused by the apparatus. Instead, Rossetti and his collaborators observed that the bias was about one-third of the predicted prismatic shift (Figure 3.3b). They also analysed the initial path of the movement, and again found that this deviated

(a)   (b)

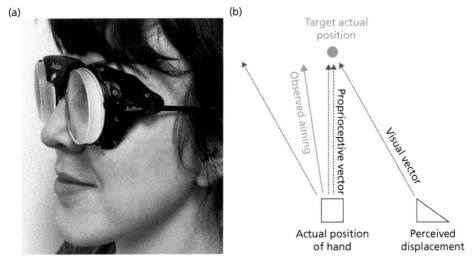

Figure 3.3 Prismatic shifts in pointing. (a) Wedge-prism spectacles. This particular specimen deflects the optical input by 10 degrees to the right of the wearer. (b) Typical results in the study by Rossetti, Desmurget, & Prablanc (1995). Note that aiming (green arrow) is a compromise between the predictions based on the visual and the proprioceptive vectors (blue arrows).

(a) © Nicola Bruno.

(b) Data from Y. Rossetti, M. Desmurget, and C. Prablanc, Vectorial coding of movement: vision, proprioception, or both?, *Journal of Neurophysiology*, 74 (1), pp. 457–463, 1995.

less than predicted by the prismatic shift. They therefore concluded that the movement was computed by performing a weighted fusion of the visual and proprioceptive signals about the initial hand position. In contrast to Woodworth's intuition, we now know that this is typical in guiding an aiming movement, and that it happens in many other forms of multisensory interaction, not only in relation to movement. The brain takes into account all available sensory signals, but gives more weight to some in comparison to others.

In the case of Rossetti's experiment, we know that proprioception must have been more important than vision in their conditions because the response was only one-third of the visual prediction. This makes good sense in this case, because vision of the hand was removed at the onset of movement whereas somatosensory signals remained available until its end. But how are sensory weights determined in general when the brain performs multisensory fusion? Several more recent studies have investigated this issue, and there is now a growing consensus that, in many cases, the weights depend on the precision of the signals themselves. For instance, it has been shown that localization of a visual target is more precise in the direction orthogonal to the line of sight, whereas localization of a proprioceptive target is more precise in the direction parallel to it (van Beers, Wolpert, & Haggard, 2002; see Figure 3.4). One would predict therefore that vision would be given more weight when adapting to an orthogonal optical shift, but that proprioception would be given more weight when adapting to a parallel shift. This is precisely what van Beers and collaborators observed when they used a virtual reality set-up to displace visual

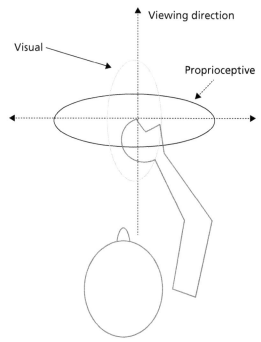

Figure 3.4 Relationship between target localization and sensory precision for visual and proprioceptive signals. Ellipses represent variability of localisation (the narrower along a given direction, the higher the precision).

Adapted from *Current Biology*, 12 (10), Robert J van Beers, Daniel M Wolpert, and Patrick Haggard, When Feeling Is More Important Than Seeing in Sensorimotor Adaptation, pp. 834–7, Figure 1, doi: 10.1016/S0960-9822(02)00836-9. Copyright © 2002 Cell Press. Published by Elsevier Ltd. All rights reserved.

signals in the two directions and measured after-effects. (In comparison to prisms, this method has the advantage that visual displacements can be produced in both directions without distortions.) After Woodworth, it has often been hypothesized that visual signals dominate over other sensory channels. For instance, we have already encountered an example of this idea in Chapter 1 (the ventriloquist's effect), and we will encounter other instances when discussing the multisensory perception of objects in the next chapter. Earlier prismatic adaptation studies seemed also consistent with this idea, but we can now conclude that this is a special case, due to the nature of prisms that typically displace optical input horizontally. In fact, what the brain does may be better described as an adaptive process that makes optimal use of the available signals by giving more weight to those that are more informative. We will discuss this concept in greater detail in Chapter 4.

As you may recall, Woodworth also speculated that multisensory interactions in motor control are not mere modifications of sensory inputs or motor outputs, but involve a more abstract, higher-level internal representation of the movement in space, a 'sense of the extent of movement.' Important insights on the nature of this internal representation have come from studies of how prismatic adaptation generalizes, or fails to do so, to unadapted actions or acting limbs. In a classic study, Charles Harris (1963) adapted participants to using a wedge prism in an aiming task to a visual target. He then compared after-effects when aiming to a visual target to those to an auditory target (an invisible clicker behind the table top) and in a generic 'straight-ahead' movement with no target, both for the adapted and unadapted hand. His results are summarized in Table 3.1. Harris found that adaptation to a visual target readily transfers to an acoustic target and to a generic movement if the same hand is used pre-, peri-, and post-adaptation. Transfer to the acoustic target demonstrates that adaptation is multisensory and not merely visual. Transfer to the generic movement demonstrates that adaptation is not merely a motor process, because a generic straight-ahead movement is different from a specific vector displacement to a visible target. Taken together, these findings suggest that adaptation is, indeed, a change in a higher-level, multisensory representation of space. This conclusion is consistent with later studies of sound localization. After adaptation to prisms, for instance, the perceived shift of visual space has been shown to produce a corresponding shift in sound localization, with the size of shift depending both on shifted fixation eye movements and on multisensory realignment (Cui et al., 2008).

However, Harris also observed essentially no transfer to the unadapted hand. This seems to suggest that the multisensory processes for motor control are effector-specific. This notion underscores the link between these putative processes to concepts that have been described in Chapter 2 on the multisensory perception of our own body, and to related ideas that we will encounter in Chapter 7 on the multisensory perception of space. It is perhaps not surprising, therefore, that the question whether adaptation of one hand movement generalizes to the unadapted hand, or to other limbs, has attracted the attention of other laboratories after Harris' classic study. These studies indicate that prismatic adaptation may transfer from the adapted hand to the unadapted hand, or even to another limb, but only under certain conditions. For instance, Redding and Wallace (2009) observed transfer of adaptation from the non-dominant left hand to the dominant right hand, but not from the right to the left (see also Choe & Welch, 1974; Redding & Wallace, 2008). Note that Harris could not have detected this asymmetry, because he tested both hands in each participant and averaged the results. Redding and Wallace interpreted this asymmetric transfer as due to the cortical organization of space, attention, and motor control. In this model, the left hemisphere represents the right visual hemispace, whereas

Table 3.1 Size of after-effects (average difference between pre- and post-adaptation aiming, in cm) in the six conditions of Harris' experiment (1963).

	Adapted hand	Unadapted hand
Aiming to visual target	5.8 cm	1 cm
Aiming to acoustic target	5.1 cm	−0.5 cm
Generic forward movement	5.6 cm	0.5 cm

the right hemisphere represents both the left and the right hemispaces (for a review of neuroimaging and patient data supporting this asymmetry, see Redding & Wallace, 2009). In contrast, motor control is symmetrical, with the right hemisphere controlling only the left hand and the left hemisphere controlling only the right hand. Because of cortical asymmetry in spatial attention, but not in motor control, sensorimotor adaptation using the right hand will engage only the left hemisphere, preventing transfer to the unadapted left hand. In contrast, adaptation using the left hand will engage the right hemisphere for motor control, but both hemispheres for representing target position and hand position in space, creating the conditions for transfer to the unadapted right hand.

Even this elegant model is likely to be incomplete, however, for yet other studies have reported transfer both to the left and to the right unadapted hands (e.g. Mostafa et al., 2014). Presumably, these inconsistencies depend on methodological differences between adaptation paradigms, for instance, in the use of prism or of computer-controlled visual stimuli, or in the availability of both terminal and online feedback in comparison to terminal feedback only. In any event, it seems safe to conclude that prismatic adaptation can be highly specific in certain conditions, as shown also by studies suggesting specificity for fixation, initial posture, and movement velocity (discussed in Tutorial 3.1), but can generalize in other conditions, as shown by intermanual transfer. But what about different actions? For instance, it is known that prismatic adaptation also occurs for walking towards a target (Michel, 2008). Will adaptation of aiming generalize to locomotion, and will locomotion generalize to aiming? To answer this question, Morton and Bastian (2004) adapted participants to prisms during either aiming or walking to a target, and then tested them for generalization to the other movement. Their results revealed another interesting asymmetry: walking generalized extensively to aiming, but aiming did not generalize to walking. They then repeated the study with cerebellar patients (recall that the cerebellum is believed to be a key structure in spatial realignment during adaptation, see again Tutorial 3.1). Patients showed reduced adaptation and, most crucially, no generalization in either condition. These results may be interpreted as evidence that the multisensory control of whole-body actions in distant space involve a more general representation than isolated-limb actions. The former may affect higher-order, effector-independent brain regions more than the latter. This would make good adaptive sense, as walking towards an object often entail a later hand-based interaction with that object, whereas merely aiming towards an object does not necessarily entail a related action after walking away from it.

3.3 Multisensory interactions in grasping

One type of visually guided reach-to-grasp movements has been especially studied over the last 40 years. This is the act of picking up relatively small objects with the thumb and index finger, the so-called *precision* or *pincer* grip. Precision grips are easy to record because they unfold over a small spatial extent and require tracking the trajectories of only two fingers. Thus, a complete picture of the kinematics can be obtained by tracking only three markers, usually attached to the fingertips and to the wrist, within a manageable laboratory portion of lab space. The trajectory, velocity, and acceleration of the wrist marker describe how the hand moves towards the object (the *transport* component of the grip). The relative position of the fingertip markers over time describes how the configuration of the hand evolves over the course of this movement (the *manipulation* component of the grip). A simple-minded expectation could be that these components should unfold in sequence. The hand will be transported near the object first, and then the fingers will open to perform the grip. You might agree however that this evokes the movement of the clunky, buzzing robotic hands of the famous *Star Wars* droid C-3PO. When we pick up an object, we usually perform a much more fluid, smooth action. Our hand assumes an appropriate configuration *while* it approaches the object, not after the approach is complete. Now-classic kinematic analyses of precision grips have revealed that this involves a sophisticated use of the muscles controlling the shoulder and the elbow (transport) with those controlling the hand (manipulation). Their coordination results in an efficient movement whereby the fingers open while the hand accelerates, reach a point of maximum aperture near the target object, and then initiate a deceleration phase which brings the fingers into contact with the object surface (Figure 3.5). The accelerating phase is mainly based on spatial representations computed before movement onset (you may recall Woodworth's initial impulse). For instance, it has been shown that the grip configuration depends on the shape of the object (Santello & Soechting, 1998), and that the aim-points of the fingers on the object surface depend on the perceived position of the centre of mass (Lukos, Ansuini, & Santello, 2007). The decelerating phase, conversely, involves finer adjustments that are based on online sensory feedback (Woodworth's current control). For instance, it has been shown that changing the shape of the object after movement onset results in a rapid reorganization of the trajectories of the fingers (Ansuini et al., 2007). As we shall soon see, both phases are not necessarily based on vision only, and can be affected dramatically by multisensory interactions.

The main sensory and motor areas controlling reach-to-grasp movements are relatively well understood (Binkofski et al., 1998; Cavina-Pratesi, 2010; Connoly, Andersen,

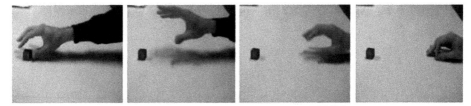

Figure 3.5 A typical reach-to-grasp movement involving a precision grip. The movement unfolds from right to left and starts with the index and thumb touching. In the initial phase the fingers open and the hand accelerates. Near the object, the fingers reach their maximum aperture and at approximately the same time the hand reaches its peak velocity. In the final phase the hand decelerates and the fingers close to contact the object.

& Goodale, 2003; Fattori et al., 2017; Jeannerod et al., 1995). There is less of a consensus as to whether the computations implemented by these brain networks explicitly coarticulate separately coded transport and manipulation components (Jeannerod, 1981; van de Kamp & Zaal, 2007; Wang, 1999), or simply control the trajectories of the two fingers in parallel, with the observed kinematics emerging spontaneously from the interaction of the two movements (Smeets & Brenner, 1999; Smeets, Brenner, & Biegstraaten, 2002). Whatever the neurally implemented algorithm, it is clear that the key aspect driving the initial phase is an anticipatory computation of relevant features, such as object position, size, and shape, of the to-be-grasped object. For instance, assessments of grip kinematics have revealed, among other things, a precise scaling of the maximum grip aperture (usually abbreviated to MGA, the maximum in-flight distance between the thumb and the finger) to object size and of the relative time to the peak velocity (TPV, the duration of the acceleration phase scaled to the total duration of the movement) to object distance (Marteniuk et al., 1987; Marteniuk, Leavitt, MacKenzie, & Athenes 1990). These results pose the problem of understanding how perception actually performs this anticipatory computation. In other words, how does the brain 'know' the appropriate hand trajectory, speed, and shaping for a given object in a given position, *before* the hand actually touches the object?

One seemingly obvious answer to the question above is that the brain knows all of that from *seeing* where and what the object is. This answer, however, merely moves the problem one step up in a conceptual hierarchy. How does the *visual* brain know where and what the object is? It is known that humans respond to a variety of visual sources of information about the layout of objects in the environment (e.g. Bruno & Cutting, 1988; Cutting & Vishton, 1995) and about their three-dimensional shape (Biederman, 1987). There is evidence that among these a key role in grasping is played by binocular spatial mechanisms. When we fixate on an object, we rotate the eyes towards it. This is called *binocular convergence,* and the convergence angle contains potential information about the position of the fixated object. The bigger the angle, the closer the object, in accord with a simple trigonometric relation. In addition, when we fixate on an object its projections on the two retinas always occupy corresponding locations: the projection falls on the centres of both the left and right retinas. This, however, is true only for the fixated object, and for other objects on a theoretical locus of points called the *horopter* (exact definitions vary somewhat on assumptions—think of a circle passing through the centres of the eyes and the fixation point). All other non-fixated objects occupy non-corresponding locations on the retinas. The difference between these non-corresponding retinal locations is called a *retinal disparity,* and retinal disparities also provide potential information about positions in depth as well as three-dimensional structure, relative to non-disparate locations (see Practical 3.1). A relevant feature of both convergence and disparity is that as information about space they are mostly useful up to about 1–2 metres from your body, which of course is roughly correspondent with the portion of space where we reach for objects to pick them up. There is some evidence that the brain, indeed, makes good use of this information to guide grasps.

Practical 3.1 Binocular vision and grasping

To understand binocular convergence and binocular disparities, no special equipment is needed. Let's start with convergence. Raise your index finger, arm fully stretched, in front of your nose. Fixate the tip of the finger. Slowly move the finger toward your nose following a straight line, maintaining fixation. Grab your smartphone, hold it at about 45 degrees on the side, and make a video of yourself while you maintain fixation on your finger going back and forth. Finally, look at your eyes in the video (in the unlikely event that you don't have a smartphone handy, you can ask a friend to do the experiment and look at your friend's eyes). You will readily notice that the convergence angle changes a lot when the finger is near your nose, and then less and less. When the arm is fully stretched (that is, a little less than one metre away), the angle is rather small. A little trigonometry, which we spare you, gives approximate angles of 35, 7, 3.5, <1 degrees for 10, 50, 100, and 400 cm distances. Now to disparities. Hold both index fingers in front of your nose. One arm should be fully stretched, whereas the other should place your finger at about midway between the first finger and the nose. Fixate the nearer finger first. Close one eye, open it, close the other eye. Repeat a few times. You will notice that the other, nonfixated finger 'jumps' sideways as you alternate the eyes. Try again while fixating the farther finger. Again, the nonfixated finger will jump sideways. The jumps are due to binocular disparities. When you look with two eyes, your brain fuses two slightly different images and converts them into perceived locations in depth. When you look with one eye, no binocular disparity is available and the brain localizes the finger according to the retinal position. We leave as an exercise to the reader to figure out how the direction (left or right) and extent of the jump depends on fixation and on the distance between the fingers.

To explore the role of binocular vision in grasping you can't simply use your fingers. For instance, try holding again your index in front of your nose. Close one eye to remove disparities and grasp the fingertip with the other hand. You will notice that you can do that rather accurately. This is not particularly telling, however, because there are other sources of information about the position of the target fingertip besides binocular vision. For instance, there are proprioceptive signals telling your brain where your hand is, although they are not as precise as binocular vision. Crucially, there is visual feedback about the positions of both your hands while you are moving one towards the other, and you can monitor that to guide the approach. So let's use another target and complicate the experiment just a little bit. Go near a window and open it by 90°, placing yourself so that the open window is more or less parallel to your line of sight and you are at about arm's length from the window handle. Close one eye. You job will be to grasp the handle, but at the very instant you decide to move you should close the eye and quickly perform the grasp without vision. Most likely, you will find that you ended up too short. Repeat but this time look at the handle with both eyes, close, and grasp. Most likely, you will find that you could grasp the handle just fine. Repeat a few times. There may be some conscious correction once the systematic error is salient, but the tendency to overshoot should still be noticeable. The systematic error is a symptom that binocular disparities are critical for the motor programme that attempts to bring the hand to the appropriate location.

The basic idea in studies investigating the role of binocular spatial mechanisms in grasping is to compare the kinematics with and without binocular information available. It has been reported that monocular grasps have lower peak velocity, longer deceleration phases, and larger grip apertures, in comparison to binocular grasps (Melmoth, 2006; Servos, 2000). These changes in the kinematics of the action cannot be attributed to restricting the field of view from two eyes to one eye, because an equivalent effect occurs when wearing a special device that presents identical 'images' to both eyes (Bradshaw et al., 2004). In addition, the effect appears not to depend on a conscious misperception of space. Direct comparisons of grasp parameters and verbally reported depth judgments suggest that visuo-motor differences between monocular and binocular grasps are not necessarily mirrored by comparable differences in space perception (Watt, Bradshaw, & Rushton, 2000). These findings are corroborated by developmental and patient observations. During development, infants showing sensitivity to binocular disparities perform more frequent and more accurate reach-to-grasp movements than infants showing no sensitivity (Yonas & Granrud, 1985). In one of the many studies of visual form agnosic patient D.F., it has been shown that D.F. could perform successful grasps under binocular, but not monocular conditions, even if her ability to verbally report the size or three-dimensional shape of the grasped object was severely impaired by her neurological condition (Marotta, Behrmann, & Goodale, 1997). Taken together, these results provide strong evidence that binocular vision is critical for visuo-motor control in grasping.

An interesting aspect of the above studies is that effects of binocular vision seem to be specific for a grasping response and do not affect conscious judgments of size. However, these findings do not rule out that other sources of information may also be taken into account to guide grasps. For instance, a study by Gentilucci, Benuzzi, Gangitano, and Grimaldi (2001) reported subtle effects of target colour on grasp kinematics for objects that were identical in shape and size, with red targets yielding larger MGAs than green targets. However, a qualitatively similar difference was found in a perceptual matching task. This latter finding is consistent with a much older study (Warden & Flynn, 1926) that had already reported that red objects were judged to be slightly bigger than otherwise identical green objects. Thus, this effect may depend on a different mechanism than the binocular effects described above. Assuming that, in the ecological niche typical of the evolution of our species, reddish colours (say, fruits and tree branches) were statistically associated with larger objects than greenish colours (say, leaves), it would be plausible that visual systems incorporate a sort of hard-wired assumption that is entered in the anticipatory computation of the object size before grasping it. A direct test of this general idea has been provided by a more recent study by McIntosh and Lashley (2008). This study used two match brands commonly sold in Scotland, *Swan Vestas* and *Scottish Bluebell*, which come in boxes of different sizes. McIntosh and Lashley recorded precision grips to the larger *Swan Vestas* and the smaller *Scottish Bluebell,* and compared these to grips of experimental replicas which inverted the normal sizes, such that the *Swan Vestas* were now smaller and the *Scottish Bluebell* larger. They found that when sizes were inverted, both the transport and the manipulation components of the grips were modified in the direction of the familiar size of the matches. Crucially, although these effects were stronger under monocular viewing, they were still detectable although smaller under binocular viewing. It seems, therefore, that binocular vision is important for guiding grips, but top-down knowledge about a recognizable seen object can also be taken into account.

In principle, top-down knowledge could be activated not only visually, but also from signals coded within other sensory channels. One study performed in the context of a collaboration between groups at the universities of Padua and of Parma (Castiello, et al., 2006) asked if grasping can be influenced by odours. Participants were presented with an odorant and were then requested to grasp a small (e.g. a strawberry) or a large (e.g. an orange) object. The odorant could evoke an object of similar size, or a different size.

Castiello and his collaborators observed that both the MGA and the TPV of the grasp were influenced by the odour. For small objects, the MGA was larger and the TPV was later when the size suggested by the odour was incongruent with the visual size, in comparison to when it was congruent with it or in a baseline no-odour condition. For large objects, conversely, the MGA was smaller and the TPV was earlier in the incongruent condition, in comparison to congruent or no-odour. Other studies from the same groups have confirmed this finding, extending it to the selection of a precision two-finger grip more appropriate for small objects vs a whole hand power grip appropriate for larger objects (Tubaldi et al., 2008), and to retronasal olfactory signals from drinking a sip of a flavoured solution (Parma, Ghirardello, Tirindelli, & Castiello; 2011a, Parma et al., 2011b; for a discussion of retronasal olfaction and its role in flavour perception see Chapter 5). These studies confirm that the kinematics of grasping can be modulated by information coded within olfaction.

Yet other studies have revealed effects of acoustic signals. Studies of acoustic effects have adopted different approaches from those studying olfaction. This is understandable, as graspable objects do not typically emit sounds. Sounds are instead produced by some interaction with the object, such as, for instance, hitting or rubbing it. With this in mind, the Padua group of Umberto Castiello recorded sounds produced by finger contact when participants grasped objects covered with different materials. They then delivered these sounds either before or following the onset of grasps of objects covered with congruent or incongruent materials (Castiello et al., 2010). They observed that the total duration of the grasps as well as the duration of the deceleration phase (or, alternatively, the roughly equivalent duration of the closing movement of the fingers) were longer in the incongruent condition and shorter in the congruent condition, relative to a baseline with a synthetic control sound. Interestingly, these effects were present irrespective of when the sounds were delivered (before or following grasp onset). These results indicate that sound congruency facilitated the action, whereas sound incongruency interfered with it, and this could happen during motion preparation but also online during its execution. This possibility has been confirmed by a later study documenting online corrections when visual targets were switched to auditory displaced targets during execution (Holmes & Dakwar, 2015). Finally, a different kind of auditory influence has been observed recently in the lab of Tzvi Ganel in Israel (Namdar & Ganel, 2015). In this study, participants were presented with short (half a second) or long (two seconds) auditory tones and were then requested to grasp a target object that was presented immediately after the end of the tone. They observed that, on average, participants opened their fingers more in the initial part of grasp (up to 50 percent of the total movement) after the long tone in comparison to the short. This intriguing result could be interpreted as due to the activation of a high-level, crossmodal mental representation of magnitude. The reasoning behind this interpretation is as follows. There is evidence that the human brain processes space, time, and quantities within a shared set of cortical areas in the parietal lobe (Walsh, 2003). It turns out that these areas largely overlap with those involved in grasping. Perceiving magnitudes, such as on object's size, are of course critical for planning and executing grasps.

It would make sense therefore if these tapped on common, modality-aspecific representations, to some extent, and therefore that a seemingly irrelevant dimension like the duration of a tone could influence magnitude processing for grip aperture. This speculation
opens up interesting potential links with other possible multisensory interactions, such as
grip aperture and pitch, or grip aperture and loudness. We return to other aspects of these
potential interactions in Chapter 6 on the multisensory phenomenon called synaesthesia.

Olfactory and auditory signals can in principle provide information about an object
even if there is no direct contact with the hand. It makes sense therefore that they might
be used in the preparatory phase of a grasp. But what about somatosensory signals? In this
case, one might expect that hand contact is necessary and therefore that they would be not
relevant in grasping per se but only in the haptic perception of the object once touched.
Some studies, however, have revealed that multisensory influences on grasping do extend
even to somatosensation in some conditions. Suppose that for some reason you need to
grasp an object with the right hand, but you have the opportunity to feel the same object
with the left hand at the same time. In a study by Patchay, Haggard, and Castiello (2006),
participants were asked to grasp an object positioned over a table top, while they touched
a similar object *under* the table top with the other hand. They observed that the kinematics of the grasp were influenced not only by the perceived size of the to-be-grasped
objects, but also by the size of the felt object. Interestingly, this effect was detectable not
only when the felt object was exactly underneath the seen object, but also when it was displaced laterally relative to it. Thus, grasping was based on an integrated representation of
size, shared between different effectors as well as visual and somatosensory signals, and at
least in these conditions independent of spatial coincidence.

This conclusion is consistent with findings we have already encountered when discussing aiming. In some conditions, it might be advantageous to share object representations across effectors or between spatial locations. One such condition is bimanual
haptic exploration, where the perception of three-dimensional shape implies some combination of sensory signals from the two hands. Or consider the class of grasps that have
the goal of bringing an object to the mouth, to eat it or, as in early development, for oral
exploration. It has been shown that participants adopt a specific pattern of oculomotor
behaviour in this type of grasp. They converge the eyes to the target object to prepare the
grasp, but once they pick up the object they deactivate oculomotor control and switch
to proprioceptive control to bring the object to the mouth (de Bruin et al., 2008). This
suggests the possibility of a shared representation between the hand and the mouth, and
there is indeed evidence that this shared representation exists. Castiello (1997) studied
grasp-to-eat actions in a group of participants that were presented with cheese morsels of different sizes. Castiello observed the usual scaling of the MGA and the TPV in
the hand kinematics, but also similar kinematic signatures for the mouth. As for the
hand, the maximum aperture of the mouth was scaled to morsel size, and it occurred
earlier for smaller in comparison to larger morsels. This finding has been extended by
a later study to non-ingestive mouth movements (Gentilucci, Benuzzi, Gangitano, &
Grimaldi 2001). Gentilucci and collaborators recorded both hand and mouth apertures

in two tasks. In the first, participants were required to grasp objects of different sizes while opening their mouths (they were left free to open it as they wish, but were required to keep the aperture constant in all trials). In the second task, they were required to grasp objects while pronouncing syllables (the syllables were printed on the objects themselves). They observed that mouth opening and even the production of sound were affected by the object size. Participants opened their mouths more (despite the instructions) and also pronounced slightly louder syllables when grasping larger objects, in comparison to smaller. This last result hints at a possible shared representation not only between two performative actions, grasping and biting food, but also between grasping and a communicative action, voicing. And there is evidence that the link between grasps and communication is more than a wild speculation. In a later paper, Gentilucci (2003) asked participants to pronounce syllables while they *watched* (mind you, not performed) videos of hands grasping small or large objects. Again, he found that participants opened their lips more and voiced louder syllables when watching grasps of larger objects, in comparison to small. It seems, therefore, that the link between hand, mouth, and voice may go beyond the execution of actions, extending to the perception of grasps performed by someone else.

We have started our discussion of multisensory interactions in grasping with the act of picking up a small object with two fingers. Our quest has now taken us very far from this humble beginning. We use hands for many purposes and among those is gestural communication. Thus, evidence of possible links between grasping and voicing suggests an exciting speculation about the possible origin of language. Perhaps, common representations between hand movements, mouth movements, and voicing exist because communicative sounds evolved from communicative gestures. In an influential review paper, Gentilucci and Corballis (2006) set forth several arguments in favour of this speculation. Among these, one of the most convincing is the existence in monkeys of motor neurons that fire both during grasps with the hand and with the mouth (Rizzolatti et al., 1988). These neurons are located in the monkey premotor area F5, which is generally believed to correspond to Broca's area—a key area for language processing in humans. Shared motor representations for the hand and the mouth in these neural substrates may have triggered a gradual transition from gestural to vocal communication. In turn, this transition may have been further facilitated by neural mechanisms encoding actions at an even higher-level of abstraction, that of a common neural representation for actions that are performed and actions that are observed. These neural mechanisms, widely known as 'mirror' neurons, are now known to exist in monkey F5, as well as other cortical areas, and in the human brain (although this is somewhat more controversial). The discovery of mirror neurons (di Pellegrino et al., 1992) by the group of Giacomo Rizzolatti at the University of Parma has been arguably one of the most influential findings in contemporary cognitive neuroscience, and we discuss it in greater depth in Tutorial 3.2. Its relevance for the hypothesis that language might have evolved from hand gestures lies in the fact that shared mechanisms for action production and perception provide a potential substrate for understanding actions performed by conspecifics, and therefore between the sender and the receiver of a message. This may well be one of the bases of verbal communication (Rizzolatti & Arbib, 1998).

Tutorial 3.2 Mirrors in the multisensory brain

The existence of mirror neurons was first reported in 1992 by a team of Italian physiologists led by Giacomo Rizzolatti. Reportedly, the discovery happened by accident. Working in his lab in Parma, Rizzolatti and his colleagues were recording from neurons in the premotor cortex of the monkey. These neurons seemed to be ordinary motor neurons: they discharged during goal-directed hand movements such as grasping, holding, or tearing. For instance, certain neurons fired when the monkey moved the hand to grasp pieces of food. To do the recordings, naturally food had to be moved back and forth in the area within reach of the monkey's hand. Therefore, the experimenter also had to perform several grasping movements. In one instance, the team realized that the same neuron that had just been recorded while the monkey performed the grasp was now firing again while the experimenter was doing a grasping movement. Digging deeper, they were able to convince themselves that there was a clear link between the observed and performed movements. In many cases, this link was so specific that the neurons fired only when the observed movement was exactly the same as that previously performed! Apparently, these neurons were more than ordinary motor neurons. The activity that was elicited by the motor action mirrored the activity that was elicited by the perception of that same action, as if knowing what someone else is doing recruited the same internal model as actually doing it. The term mirror neurons was proposed for this notion, and it stuck.

Initially, Rizzolatti sent the report of his findings to the journal *Nature,* which declined to publish it for its 'lack of general interest.' He therefore resubmitted to *Experimental Brain Research,* which soon thereafter published it (di Pellegrino et al., 1992). After this initial report, several other microelectrode studies have documented the existence of mirror neurons in the monkey brain. For instance Gallese, Fadiga, Fogassi, and Rizzolatti (1996), recording from premotor area F5 of the macaque, reported that about 20 percent of neurons in this area responded while the monkey was performing an action as well as while it was seeing it, but not when merely seeing the acted-upon object or the agent of the action. Moreover, about 30 percent of these mirror neurons responded only when the observed and performed action were exactly the same (for instance, both precision grips, or both power grips). These are now known as 'strictly congruent' mirror neurons. The others responded also when there was a more general similarity between the actions (for instance, both a grasp). These are known as 'broadly congruent' mirror neurons. Umiltà et al. (2001) reported that a subset of these neurons became active even when the final part of an observed action was hidden behind a screen, such that the full perceptual representation of the action required a form of perceptual completion. Other studies have documented the existence in monkey F5 of neurons that discharge when an action is performed, seen, but also heard but not seen (Kohler et al., 2002; Keysers, 2003). Yet another study has found mirror neurons in the inferior parietal lobule of the monkey brain (Fogassi et al., 2005). This study also showed that these neurons may not respond to the specific kinematic characteristics of a movement, but to its underlying intention: Fogassi and colleagues observed markedly different activations when the same grasping kinematics were aimed at bringing the food to the mouth (eating) in comparison to moving the food to another location (placing). Still another study (Caggiano et al., 20009) reported that mirror neurons in the monkey premotor cortex are differentially modulated by location, responding preferentially to actions in near or far space (see Chapter 4). Crucially, Mukamel, Ekstrom, Kaplan, and Iacoboni (2010) recorded from single neurons of human patients before these patients received brain surgery for intractable epilepsy. They observed 11 neurons that behaved exactly like broadly congruent mirror neurons in monkeys. Specifically, these 11 neurons discharged both while patients observed or executed specific actions, but not when they read a word describing that action. These findings provided the first conclusive evidence that mirror neurons exist not only in non-human primates, but in the human brain as well.

In addition to microelectrode recordings, considerable evidence bearing on the issue of human mirror neurons has accrued from non-invasive techniques such as EEG, EMG, PET, and fMRI. In an early study, French neurologist Henri Gastaut observed that mu-rhythm desynchronization, an EEG pattern that is typically recorded over the motor cortex during action execution, also takes place when participants are shown short films showing the same actions (Gastaut & Bert, 1954). This finding has later been confirmed and extended (Cochin, Barthelemy, Roux, & Martineau et al., 1999), and it is regarded by many as a signature of mirror systems in the human frontal lobe (Altschuler et al., 2000). Using EMG to record electric potentials from hand and arm muscles after the application of magnetic stimulation to the contralateral motor cortex, Fadiga, Fogassi, Pavesi, and Rizzolatti (1995) observed that these potentials could be evoked by mere action observation. This supports the idea that viewing the action being performed activated motor mechanisms even without overt movement. Finally, numerous imaging studies using PET and fMRI have observed activations of motor cortical areas during action observation (Rizzolatti et al., 1996; Grafton, Arbib, Fadiga, & Rizzolatti, 1996; Grèzes, Armony, Rowe, & Passingham, 2001; Buccino et al., 2001). Although there are disagreements in the interpretation of some details, all these studies agree that these areas include the anterior part of the inferior parietal lobule, the inferior part of the precentral frontal gyrus, and the posterior part of the inferior frontal gyrus which largely coincides with Broca's area. Although homologies between human and monkey areas are always tricky to ascertain, there is a reasonable correspondence between these areas and the parietal and frontal areas where mirror neurons have been recorded in monkey. In particular, it is generally believed that Broca's area can be considered the human homologue of monkey area F5. Thus, these studies provide support for the conclusion that there are functional mechanisms in the human brain providing a common representation for action execution and action observation.

The importance of these reports has been underplayed in some contributions to the literature (see Dinstein, Gardner, Jazayeri, & Heeger, 2008; Pascolo & Budai, 2013). The strongest criticism was that, due to the poor spatial resolution of imaging techniques, one can never be sure that activations in the observation and execution conditions are from the very same neurons. For instance, one could observe activation for both execution and observation if an area contained separate populations of motor and visual neurons relatively close to each other. The strength of this objection is, however, much reduced if one considers that we would then need to specify what visual neurons are doing in the middle of the motor cortex, prove that these do not communicate with the motor neurons, and explain why the observed activations are congruent to specific motor acts (Rizzolati & Fabbri-Destro, 2010). In addition, as mentioned earlier, there has been at least one report of single-unit recordings in humans (Mukamel et al., 2010). One problem that has been raised with this study is that Mukamel and colleagues had to record from the areas that had been targeted for surgery, which included the cingulate cortex, the supplemental motor area (SMA), and the medial temporal lobe. While they managed to find some seeming mirror neurons there, these areas do not correspond to the typical mirror areas in the monkey. It should be noted, however, that these areas are not in contrast with areas showing mirror properties in human fMRI studies. Rather than discarding these findings, it could be suggested that they may provide evidence that mirror systems are not limited to supplemental motor and inferior parietal areas, but represent a general organizational principle of human higher level multisensory perception.

Finally, another potential problem regards the interpretation of studies that used a technique known as fMRI adaptation to study mirror properties of human cortical areas (Dinstein, Hasson, Rubin, & Heeger, 2007; Lingnau, Gesierich, & Caramazza, 2009; Chong et al., 2008). This technique takes advantage of the fact that standard sensory neurons reduce their firing rate under repeated presentations of their preferred stimuli, causing fMRI activations to similarly reduce over successive repetitions ('repetition suppression'). To the extent that mirror neurons can be equated to sensory neurons, one might predict that they should show crossmodal adaptation, that is, reduced activation during action observation following action execution, or during action execution following action observation. The evidence supporting this prediction is, at present, rather mixed. Dinstein and collaborators readily found areas that adapted under visual or motor repetitions, but no hint of crossmodal adaptation. Lingnau and collaborators found visual-to-motor adaptation, but no motor-to-visual adaptation. Chong found motor-to-visual adaptation, but no visual-to-motor adaptation. What is going on here is, therefore, still not well understood, and may depend on limitations of the technique more than on actual inconsistencies in the data (see Logothetis, 2008).

Disagreements on specific features of the evidence notwithstanding, mirror neurons are now widely regarded as one of the most important discoveries of cognitive neuroscience in recent decades. This said, while the existence of mirror neurons in the primate (non-human as well as human) brain is today largely undisputed, much debate remains on the interpretation of the observations, on the assessment of their implications for theories of human cognition and perception, and on their clinical relevance. Glenberg (2011) grouped the issues under debate into six questions: i) whether mirror neurons are for action understanding; ii) whether they are for imitation; iii) whether they contribute to speech perception; iv) what is the role of associative learning for mirror neurons; v) whether they are part of what causes autism; and finally vi) to what extent mirror neurons contribute to social cognitive processes. A thorough discussion of differing opinions on each of these is beyond the scope of this tutorial, and we refer interested readers to more specialized papers (for instance, Gallese et al., 2011).

From the perspective that motivates this book, however, we feel that another speculation should be added to Glenberg's list. Perceptual mechanisms exploiting mirror neurons represent a prime example of multisensory process in perception and action. This not only for the obvious reason that the equivalence of motor and perceptual coding seems to generalize across perceptual modalities (Kohler et al., 2002; Keysers, 2003), but perhaps also for a more fundamental reason. One of the key questions in multisensory perception is the binding problem. Given two incoming sensory signals, how does the brain decide that they should be bound together, resulting in a unified percept, or rather they should be kept separate and attributed to distinct percepts? As we shall see in Chapter 4, several hypotheses have been advanced on how the brain might solve the binding problem. A mechanism such as that embodied by mirror neurons suggests that one of these strategies might exploit action-related neural codes that are somehow linked to signals from several sensory channels (Fogassi & Gallese, 2004). Whether this proposal will prove fruitful in future research on multisensory perception, it is probably too early to determine. Nonetheless, it is an easy prediction that the functional interpretation of mirror neurons for human perception and cognition will remain one of the key theoretical issues in psychology and cognitive neuroscience in future years.

3.4 Multisensory interactions in walking and standing

The role of multisensory perception in guiding motor behaviours is not limited to hand actions, but extends to all bodily movements. Another interesting case is how we control how we walk and maintain our balance when standing. Our discussion of these two topics will offer an opportunity to evaluate the interplay between higher-level perceptual processes, which involve the cortex, and lower-level motor responses that are generated and modulated subcortically. The rhythmic organization of walking is illustrated in Figure 3.6. The gait cycle in human locomotion can be divided into two main phases: stance (about 60 percent of the cycle) and swing (the remaining 40 percent). These in turn can be further divided into several subphases. As illustrated in the figure, these correspond to a series of movements that cause your bodyweight to be transferred from one foot to the other foot. This is achieved by swinging one foot forward while the other supports your weight, while the centre of mass of the body is also moved forward. One way to picture this process is in terms of a series of small, controlled falls that propel the body in the desired direction.

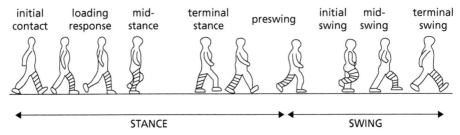

| initial contact | loading response | mid-stance | terminal stance | preswing | initial swing | mid-swing | terminal swing |

STANCE | SWING

Figure 3.6 The gait cycle of human locomotion. The whole cycle comprises two steps (one stride) and is divided into two main phases (stance and swing). These in turn can be further divided into eight sub-phases for each foot. The classification in the upper row refers to the right foot (identified by hatching).

Walking involves the whole body, although at normal walking speed most of the work is done by the legs, with the arms and trunk mostly acting as stabilizers. As speed increases, the legs produce greater ranges of motion and the upper body increasingly contributes to propulsion. Whatever the speed, it is clear that walking requires controlling the trajectories of several body segments as well as jointly regulating forces applied on the ground. In the classic view, this sophisticated work of coordination is managed by efferent, hardwired motor configurations that are elicited automatically, but that can be modified by afferent feedback eliciting reflex behaviour (Dickinson et al., 2000). Efferent motor configurations are generated by neural circuits at the level of the spinal cord (sometimes called *pattern generators),* whereas reflexes that can activate or modulate these motor commands are controlled by the cerebellum. It is generally believed that the interaction of automatic motor efference and afference-based reflexes are key for the efficient control of locomotion, in that it allows for rapid adjustments in the presence of sudden changes in environmental conditions (Schmidt & Lee, 1999).

Evidence for the existence of pattern generators modulated from muscle afferents comes from physiological data in animal models as well as behavioural data in human infants. Recording from the spinal cord of animal preparations have revealed clear periodicities of neural activity (Grillner, 1975; Marder & Calabrese, 1996). In studies of the cat nervous system, for instance, investigators have blocked both the efferent connection from the cortex and the afferent connections from the muscles. These studies have revealed rhythmic activity, after applying electrical stimulation, in the efferent fibres of the spinal cord. Given that in this preparation the spinal cord is disconnected from any external input (be it afferent, or efferent), this observation suggests that motor patterns can be generated within the spinal cord itself. Other studies have investigated whether cortical efferences are necessary for an animal to exhibit locomotor behaviour. One especially suitable technique is to surgically interrupt all efferences and afferences at the level of the midbrain, and then test the animal on a treadmill. This has been done for instance in the cat. After the treadmill starts to move, the legs of the animal soon begin to execute step sequences resembling natural locomotion. If the speed of the treadmill is increased, the step frequency also increases and the animal can even transition to a run at higher speeds.

Thus, muscular afferents from the legs seem to be sufficient to activate motor patterns and to modulate them, even without any cortical efferent command. Similar conclusions can be drawn from studies of the stepping reflex and of the development of walking in infants. Most newborns show stepping movements when held upright, suggesting the presence of an innate motor programme for walking. This stepping reflex however disappears after about two months of age. At the same time, when in a supine position infants tend to show an increase in frequency of spontaneous kicking. It has been shown that these kicking actions recruit the same muscle groups as stepping (Thelen & Fisher, 1982) and that seven-month-old infants, although they no longer show the stepping reflex and do not yet walk, nonetheless perform step sequences if supported on a small treadmill (Thelen, 1986). Based on these observations, the influential developmental psychologist Esther Thelen proposed that the stepping reflex does not disappear, but is merely not expressed in the upright posture if the increment in muscle mass is not yet matched by a corresponding increment in muscle strength. She therefore proposed that adult walking emerges gradually from the interaction of an inborn motor pattern with the neural structures responsible for posture and balance, within the biodynamic constraints of bone and muscle development (Kamm, Thelen, & Jensen, 1990; Thelen & Cooke, 1987).

A combination of reflex-like behaviour, controlled at the spinal level, and cerebellar modulations is also found in the control of posture. A classic case in point is the stretch reflex of the gastrocnemius muscle (calf). Stretching of this muscle causes increased activity in muscle spindle receptors, which in turn increases motor neuron activity within a spinal reflex arc. The effect is that the muscle fibres contract, opening the ankle joint and thereby stabilizing the posture. In a series of classic studies, Nashner (1976) asked participants to stand on platforms that could slide backwards or rotate (see Figure 3.7).

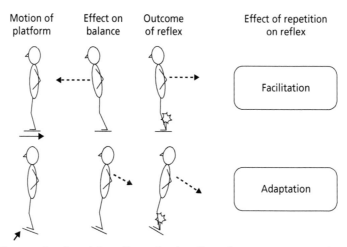

Figure 3.7 The stretch reflex of the calf muscle. The effect of repetition on the reflex depends on its postural consequences.

Adapted from *Experimental Brain Research*, 26 (1), L. M. Nashner, Adapting reflexes controlling the human posture, pp 59–72, doi: 10.1007/BF00235249. © Springer-Verlag 1976. With permission of Springer.

In both cases, the motion of the platform stretches the calf muscles and evokes the reflex, but the behavioural consequences differ. When the platform slides backwards (upper panel of the figure), the body weight is shifted forward and the effect of the reflex is to counter this forward motion, stabilizing the posture. When the platform rotates (lower panel), conversely, the body weight is shifted backwards, and the effect of the reflex is that the body weight is displaced backwards, destabilizing the posture even more. Using electromyography, Nashner observed that over repeated trials the reflex changed in different ways in the two conditions. When the outcome was stabilization of the posture, muscle activation increased as more and more trials were performed (*facilitation* of the reflex). When the outcome was further destabilization, muscle activation tended to decrease over trials (*adaptation* of the reflex). Critically, he did not observe facilitation and adaptation of the reflex in patients with lesions at the level of the cerebellum, suggesting that the reflex is indeed modulated by activity in this subcortical structure.

These observations suggest that the control of locomotion and posture recruits mechanisms that are phylogenetically more ancient than the human cortex. This does not mean, however, that these motor behaviours are based only on subcortical mechanisms. Indeed, other studies have revealed that multisensory processes, controlled by higher-level cortical mechanisms, also have a role in how we walk and stabilize posture. An experimental paradigm that can be directly compared with the studies performed by Nashner is the so-called 'moving room' set-up (Lee & Lishman, 1975). The moving room is a sort of narrow corridor, with an elongated rectangular ceiling, rectangular side walls, and a front wall. Usually there is no back wall as participants enter the room from the back. Most importantly, and this is what makes this an unusual 'room,' there is no floor and the walls are in fact slightly raised from the laboratory floor. The moving room is suspended with cables on the real ceiling of the laboratory, or fitted with small wheels. (Classic footage from David Lee's laboratory at the University of Edinburgh can be seen on You Tube at https://www.youtube.com/watch?v=F4xenIulg_8.) In a typical experiment, a participant enters the room and is asked to stand with her feet on a narrow beam. This is not strictly necessary but makes the effect of the room more obvious as the participant's balance is already slightly more precarious than normal. The participant has to look at the front wall, and the experimenter simply moves the room slightly towards the participant. The outcome of this simple manipulation is that the participant will tend to fall backwards (Figure 3.8) and will stumble to avoid a fall. Children who have just learned to walk, when tested in the moving room, do actually land flat on their bottoms. If posture were controlled only with reflexes modulated by proprioceptive signals from the legs, these effects should not be observed. The room is suspended, but the feet of the participant are not. Thus there is no mechanical disturbance that could stimulate stretch receptors in the calf muscles (or any other muscle). The key sensory signals that cause the falls are visual, not proprioceptive.

The visual signals that come into play in the moving room set-up are an instance of *optic flow*. Consider what happens on an optical projection plane (the retina in the back of

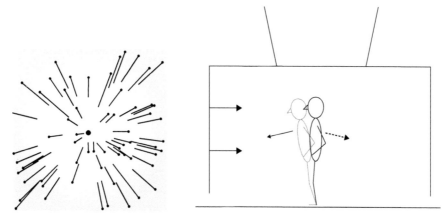

Figure 3.8 The moving room. Radial optic flow specifies forward movement of the body. The multisensory process that controls posture responds by displacing the body weight backwards, despite contrasting proprioceptive signals, and participants tend to lose their balance.

your eye is not flat, but for the present purposes, we can consider it as a projection plane) when this is moved relative to stationary objects in the environment (the retina, of course, moves with you as you move in the environment). As the position of the plane changes relative to these objects, so do their projections in accord with the rules of projective geometry. In particular, if you are fixating ahead in the direction of your own movement, all the projections of points in the external environment move radially from a central point which corresponds to fixation. This central point is the *focus of expansion* (FOE; Figure 3.8 left) and it is the only point whose projection does not move. Psychophysical studies have demonstrated that information in optic flow is sufficient, although not necessary, to perceive one's heading direction (Bruggeman, Zosh, & Warren, 2007; Warren et al., 2001; but see Loomis et al., 2006) and that a specific parameter (the inverse of the rate of radial expansion, called *tau)* contains information about time-to-contact with an object, or a wall, that we are approaching. Monkey studies (Britten & van Wezel, 1998) have located the neural structures responsible for optic flow analysis in the superior medial temporal area (MST), and functional imaging studies have revealed that the human homologue of monkey MST is selectively activated by radial optic flow (Morrone et al., 2000). In the moving room set-up, radial optic flow is produced by the movement of the room towards the stationary observer. This is interpreted as forward motion, causing a postural adjustment. Because the body did not really move forward, this has the undesired result of destabilizing the posture.

The moving room paradigm provides evidence that postural control is not managed only by reflex-like mechanisms based on muscular afferents, but is also based on visual signals. In fact, vision appears to be much more important than one would expect. When you stand in the room with your feet firmly placed on the floor *of the laboratory,* your brain is getting abundant information, from proprioceptive and vestibular signals, about your true posture—no matter how the room is moving. The optic flow information nonetheless seems to overwrite this, and you can't help responding with a 'wrong' postural adjustment. Do we in fact control posture on the basis of vision, resorting to the other channels only when vision is not available? Not quite. In a recent study, Kabbaligere, Lee, and Layne (2017) measured body sway in participants that were exposed to conflicting optic flow and proprioceptive signals. The visual signal was always a contracting flowfield (note that this corresponds to backwards body motion, so it is the opposite of the moving room situation), whereas the proprioceptive signal was a vibration applied bilaterally at the Achilles' tendons (the Achilles' tendon serves to attach the calf muscle to the heel bone). As we have already seen in Chapter 2 in the context of Pinocchio's illusion, tendon vibration activates stretch receptors. Thus, a sensory signal specifying stretching of the calf muscle is issued, which in turn implies that the body centre of mass is being displaced forward. Kabbaligere and collaborators observed that the amount of sway reflected a compromise between vision (i.e. sway to compensate a backward fall) and ankle proprioception (compensate a forward fall). To investigate the nature of this compromise, they estimated the variability associated with postural responses when presenting only the visual or proprioceptive signals. The inverse of these variability estimates can be interpreted as a measure of sensory precision (the lower the variability, the higher the precision). They therefore used sensory precision to weight the relative contribution of visual and proprioceptive components to sway. This model predicted their data very well. Thus, visual—proprioceptive interactions in the control of posture appear to be a form of optimal multisensory fusion, akin to visual and proprioceptive interactions in aiming (see our discussion of van Beers, Wolpert, & Haggard's paper in section 3.2).

That visual signals alone can cause the perception of one's own movement even without corresponding proprioceptive and vestibular signals should come as no surprise. Many of us experience *vection* (the technical term for the illusion of body movement in space) when sitting in a train at the station, waiting for the train to leave. If at the same time another train arrives on a nearby track, in certain conditions it feels as if our train is finally departing. The perception of one's own movement is entirely convincing—until we look directly out of the window. The optic flow (in this case, *lamellar* rather than radial) that becomes available in the periphery of the retina when we sit in our train looking in front of us and another train enters the station on the nearby track is indeed equivalent to that available when our train is moving and there is a stationary train at its side. An interesting apparatus for studying multisensory interactions in vection is the so-called *optokinetic drum*. This is a circular platform that can be rotated around a central bar (usually, with a handrail mounted on the bar). All around the platform there is a cylindrical surface, such that the platform becomes a sort of floor to a circular room with round walls. The cylindrical surface can also rotate, independently of the platform. The optokinetic drum provides a convenient set-up for investigating the interaction of visual, muscular, and vestibular signals when we walk. For instance, imagine that you have to stand on the platform holding the handrail (you need to do that, for reasons that will soon become obvious). Now both platform and walls begin to move at the same speed, but in different directions. The platform rotates towards you, whereas the walls go the other way. If you stand still, you will be carried around as in a merry-go-round, but your task is to walk forward against the platform. Initially, this will be unsettling. You will feel the platform starting, the walls will appear to move, and you will need to support yourself on the handrail. But soon thereafter the whole situation will stabilize. You will perceive yourself walking around a stationary room (see Lackner & DiZio, 2000). The correct alternative solution, perceiving that you are walking in place within moving walls and platform, becomes almost impossible to achieve.

This surprising outcome raises two questions. The first is why we discard the vestibular signals that should provide information about the lack of forward acceleration of the body. This is easily answered. The mechanoreceptors in the otolith organs of the inner ear respond best to linear accelerations of the body, and stop responding when we move at constant velocity. Thus, once you have started moving, and provided that velocity remains approximately constant, for vestibular signals there is little difference between walking in place and walking forward. Now recall that the visual and muscular signals are also the same in both conditions. This therefore introduces the second question, which is less easy to answer. Why does the brain perceives forward walking over the equally supported walking in place, if these are equivalent in terms of sensory signals? It is tempting to speculate that the choice depends on a sort of internal prediction of the expected consequences of one's own movement. Given that I am stepping, my brain expects optic flow consistent with forward movement. This is what it is getting, so the walls must be stationary and I perceive myself moving. Phenomena that may be consistent with the same speculation do occur in real life. Consider again the train effect that we described above. Perhaps, what makes the experience of vection compelling is precisely that we are sitting there, expecting our train to finally depart. Or consider broken escalators, a frustrating encounter many of us have experienced in subways or supermarkets. Many of us, when forced to climb an escalator that has stopped working, experience an odd sensation of imbalance despite full awareness that the escalator is not moving. Data on after-effects observed when participants attempt to walk on a stationary treadmill after adaptation to standard treadmill walking (Reynolds & Bronstein, 2003) suggest that this real-life illusion may indeed involve predictive mechanisms for motor control. But perhaps the strongest evidence for the existence of predictive internal mechanisms comes from studies of a deafferented patient (see Box 3.1). As we will see in the next section, this idea will also prove useful in understanding the last topic of this chapter, how we perceive that our own minds are the agents that will our actions to take place—the perception of *agency*.

Box 3.1 Living with a deafferented body

Suppose you had to choose: would you prefer to become blind or to loose somatosensation? In our experience, when presented with such a thought experiment, most people do not hesitate and they declare that they would prefer to retain their ability to see. This is justified by the importance of vision to move in space, to recognize objects at a distance, and of course to communicate. Another plausible reason for this preference is that most of us are not aware of the importance of proprioception for controlling locomotion and posture. But what is it really like to lose all somatosensation? A detailed answer to this question is found in a wonderful book written by English neurophysiologist Jonathan Cole (Cole, 1995). At age 19 the protagonist of the book, Ian Waterman, was diagnosed with a rare neurological illness that deprived him of all somatosensory signals, including information about limb position, muscle stretching, and mechanical events on the skin, from the neck down. After months in the hospital he was judged incurable. *Somatosensory deafferentation* causes damage at nerve fibres at the level of the spinal cord. In the case of Waterman, this involved the large myelinated fibres in the dorsal root, which carry sensory inputs from neuromuscular spindles, tendon receptors, and cutaneous receptors. Patients with this condition are typically condemned to a life of wheelchair dependence. Thanks to the efforts of excellent physiotherapists, and to his young age that gave him a strong motivation to recover, Waterman instead has been able to relearn how to stand, walk, and go about his daily activities in a quasi-normal way. This has been no easy feat. As was originally diagnosed, there was no cure that could reinstate the normal sensory inputs. With incredible effort, he taught himself how to compensate for his deficits using his spared sensory inputs and effortful attentional strategies. His is a life of constant, intense concentration to monitor his movements and posture by vision and to exploit whatever additional information he has about objects he manipulates, a marathon that he has to run every day armed only with his pride and determination.

The compensation strategies used by Waterman are instructive. To walk, for instance, Waterman constantly monitors his body movement by vision and by vestibular inputs. As a consequence, he tends to walk from the hips, keeping his knees straight to reduce the amount of relative movements between limb segments he needs to control. He cannot walk in the dark, and if he stands still a sudden disturbance of his balance, as when someone accidentally bumps into him from the back, can cause a fall. Luckily for him, fibres responsible for coding cold, warmth, pain, and muscular fatigue have been spared. He uses these in conjunction with visual signals to manipulate objects. When he presses a shirt, for instance, changes in temperature inform him about the position of his hands on the ironing board. When he wakes up in the morning, temperature gradients help him to locate his limbs as he gets out of bed in conditions of reduced illumination. When he grasps a plastic cup, he must carefully monitor temperature and visual information about his hand and the cup to avoid squeezing too hard. Waterman's condition is rare and quantitative data on grasping with somatosensory deafferentation are hard to find. However, experiments about the grasping

Box 3.1 Continued

behaviour of a similar patient have confirmed that the kinematics of grasping are relatively normal in the initial, visually driven phase, whereas they are profoundly altered in the final, feedback-based phase, requiring longer and laborious adjustments (Gentilucci, Toni, Chieffi, & Pavesi, 1994). These results underscore the importance of somatosensory afferents in the final phase of a grasp.

The range of Waterman's visually based abilities is also surprising, and instructive. Despite his condition, Waterman has obtained a driving license and can drive a car. His driving ability is testimony of the importance of visual signals for monitoring one's direction and speed of movement. Even more surprisingly, he can also estimate the weight of objects when he picks them up. For instance, when he grabs his briefcase he can tell whether it is full or not ('How do I know? Good question. I just know.'; Cole, 1995, p. 133). Presumably, Waterman uses visual information about the kinematics of his own movements to estimate the force needed to raise it from the ground. This echoes a well-studied visual process, known as *kinematic specification of dynamics* or KSD (Runeson & Frykolm, 1981). In studies of KSD, participants are shown movies of biological motions, such as individuals lifting weights, walking, or dancing. The motion stimuli are deprived of information about form and colour by applying luminous dots to the actor's joints and by shooting the film in the dark. When watching the movies, the only available information is therefore contained in the trajectories and velocities of these dots. In typical studies, participants have no idea of what they are seeing when shown still frames from the movies, but immediately recognize a dynamic event when shown the motion sequence. A simple test of the hypothesis that Waterman uses KSD is to compare weight perception with or without vision. This test has been performed on another patient (Fleury et al., 1995) and it has indeed been shown that this patient's ability to discriminate weights is comparable to that of controls if vision is allowed, but is severely reduced if the light is turned off. In addition, limb peak velocity while raising the object was observed to be highly correlated with perceived weight in this patient, whereas this was not observed in controls. These results therefore confirm that deafferented patients not only learn to use vision to compensate missing somatosensory signals, but also develop seemingly inefficient movement strategies that are, in fact, useful to enhance kinematic information about objects.

3.5 The multisensory perception of agency

A famous anecdote about Wolfgang Metzger, one of the great perceptual psychologists of the past century, nicely illustrates the final topic of this chapter. Metzger had to serve in the German army during World War Two and was once quartered in military barracks near Cassino, in Italy. The story goes that he needed to go to the barrack bathroom, and, having completed the necessary operations, he flushed the toilet. Exactly in that instant, enemy artillery opened fire, a grenade hit the barracks, and there was a loud explosion.

To his astonishment, Metzger had the most compelling impression that *he* had caused the explosion, by his very gesture of pulling the chain! Phenomena such as these are not rare, are easy to reproduce, and can be great fun. For instance, when lecturing one of us used to point to projected slides using a short wooden stick. During one lecture, it so happened that he was explaining a particular graph and touched the screen to draw attention to one particular detail of the data. Exactly at that moment, an electrical blackout occurred, the projectors switched off, and the slide disappeared. The teacher perceived that he had caused the slide to disappear with a magic wand. Even more interestingly, *the students* perceived that he had magically made the slide disappear. Everyone laughed. Or try this trick, studied in detail in a little-known Italian paper (Spizzo, 1984). Find a device that can flash a small light on and off at regular intervals. For instance, most digital metronomes do that. Or washing machines sometimes have small flickering lights to signal the end of the washing cycle. Observe the light, and try to synchronize a gesture to the flickering. For instance, try snapping your fingers in synch with the light going off. You will find that it is not difficult to feel that your gesture *causes* the light to go off.

The problem of causality has long attracted the attention of philosophers. From Aristotle, to Hume and Kant up to contemporary epistemology, they have traditionally divided into two camps. In one view, causality is grounded in human rationality: we experience causality because we deduce effects from their causes by logic. According to the alternative view, causality instead stems from empirical data: we learn to associate effects with causes due to statistical covariations that trigger associative learning. But think of Metzger's war mishap. Within both conceptions of causality, a phenomenon like this is deeply puzzling. Try to deduce bombs from toilets by logic, or to assume statistical covariations between toilet flushing and artillery explosions. From the standpoint of perception science, these phenomena are instead interesting because they demonstrate that the relationship between conscious intentions, actions, and the observable consequences of actions are much more complicated than one would initially assume. Researchers interested in these problems have coined the term *agency* to refer to the perception of one's self as the originator of an intention to act, that is, of being the cause of a performed action and of its consequences. As we shall soon see, the psychological mechanisms that are involved in the perception of agency are inherently multisensory and imply predictive motor representations. This makes them a fitting topic for the last part of this chapter.

Interest on the perception of agency within the cognitive neurosciences was spurred by a controversial study conducted by University of California physiologist Benjamin Libet (1916–2007) at the beginning of the 1980s (Libet, Gleason, Wright, & Pearl, 1983). In each trial of this study, participants were requested to perform a peculiar task: lift one of their hands, *whenever they felt the urge* to do so. In other words, they simply sat with their hand on a table, made the decision to lift the hand, and lifted it for a certain number of times. It may sound strange that Libet decided to use such a seeming haphazard task, but his motivations will become clear soon enough. While participants performed this task, Libet collected several different measures. One group of data was physiological. He applied EEG electrodes on the skull of participants to measure variations in electric potentials due to brain activity. In particular, he was interested in measuring the *readiness potential,* an EEG feature that is reliably observed before voluntary movement (see, for instance, Shibasaki & Hallett, 2006). He also used electromyography (EMG) electrodes applied to the participant's arm to record variations in potentials due to muscle activity. From this data he could time-stamp neural signatures in cortical activity as well onsets of neural activations related to muscles producing movement. A second group of data was instead psychological or, if you wish, introspective. Participants were required to report two times, the time at which they had become aware of their intention to move, and the time at which they had become aware that the arm had actually started moving. Libet called these the W (for Will) and the M (Movement) judgments. To measure these times, Libet adapted a classical technique that dates back to Wilhelm Wundt's pioneering psychological laboratory in Leipzig (Wundt, 1908). He built a clock-like device with a rotating arm that completed one revolution in a little less than three seconds. This was placed in sight of the participants while a trial was running. The participants were required to pay attention to the rotating arm and to report its position at the time they decided to move (W) or, in other trials, when they saw the arm beginning its movement (M). Thus, Libet was able to compare the time courses of neural signatures for motor preparation with those of actual movement, and to relate these to underlying physiological events.

Let us consider first how these physiological events related to each other. On the average, the EEG readiness potential was observed first, and the initial contraction of the muscles followed. This is in accord with everyone's intuition. The brain processes the intention to move, and actual movement follows. But what about the W judgements? The natural expectation is that these should precede the readiness potential. First, the self (whatever that is) makes the decision, then the brain machinery processes it, and finally a command is issued to the muscles and the hand moves. In accord with the natural expectation, Libet found that on the average W judgments preceded actual movements. Surprisingly, however, he found that W judgments did not occur, on the average, before the onset of the readiness potential. Instead, the readiness potential began its course well before W. In Libet's data, brain activity related to the preparation of the movement began about half a second *before* participants experienced the conscious intention to move (Figure 3.9). This feature of Libet's results seems to runs counter to everyone's conception of intention and

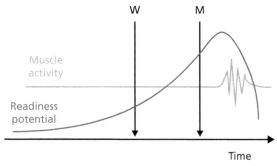

Figure 3.9 Summary of Libet's results. The onset of the readiness potential (EEG signature of movement preparation) occurred before the time of conscious intention (W judgment). In contrast, the onset of actual movement (burst of muscle activity towards the end of the graph) occurred only *after* participants reported awareness of movement (M judgment).

causality, and it has been heavily discussed and criticized. Some critics have even argued that Libet's introspective measures are subject to systematic errors (Danquah, Farrell, & Boyle, 2008; Joordens, van Duijn, & Spalek, 2002). An influential philosopher (Dennett, 2006) has argued that the self emerges from a variety of competing and dynamically evolving brain processes, which could well create temporal misalignments between separate internal representations. Everyone must however concede that the finding has been replicated by several other studies (Haggard & Elmer, 1999; Lafargue & Duffau, 2008; Sirigu et al., 2004; Trevena & Miller, 2002).

That brain activity precedes conscious intention is deeply counterintuitive. As Libet and many others have noted, this conclusion seems to negate the very notion of free will by a conscious self. But this is true only up to a point. Although neural activity seems to come first, W judgments still precede actual movements (by about one fifth of a second). This observation suggests another possibility. Perhaps, the perception of agency emerges not from the neural substrate of movement preparation, but from a later brain process. In that one-fifth of a second separating intention from execution there is still time to process how the movement will be executed—for instance, with the right or the left hand—or to stop it altogether. If this interpretation is correct, then what we consider free will is in fact 'free don't' (Brass & Haggard, 2007; Ohbi & Haggard, 2004). Supporting this speculation, a study from the group of Patrick Haggard in London revealed that W judgments correlate with a later EEG feature, the *lateralized readiness potential* (LRP; Haggard & Eimer, 1999). The LRP is generally believed to reflect an action selection process, i.e. the choice of the effector for executing an action (Brasil-Neto et al., 1992; Ammon & Gandevia, 1990). Haggard (2008) incorporated the free-will as free-don't idea into a five-stage model of human volition. The hypothesized process begins with an early 'whether' stage, which is based on the initial motivation to act, followed by task selection and action selection stages which jointly implement a 'what' decision. Before reaching the final execution stage, however, Haggard postulated a second, late, 'whether' stage when the action can still be modified or stopped. Only at this late stage, after the full details of the action have been specified, consciousness of will emerges. Interestingly, this late stage is hypothesized to involve a check of the consequences of the intended action. In other words, it implies a predictive mechanism comparing the predicted outcome with internal goals (Box 3.2) As we will now see, this predictive component seems to be also an important part of the perception of agency.

The timing of W judgments relative to the readiness potential was not the only counterintuitive feature of Libet's results. Recall that the experiment also involved recording M judgments—the times at which participants became aware that their hand had started moving. Surprisingly, Libet found that the average timing of M was approximately one tenth of a second *before* the beginning of electromyographic activity. This suggests that, when we become conscious of the sensory consequences of our decision to move (i.e. when we feel and see the hand moving), we are in fact perceiving the future. The arm will begin to move only after another fraction of a second! Of course, we are not claiming that this is a case of supernatural precognition. This second result of Libet's

Box 3.2 Sensorimotor predictions

One of our common threads in this chapter has been that motor control involves monitoring multisensory *afferent* signals while moving, but also computing preparatory *efferent* motor programmes before movement onset. This is, of course, the classic two-phase model of motor control that dates back to Woodworth's studies of more than a century ago. However, we have also repeatedly encountered the idea that sensorimotor *predictive* mechanisms may be important to multisensory motor control, and to multisensory perception as well. The idea here is that motor programmes can be useful for more than issuing efferent signals to the muscles. Such programmes implicitly also contain information on the movement that is expected to take place, which in turn is useful to formulate internal models of anticipated *afferent* sensory signals, given the programmed movement (for technical details, see Wolpert, 1997; Wolpert & Gharamani, 2000). These internal predictions can be put to good use in two ways. Predictive mechanisms can be used to create a form of 'current control' even with very rapid movements. In addition, internal predictions can be used to stabilize perception in the face of continuously varying proximal stimuli. Let us examine each function in turn.

In the traditional, two-phase model, very rapid movements can only be ballistic (i.e. guided entirely by a preparatory programme) as sensory delays will cause afferent signals to reach control mechanisms at a time when movement correction is no longer useful. Accurate rapid movements, therefore, were assumed to be based on accurate motor programmes, and executed without sensory feedback. This, however, is computationally expensive and sometimes neurally implausible. But what if motor programmes did not remain unaltered, but could be updated during the movement within an *internal control loop*? For instance, predictive control could be attained by comparing predicted limb positions with their predicted sensory consequences. Such an internal control loop would be very fast, because it would not have to wait for afferent signals to actually arrive at control centres. Alternatively, predicted limb positions could be compared to actual sensory afferents. This would not be so fast but still faster than a classic feedback loop. Either form of control would lessen the requirement of having super-accurate motor programmes—an approximate initial programme will still do, as it will be amenable to further revision while the action unfolds. There is evidence that predictive mechanisms of this type might be involved in the control of eye movements, hand aiming, reaching, and interjoint coordination (for a review, see Desmurget & Grafton, 2000) as well as in the processing of vestibular sensory signals (for a review, see Klinger, 2016).

Predictive models can also be used to cancel the sensory effects of predicted movements. This is probably strange to read if you are not a specialist in cognitive neuroscience. Why would the brain want to cancel out sensory signals? The reason is that sensory signals are continuously varying, and most of these variations are not due to anything changing in the world, but to our own movements. Saccadic eye movements are one much-studied example. When we look at a scene, we perform a series

Box 3.2 **Continued**

of successive ultrarapid eye movements, called saccades. Thus, at each saccade a new target is fixated, and the whole scene is displaced rapidly on the retina. Despite this, the scene looks completely stable, and no environmental motion is perceived. Although there is still debate on how exactly the brain achieves such perfect stabilization across saccades (for a recent review, see Bridgeman, 2010), it is clear that a key role is played by a predictive mechanism which subtracts the actual motion sensory signals on the retina from the expected sensory signals, computed from the oculomotor programme (von Holst & Mittelstädt, 1950). Vection phenomena, as seen in an optokinetic drum or related paradigms (see section 3.4) may also be interpreted as situations where sensory signals interpreted as due to one's own motion are cancelled out. But the range of applicability of the general principle is even broader than this, and you will find it at work again in our account of ticklish laughter (Box 3.3), and of multisensory interactions in the perception of agency (section 3.5).

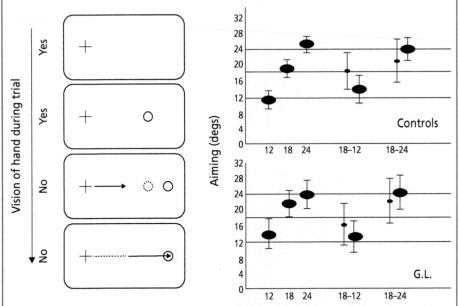

Figure 3.10 Performance of G.L. in double-step aiming. Left: basic structure of experimental trials. Note that participants could see their hand when viewing the initial target, but could not when the target was later displaced. Right: aiming perfomance of G.L. in comparison with control participants. Horizontal lines mark the three possible initial positions of the target. The first three labels on the horizontal axis identify single-step trials. Trials labelled 18-12 are double-stepped backwards. Trials labelled 18-24 are double-stepped forwards as in the trial exemplified in the left panel. Squares identify final hand positions. Ellipses identify the locations at which the peak velocity occurred.

Adapted from *Experimental Brain Research*, 125 (4), C. Bard, Yvonne Turrell, Michelle Fleury, Normand Teasdale, Yves Lamarre, and Olivier Martin, Deafferentation and pointing with visual double-step perturbations, pp 410–416, Figure 1, doi: 10.1007/s002210050697 © Springer-Verlag Berlin Heidelberg 1999. With permission of Springer.

Box 3.2 Continued

The best evidence for a predictive mechanism in the visual guidance of an action comes from a much-cited study of deafferented patient G.L. (Bard et al., 1999). Similarly to Ian Waterman (see Box 3.1), patient G.L. lost all tactile or proprioceptive afferences from the neck below, and learned to control hand movements from vision alone. Bard and colleagues tested her using an ingenious paradigm known as *double-step* aiming. In double-step aiming, participants are initially presented a peripheral target dot and initiate a pointing response to that target. At this point, the apparatus prevents vision of the hand, and the target, which remains visible, is rapidly displaced forwards or backwards. Because it occurs in between two saccades (the experiment also involves measuring eye movements) participants remain unaware of the displacement (this is called saccadic suppression). Even if they do not notice the double step, participants correct the trajectory and end up at the second position of the target (see Figure 3.10). These rapid online adjustments would be most efficiently attained by a predictive control mechanism matching expected hand positions to current sensory afferents (the second kind discussed earlier). In a neurologically healthy participant, however, it cannot be ruled out that the double step is managed within a traditional afferent feedback loop, by comparing visually monitored positions of the target with proprioceptively monitored hand positions. G.L. however cannot monitor hand positions by proprioception, and this is what makes testing her on this task so interesting. The right panel of Figure 3.10 compares the performance of G.L. with that of controls. As you can see, she is almost as good as the controls despite her neurological condition that rules out any proprioceptive input. This is strong evidence that she must be using predictive control. As Holmes famously tells Watson in *The Sign of the Four,* once eliminated the impossible, whatever remains must be the truth.

Box 3.3 Are you ticklish?

Everybody knows what it is like to be tickled. But what form of perception in involved? To sketch an answer, we must first draw a distinction between two forms of tickle (see Selden, 2004). The first, known as *knismesis,* is the mixed sensation that stems from lightly moving a small object almost anywhere across the skin. Knismesis stimulates you to rub your skin, for it can be pleasant but is also similar to itching in certain respects. The second form, known as *gargalesis,* is the peculiar feeling that arises from rougher and deeper pressure or vibration in a few areas only, mostly in the soles of the feet, armpits, and on the sides of the waist. Gargalesis causes you to experience ticklish laughter, an intermittent, incontrollable, and playful response having mostly pleasant but also some bordering on unpleasant connotations. An important difference between knismesis and gargalesis is that knismesis can be self-produced, although the

Box 3.3 Continued

externally produced experience is more salient (read on). In contrast, gargalesis cannot be self-produced. No matter how and how long you try, you will never provoke ticklish laughter to yourself. Besides the simple self-test, this conclusion is supported by many rigorous studies (for instance, Weiskrantz, Elliot, & Darlington, 1971, Chronicle & Glover, 2003; Pridmore et al., 2006). Recently, Van Doorn, Hohwy, and Symmons (2014) even went as far as asking whether one can tickle oneself when viewing one's own body from another person's perspective, a multisensory situation that induces a body swapping illusion (see Chapter 2). They observed that even in these conditions it was not possible for participants to tickle themselves.

Tickle is a bit of a mystery: we still do not have a satisfactory explanation for the phenomenon, although some proposals have been advanced. According to Charles Darwin (1872), for instance, tickle is essentially intergroup social communication. We tickle and are tickled by friends, family, and lovers, and dislike the idea of being tickled by total strangers (Provine, 2001). Darwin suggested that the behaviour derives from earlier forms of social communication that had adaptive functions. The reasoning is that knismesis may occur during grooming, an important component of social interactions in primates, and that gargalesis might have evolved from knismesis within the context of social play. Consider the typical game of 'I'm getting you—no, you're not' that takes place in tickle battles with our children. Games of this sort may have been originally a way of teaching our offspring defence strategies for actual combat (Provine, 2004; Selden, 2004). In this line of explanation, it is critical that the tickler be a conspecific and be different from the tickled—which might explain why you can't tickle yourself. According to a different hypothesis, however, tickle is a sort of startle reflex, presumably evolved from defence mechanism to protect the body from sudden noxious stimuli (Harris, 1999). In support of this idea, Harris and Christenfeld (1999) reported that participants could be tickled by a make-believe 'tickle machine,' which was in reality an experimenter providing the same stimulation as in a control 'human' condition. This finding seems to run counter Darwin's theory, suggesting that the reason that one can't tickle oneself is that self-produced stimulation is predictable (by definition). The two proposals however need not be mutually exclusive. Tickle may well be the remnant of social interactions that had specific adaptive functions for our ancestors. At the same time, unpredictability may be a key ingredient of those interactions. Let us see why.

With regard to the first proposal, note first of all that tickle battles take place near the body, where close proximity bears social implications (we return to these in Chapter 7, which discusses the multisensory perception and representation of space). There is evidence that the neural representation of the space near the body recruits multisensory neurons (Hyvärinen & Poraren, 1974; Graziano & Gross, 1993). These neurons are peculiar in that they do not respond to visual stimuli in a specific location of the visual field. Instead, they respond to visual stimuli that are presented in the proximity of the

Box 3.3 Continued

region of the skin where touches elicit responses. Thus, these neurons fire even before touch occurs, provided that there is a visual stimulus that, so to speak, 'warns' them of a forthcoming contact with the skin. This warning, however, cannot work well for regions of the skin that are not easily seen, such as the armpits, the sides of the trunk, or the soles of the feet. Interestingly, these are precisely the regions that elicit stronger gargalesis (Ruggieri & Milizia, 1983). In contrast, regions of the skin that are never seen directly, such as the back, the buttocks, or the top of the skull, do not elicit it at all. Thus, gargalesis appears to be related to the limits of anticipatory visual signals in the representation of one's personal space. In the original social play of our ancestors, this may have represented an efficient way to teach offspring about these limits.

With regard to the second proposal, one cannot avoid noticing that learning to respond to stimuli in personal space will be most efficient with manipulations of stimulus predictability, and that developing defence strategies will be greatly facilitated by neural mechanisms that enhance unpredictable, novel stimuli over predictable ones. A simple way to accomplish this would be to recycle a functional mechanism that we have already discussed in the context of the multisensory control of actions (see sections 3.3 and 3.4 of this chapter). The mechanism in question makes use of predictive, efferent models of one's movements and of their sensory consequences. As we have seen, such predictive models are critical to guide fast movements, which are controlled mostly using preparatory motor programmes; but are equally critical in keeping perception stable during one's own movement in spite of the consequent changes in proximal stimulation. It has long been known that the basic principle underlying such stabilization is the attenuation of those sensory signals that are predictable on the basis of one's efferent motor models (von Holst, 1954). Blakemore, Wolpert, and Frith (2000) reviewed several studies demonstrating that predictable sensory signals are attenuated, that as the discrepancy between predicted and actual signal increases this attenuation is reduced, and that such attenuation is observed with stimuli that may be classified as inducing knismesis (see also Blakemore, Wolpert, & Frith, 1998, Carlsson et al., 2000; Bays, Wolpert, & Flanagan, 2005). Attenuation of self-generated sensory signals therefore provides a powerful mechanism for highlighting unpredictable stimuli, while at the same time providing a means for categorizing actions as due to the self or to an external agent.

study is interesting because it suggests that processes related to motor intentions impact on perception, and most notably on multisensory and sensorimotor integration. An especially relevant phenomenon with this respect is *intentional binding* (Haggard, Clark, & Calogeras, 2002). In a typical study revealing intentional binding, participants move one finger, and the movement causes the presentation of a tone. Using a Libet-type clock, they are instructed to report when they had become aware of the onset of movement (this is Libet's M judgment) or, in other trials, when they had become aware of hearing the tone (let's call this the T judgment). Critically, two conditions are compared. In the first, participants intentionally move the finger (this condition is therefore analogous to Libet's task). In the second condition, the movement of the finger is provoked by magnetic stimulation applied to the motor cortex, using TMS. Thus, motor output is comparable in the two conditions, except for a key difference: intention. In the first condition, participants have to decide they want to move the finger. In the second, they don't—the finger just moves due to the applied stimulation. These studies have revealed that this difference has surprising consequences for the perceived timing of M and of T. When movement is intentional, M is delayed and T is anticipated relative to a baseline (this is the timing of M or T when these are not paired in the same trial but presented in isolation). When movement is provoked by TMS, instead, M is anticipated and T is delayed. Thus, intention seems to bring T and M closer in subjective time, whereas the lack of intention seems to push them apart. This demonstrates that the timing of conscious awareness can be modulated, presumably up to a point, by internal predictive processes, independently of the physical times of the perceived events.

After the initial report, intentional binding has been observed in other studies by Haggard's group (Engbert, Wohlschläger, & Haggard, 2008; Haggard & Clark, 2003; Tsakiris & Haggard, 2003). Another important implication of these results is that the perception of agency cannot be explained by a cognitive inference, drawn a posteriori on the basis of witnessed correlations between percepts of one's own movement and of its consequences in the environment. The perception of agency seems instead to emerge from multisensory interactions between sensory signals about limb movements and predictive efferent representations associated with the processing of intention. But how specific is the involved representation of the intention? Is it related to the actual intended movement, or to the more general goal of the action? Based on anecdotes such as Metzger's war misadventure, it would seem that what is critical for agency is specificity at the movement level, not the goal level. If this is correct, then one should be able to demonstrate experimentally that the perception of agency is not disrupted when the outcome of a movement results in sensory consequences that differ from those that the agent expected. This hypothesis has been tested in a study by Sato & Yasuda (2005).

In the first study of Sato's comprehensive work, participants learned the association between two arbitrary actions (pressing a key on the left or right of the keyboard) and two sensory consequences (a high or a low tone). After this preliminary phase, they were requested to perform the actions over several trials. With each action, a tone was presented that could be either consistent with the learned association or not. In addition, Sato & Yasuda varied the temporal lag between the keypress and the presentation of the tone (the delay between the action and its sensory consequences). Finally, in some blocks, participants provided the motor responses freely as in Libet's task, whereas in other blocks they did so in response to an external *go* signal. After each trial, participants provided an introspective report of how convincing was their impression of having caused the sound (on a 0–100 scale, 100 meaning full perception of agency). Results revealed that agency reduces from about 100 to about 75 if the sound is incongruent with the learned association. This indicates that the perception of agency is not completely immune from violations of the predicted sensory consequences of an action. However, it is not completely disrupted by these violations—at least when these are relatively mild such as substituting a single tone with another. A dramatic effect is instead revealed by increasing the delay between action and sensory consequence. When the delay is increased from zero to half a second, the perception of agency plummets from around 100 to less than 20. This is nicely consistent with the Metzger anecdote that opened this section. If the explosion is well synchronized with the chain pulling action, one expects a strong percept of agency even if the sensory consequence is not consistent with the intended one. And to complete the picture, Sato also found that it matters little whether the action is self-paced or in response to a go signal. If you have tried finger snapping in synch with a flashing light, as suggested at the beginning of the section, this last feature of Sato's data will be nicely consistent with your experience.

In a second experiment, Sato and Yasuda investigated yet another potential contributor to agency. In this study, they modified the task of the first experiment introducing a context that caused participants to make frequent errors, that is, pressing the key that they had not intended to press. Note that this manipulation, along with the congruence between the intention and its intended sensory consequence, now varies also the congruence between the intention and its *motor* consequences. They observed that even in this latter case agency was little affected, reducing from about 100 to about 80 in the error trials. When both the motor and sensory consequences were not congruent with the intention, however, agency again dropped from 100 to about 25. This additional finding therefore demonstrates that the perception of agency is not strictly specific to sensory or motor congruence with the intention, but is highly sensitive to the interaction of these two factors. Thus this result nicely reveals the nature of multisensory interactions in the perception of agency. In a later paper, Moore & Haggard (2008) suggested that these can be ascribed to the interplay of two processes: prediction and inference. The first contributes to agency due to the predictive motor representations, as well as sensory expectations, that are used to control the action within internal feedback loops (see previous section). The second, in contrast, contributes to agency by comparing the sensory feedback expected on the basis of the intention with the actual feedback. Thus, the predictive process is intrinsic to the agent, and elicits the perception of agency even before movement onset. The inferential process is instead extrinsic to the agent and intervenes after the action has been completed—it provides a 'reconstructive' sense of agency.

Chapter 4

Object Perception and Recognition

4.1 Objects

When we use the word 'object' in our daily conversations, we have the impression of knowing exactly what we mean. However, defining what constitutes an object is tricky. One of the philosophical entries of *Wikipedia,* for instance, defines an object as 'a thing, an entity, or a being' and offers a list of examples including 'the pyramids, Alpha Centauri, the number seven, a disbelief in predestination or the fear of cats'. An object, by this definition, is anything that one can talk about or that can be conceived. In contrast, ordinary usage tends to restrict the meaning of the word to solid and inanimate entities, thereby excluding animals, immaterial entities, abstract concepts, and the representations of objects that one finds in paintings and photographs.

The notion of object adopted in this chapter is close to that of ordinary usage. In the study of perception, however, the problem is not so much defining a priori what is an object and what is not, but understanding how the brain creates representations of unitary entities that can be perceived (Peterson, 2001). Implicit to this approach is that objects can be defined as *perceptual* units that enter conscious experience, are 'given' to us, as something that truly exists and that it is not merely imagined. The great Gestalt psychologist Wolfgang Metzger called this special character of perceived objects the 'encountered' (as distinguished form the 'represented', Metzger, 1941). With this term he wanted precisely to stress that perceiving objects entails experiencing entities that are out there and that are amenable to bodily interaction—that possess a three-dimensional shape, a location in space, a size; a perceivable colour and texture; as well as several other properties such as for instance weight, a degree of rigidity, an odour, and so on. In this chapter, we will discuss perceptual processes that are responsible for the construction of such object representations, typically also culminating with access to memory and recognition. One such entity is also our own body, and we have examined issues related to the multisensory perception of our own body in Chapters 2 and 3. Here we turn to external objects in general; Chapter 5 will focus on another special category, that of edible objects. Although object perception and recognition have been extensively studied within unisensory frameworks, in recent years a growing body of empirical evidence has started to reveal that multisensory interactions play a key role in the perception of object properties. We will discuss multisensory interactions occurring in three different contexts.

First, we will examine situations whereby unit formation involves two or more sensory signals about the very same property of the distal stimulus. In this case, the signals are redundant: they potentially carry information about the same object property. In addition, in these contexts signals are typically in spatial and temporal register: they originate from the same location in distal space and become available at the same time. As we shall see, powerful formal models have been developed within the last decade to predict the outcome of multisensory interactions in these contexts. Concepts originating in these modelling efforts appear also in most other chapters of this book. Since their application originated with problems of object perception, we discuss them in full here.

Next, we will discuss multisensory interactions in global perceptual organization. Organization is a core process in the construction of perceptual representations for objects: elemental features or parts, coded from sensory signals, need to be grouped together to form meaningful units. The units are separated from other units and from visible entities that we would not call objects, such as, the ground or the sky. The principles that rule such unit formation have been studied extensively *within* vision, hearing, and to some extent passive touch. Whether similar, or different, principles apply *across* sensory signals has proved more difficult to study and to model. Although there is little doubt that multisensory processes are involved in perceptual organization (Spence, 2016), the nature of these processes remains largely uncharted territory. In particular, while it is generally agreed that *unisensory* perceptual organization leads to the formation of emergent properties, or *Gestalten,* that are different from the sum of their elements, it is far less clear whether *multisensory* Gestalten exist.

Finally, we will take a look at crossmodal object recognition. Consider a situation like this: you have seen a saxophone many times (at concerts, in movies, in music shops), but you are not a musician and never had a chance to hold one in your hands. Now suppose the lights are turned off and a saxophone is given to you, such that you get to touch it for the very first time. Will you recognize it as the same object that you saw before? In other words, will the haptic sensory signal be sufficient to generate a representation of the object that will match the representation based on the visual sensory signal? This is, as we shall see, one of the oldest issues in the study of cognition (Box 4.1), predating even the birth of scientific psychology at the end of the nineteenth century. Important new findings are beginning to shed light on crossmodal object recognition, and on applications to prosthetic devices based on sensory substitution. We will review some of these issues at the end of the chapter.

4.2 Fusing spatiotemporally aligned sensory signals

Often, perceiving objects entails a sort of 'fusion' of information that we gather through different sensory signals. Consider what happens when we pick up an object and inspect it visually. In this common situation, two sources of information are potentially available about the size of the object: the information picked up by the retina and coded by the visual channel, and the information picked up by the hand that holds the object, typically coded by the haptic channel. The case of the perception of object size is especially instructive when considering the history of research on multisensory object perception.

Box 4.1 Molyneux's questions

The Irish natural philosopher William Molyneux (1656–1698) holds a place in the history of cognitive neuroscience due to a question he posed to John Locke after reading a pre-print summary of Locke's *Essay Concerning Human Understanding*. Molyneux's diverse interests included both optics, on which he authored a voluminous treatise, and what we now call philosophy of mind. It is often reported that his wife's illness, which led to blindness, was also instrumental in orienting his interests towards perception. Locke's work so interested him, that shortly after reading the summary he decided to get in touch. His famous letter to Locke began: 'A Problem Proposed to the Author of the Essai Philosophique concernant L'Entendement. A Man, being born blind, and having a Globe and a Cube, nigh of the same bigness, Committed into his Hands, and being taught or Told, which is Called the Globe, and which the Cube, so as easily to distinguish them by his Touch or Feeling; Then both being taken from Him, and Laid on a Table, Let us suppose his Sight Restored to him; Whether he Could by his sight, and before he touch'd them, know which is the Globe and which the Cube?' Locke received the letter in 1688 but at first paid little attention. The first edition of the *Essay*, published in 1690, contained no reference to Molyneux's question. Two years later, in his major work on optics, Molyneux again discussed and praised Locke's treatise. This Locke did notice, and in 1692 he wrote Molyneux expressing his gratitude. There was an exchange of letters, and in 1693 Molyneux again submitted his question in revised form. Locke finally saw the relevance of the issue for his theory, and included an answer to Molyneux's question in the 1694 second edition of the *Essay*. This prompted an intense debate between the most important philosophers of the eighteenth century (see Degenaar, 1996), as well as pioneering empirical studies. In 1728, the English surgeon William Cheselden surgically removed the congenital cataract of a 13-year old boy. Reportedly, the boy became able to use his vision but only after extensive training—at first he was unable to recognize familiar objects by sight. This was regarded as empirical evidence that the answer to Molyneux's question is negative, in accord with the theoretically motivated negative answers given by empiricists such as Locke and Berkeley. Locke believed that no innate knowledge is present at birth, and that the source of all knowledge lies in sensory experience. He noted that visual and tactile modalities are inherently different, and therefore concluded that no link could be established between them without extensive associative learning.

Molyneux's question may be regarded as a sort of thought-experiment in crossmodal recognition (Jacomuzzi, Kobau, & Bruno, 2003). It raises important questions regarding multisensory interactions between vision and touch when we perceive objects. For instance, is the association of visual and haptic percepts the only conceivable mechanism for linking touch and vision? Suppose instead that both visual and haptic processing produce a similar, multisensory representation of object structure. Depending on whether the relevant mechanisms are assumed to be inborn or to develop early in development, one might speculate that Molyneux's hypothetical observer will pass

Box 4.1 Continued

the test, or perhaps learn it rather quickly. Suggestions along these lines were provided by La Mettrie (1745) and by Leibniz (1765), and related issues continue to be debated in contemporary philosophy (e.g. Connolly, 2013; Levin, 2008; Proust, 1997; Schumacher, 2003). Interestingly, studies of visual abilities after cataract surgery on congenitally blind patients have provided only limited evidence to constrain this debate. Early anecdotal reports were provided by Senden (1932), and until recently only about ten additional cases had been studied (reviewed in Jacomuzzi, Kobau, & Bruno, 2003). In general, these studies suggested that different visual functions gain efficiency at different speeds, with colour perception happening after as little as 1–2 weeks, form discrimination taking about a month, and depth perception taking as long as several months. However, interpreting these reports remained difficult due to differences in the degree of cataract-induced blindness in these patients, in the specification, precision, and accuracy of the perceptual tests after surgery, and in the nature of the surgical techniques employed and their related post-operative consequences.

The best evidence so far has recently come from examinations of patients treated within *Project Prakash,* a scientific and humanitarian effort to treat curable blindness in rural India initiated by the MIT vision scientist Pawan Sinha (http://www. ProjectPrakash.org/). In a recent paper (Held et al., 2011), Sinha reported a careful assessment of the ability to match seen to felt objects in five newly sighted young patients. All patients suffered from congenital cataracts, and, importantly, none proved capable of visual form discriminations when tested before surgery. Tests were performed as soon as was practical (in all five, no later than 48 hours after surgery) and care was taken to ensure that the patients wore an eye patch continuously until tests begun. Test objects were large blocks from a children's construction game and they were always presented on a white background to avoid difficulties in figure–ground segregation. The patients were tested with a simple match-to-sample procedure: one sample object was presented either visually or haptically, followed by a test pair including again the sample and a distractor object. They were requested to indicate which of the test objects was the same as the sample object. This task was performed in three conditions: haptic sample and haptic tests (HH), haptic sample and visual tests (HV), and visual sample and visual tests (VV). Critically, the conditions were always performed in this order to rule out associative learning within sessions. The results were remarkably clear. All five participants were near perfect in the HH and VV conditions, whereas their performance was at chance in the HV condition. Thus, they proved unable to match the haptically perceived shape to the visually perceived one, despite the fact that both their haptic and, most importantly, their visual discriminatory abilities were fully adequate to perform the task. All participants were also retested after some weeks. At that point, all performed clearly above chance in the HV condition, suggesting that they had rapidly acquired the ability to match vision to touch.

Box 4.1 Continued

The results of Sinha's experiment indicate that crossmodal recognition is not based on an inborn mechanism, but can develop quickly once a patient is exposed to visual signals. This conclusion begs the question of what multisensory process during exposure promotes the development of the crossmodal link. As suggested by Ghanzafar and Turesson (2008), a hint may be found in the development of speech. Auditory feedback is critical for the acquisition of speech during development, and for its maintenance in adults. However, individuals who have become deaf in adulthood continue to produce intelligible speech even though they can no longer hear what they say. Ghanzafar and Turesson proposed that this is possible because somatosensory feedback from vocal tract movements participate in a multisensory-motor neural representation of speech production. Both the auditory and the somatosensory signals contribute, and movement links them during development. In late-deaf adults, the somatosensory component remains available and this permits speech production despite the absence of auditory signals. We suspect that the combination of visual and haptics with motor behaviour is likely to be also the reason why crossmodal recognition appears to develop so quickly in Sinha's patients.

Ghanzafar and Turesson concluded their paper by stating that Molyneux's question was ill-posed—as it did not mention movement. Ironically, this is only partly true. In the revised version of the problem that Locke eventually discussed in his work, Molyneux did not mention movement. In the original letter, however, in a way he did. After the first question quoted in the initial paragraph of this box, Molyneux added: 'Or whether he Could know by his sight, before he stretchd out his Hand, whether he could not Reach them, to they were Removued 20 or 1000 feet from him?' It is quite possible, of course, that Molyneux merely meant to ask whether distances would be perceived correctly by his imaginary newly sighted individual. But his second question does mention a preparatory motor process ('..before he stretched out his Hand...'), and one could rightly ask whether visually based motor programming would be possible under his imagined conditions (Jacomuzzi, Kobau, & Bruno, 2003). For instance, whether the trajectory of the reaching hand would correctly reflect the position of the object, or whether the finger aperture would scale to its size (see Chapter 3). Perhaps, if the second question had also found a place in Locke's *Essay*, the nature of the debate on Molyneux's ingenious thought experiment would have been different, as would have been its impact on early theories of multisensory perception.

In a classic experiment (Rock & Victor, 1964), the great perception scientist Irvin Rock examined this situation and concluded that multisensory object perception is characterized by *visual dominance*. He asked his participants to touch cubes hidden behind a cloth but with their front surfaces visible in bas-relief. Participants could not see their hands, which were also behind the cloth, and wore distorting goggles that altered the visible size of the surface in bas-relief. This created a conflict between vision (distorted by the goggles) and haptics (veridical). To collect measurements of perceived size, participants were presented with a graded series of cubes and were asked to indicate which best matched the size of the cube they were currently experiencing. Rock reported that participant matches were much closer to the visually distorted than to the veridically felt size, as if vision dominated touch in the conditions of the experiment.

Later studies, however, were not completely in accord with this bold conclusion. Visual dominance was not always complete (Power, 1980), tactile dominance could occur in some conditions (Hershberger & Misceo, 1996), and attention could affect dominance (Heller, Calcaterra, Green, & Brown 1999). These findings led to a different hypothesis. It was proposed that the brain chooses which sensory channel will determine the perception of a given object, depending on the task and on the overall conditions. This has been dubbed the *modality appropriateness* hypothesis (Welch & Warren, 1980). More recent work has unified these two proposals (see Helbig & Ernst, 2008), suggesting that the perception of the spatial features of objects is always based on multisensory fusing of all available sensory signals. However, sensory signals are given different weights within the fusion process, depending on their relative reliability. This, in a nutshell, is the key idea of *optimal integration* models of multisensory fusion.

The notion of optimal integration stems from statistics and measurement theory. Given two samples of measurements, both affected by random error, if one wishes to use these measurements to estimate an unknown population parameter the best ('optimal') guess is to use the information from both samples, but to weigh this information in proportion to the sample precision. Sample statistics that are less affected by random error are more precise, and should be weighted more. For instance, suppose you wanted to estimate the unknown mean of a population and that you have collected two samples that have means M1 and M2 and variances equal to V1 and V2. (The variance is a measure of random error in the samples.) Optimal weights for combining the two means into a single estimate are derived from the precisions of the samples by taking the reciprocal of the variances, 1/V1 and 1/V2 (precision being the reciprocal of random error). Specifically, the joint estimate will be simply M1, weighted by its (relative) precision, plus M2, also weighted by precision. It can be shown that the outcome of such a weighted integration will always be more precise than the original estimates based only on M1 or M2. In this, therefore, the integrated estimate will be 'optimal'.

An advantage of optimal integration models over earlier proposals, such as visual dominance or modality appropriateness, is that we can use the idea to formulate quantitative predictions. Consider again the perceived size of an object that one can see and touch at the same time. In a seminal study conducted in the laboratory of Marty Banks at the University of California (Ernst & Banks, 2002), participants were requested to discriminate the size of two objects. The objects could be seen (vision only condition), touched (touch only condition), or simultaneously seen and touched (multisensory condition). The key feature of this elegant study was that the stimuli were not real objects, as in the earlier studies, but computer-controlled virtual reality simulations. The visual stimuli were displayed on a computer screen and seen through three-dimensional glasses, whereas the touch stimuli were presented using a mechanical device that applied force feedback on the participant's fingertips to simulate contact with a virtual object. Critically, the reliability of the visual signals could be varied from trial to trial by adding appropriate amounts of random noise to the stimulus on the screen. To compare their results with the prediction of an optimal integration model, Ernst and Banks first assessed the precision of size perception by vision (at different levels of sensory reliability) and by touch in unisensory conditions. They then used these precisions to weigh unisensory percepts and compute predicted size percepts in the multisensory condition. They found that these predictions fitted their observed multisensory percepts extremely well. When visual stimuli contained little noise (high reliability), vision tended to dominate and the multisensory percept was closer to the visually specified size. When a significant amount of noise was inserted, instead, the opposite held true. Touch dominated and the multisensory percept became closer to the size specified by the force feedback device. Their experiment therefore demonstrated that both visual and tactile dominance can be observed in the multisensory perception of size, depending on the reliability of the available sensory signals. This supports optimal integration and explains the seemingly contradictory results of earlier studies.

After the publication of Ernst and Banks' study, optimal integration has received support from several other experiments. For instance, Gephstein & Banks (2003) have shown that visual reliability can be manipulated also by varying the position in depth of a visual stimulus relative to the viewpoint. When the stimulus is oriented such that a spatial extent is parallel to the line of sight, the size of the object along that direction is perceived less precisely than when the extent is orthogonal to the line of sight. Gephstein and Banks therefore compared multisensory percepts of the size of virtual objects that were always touched in the same way but could be seen in two different conditions. In one condition, participants had to judge the extent in the direction parallel to the line of sight, whereas in the other they had to judge the extent in the orthogonal direction. In accord with optimal integration, they found that multisensory size percepts were closer to tactile size in the former condition and closer to visual size in the latter. You may recall that a similar analysis motivated a study by van Beers and collaborators (2002) on multisensory aiming (Chapter 3), and that a similar reasoning about relative reliabilities was used by these authors to interpret their results. Optimal integration predictions have been found to fit experimental results well in the multisensory perception of other object properties, such as surface slant (Ernst et al., 2000) and three-dimensional shape (Helbig & Ernst, 2007). Finally, studies of the ventriloquist effect, a case of visual dominance over sound in the perception of localization, have also successfully applied optimal integration modelling (Alais & Burr, 2004; we return to audiovisual integration in Chapter 7 on multisensory space perception).

An important feature of these cases of multisensory fusion is that the channels involved provide information about the very same object property. Integration of these signals is optimal precisely because these signals are, in fact, redundant. We can perceive size by sight and by touch. When both are available, we benefit from fusing the signals and perceive size with greater precision. There is, however, one missing element in the way this situation is understood. In a controlled experiment, we know that the signals are redundant because we designed the situation that way. In real life, it may well be that sensory signals come from different parts of the same objects (and therefore they would not be redundant but complementary) or from different objects altogether. So how does the brain of a perceiver known that sensory signals are redundant—as opposed to complementary, or even conflicting? How does the brain distinguish between cases where integration of multisensory signals is appropriate and cases in which the signals are best kept separate? One possibility is that integration occurs only for signals that are aligned in space and time. In support of this hypothesis, some studies have shown that multisensory integration does not occur if the sensory signals involved come from different locations (Gephstein Burge, Ernst, & Banks 2005) or are not presented within a common temporal window lasting approximately two-tenths of a second (Shams, Kamitani, & Shimojo, 2002; Slutsky & Recanzone, 2001). This hypothesis, however, presupposes that the brain has a way of determining if the signals come from the same location and at the same time. As we will see in Chapters 7 and 8 (on the multisensory perception of space and time), this is in itself a problem. Another possibility is that multisensory interactions are not merely determined by bottom-up sensory signals but are also shaped by top-down, cognitive constraints. This is the key idea of Bayesian models of multisensory perception, to which we know turn.

4.3 **The Bayesian framework**

Reverend Thomas Bayes (1701–1761) occupies a peculiar position in the history of modern science. After studying logic and theology at the University of Edinburgh, he served as a Presbyterian minister for most of his life, but also maintained strong interests in mathematics (especially on Newton's calculus, the subject of one of his books). However, he is mostly remembered for his work on probability, which he never published. After his death, his findings on probability theory were collected by a friend and presented for the first time to the Royal Society two years after his death. In a nutshell, Bayes' theorem (or Bayes' rule, as it is also often called) states that the probability of an event, given knowledge that a second event has occurred (this is called the *posterior* probability), depends on the product of two components: the probability of the second event, given the first (this is the inverse of the posterior, called the *likelihood),* and the overall probability of the first event (this is called the *prior* probability). The theorem has proved useful in a wide range of scientific fields. Consider, for instance, the difference between the probability of anyone having a stroke and the probability of an individual having a stroke, given that this person is 80 years-old. Bayes' theorem provides a principled way of *revising* your estimate of this person's risk, based on the additional information you have gathered. The prior probability represents the initial estimate. In the USA, for instance, about 800,000 people have a stroke each year. However, among all stroke patients the number of oldies is higher than the number of younger individuals. Thus, the fact that this person is old increases the risk. Bayes' theorem will allow you to compute this increase in the probability of stroke, relative to the prior, if the likelihood is known.

Applications of Bayes' theorem to perception assume that perceiving is essentially revising one's prior representation of the environment, and using this for a probabilistic decision (for technical discussions of Bayesian modelling, see Kersten & Yuille, 2003;

Mamassian, Landy, & Maloney, 2002). The prior representation can be thought as implicit knowledge about statistical regularities of our world, for instance, knowledge that the size of behaviourally relevant objects varies within a certain range, with a certain distribution function. This prior can be modified by information in incoming sensory signals, which is modelled by a likelihood function, for instance, the likelihood of proximal visual angles on the retina, given distal sizes in the environment. The outcome is a posterior distribution function giving the probabilities of possible object sizes, given the current sensory information. Perceived size is then chosen from this posterior distribution as the most probable value (plus, in some models, an evaluation of the cost function for possible decisions). This framework provides a powerful formalization for an intuitively appealing idea: that perception depends on sensory information, but is also influenced by top-down expectations. How important this top-down component is in perception in general has been hotly debated in the last decade of the last century (Tutorial 4.1). Bayesian modelling has provided a theoretically attractive means of resolving this debate, as well as a useful framework for devising quantitative predictions.

Tutorial 4.1 Theories of perception: indirect, direct, or directed?

Theories of perception are traditionally categorized as belonging to one of two camps: *indirect* and *direct*. Although the seeds of the idea can be traced back to the works of philosophers such as Mill, Locke, and Berkeley, the earliest formulation of an indirect theory is usually attributed to the German physicist, physician, and sensory physiologist Hermann von Helmholtz (1821–1894). Helmholtz may be justly considered one of the greatest scientific minds of all times, capable of making significant empirical, theoretical, and applied contributions to a wide range of fields. In the third volume of his monumental *Handbook of Physiological Optics* (Helmholtz, 1867), he introduced the idea that perception may be described as a form of *unconscious inference*. By this, he meant that percepts could be considered akin to conclusions inferred from premises, the premises being the given sensory signals and the (unconscious and obligatory) operations implemented in the brains' perceptual centres. Helmholtz's metaphor has been tremendously influential, and remains one of the theoretical bases of modern 'computational' models of perception. A key implication is that understanding perception requires understanding sensory processing but also (qualitatively distinct) cognitive operations. The notion of perception as direct is instead due to James J. Gibson (1904–1979), whose work we reference in many parts of this book. Gibson may be justly considered one of the most important experimentalists and theoreticians of perception of the past century. The notion of perception as direct is expounded most clearly in his last book, *The Ecological Approach to Visual Perception* (Gibson, 1979). According to Gibson, perception is direct in that it is determined by information in sensory signals, and by nothing else. To perceive is simply to record (or, as he liked to say, 'pick up') this information, with no need for further cognitive operations. The recording is, of course, done by neural mechanisms, but these are not inferential engines. The brain does not compute, it merely 'resonates' to the incoming information.

The publication of Gibson's last book sparked an intense debate between proponents of the new direct theory and defenders of the more traditional indirect one. The debate was extensive and involved a variety of additional concepts from psychology and epistemology. For instance, Irvin Rock (1922–1995), another great experimentalist and theoretician of perception science, argued (Rock, 1985) that indirect theories are *constructivist* (percepts are internal representations, built by applying specific operations on the sensory information), and distinguished between *spontaneous organization constructivism* (the hypothesized operations resemble the organization of a complex field under the action of forces—this was the key theoretical idea of Gestalt psychology; see section 4.4 and Tutorial 4.2) and *reasoning-like* (or ratiomorphic) *constructivism* (operations resemble logical operations—this is the mind-as-software metaphor often found in cognitive psychological theorizing). Direct theories, added Rock, are instead *stimulus* theories, which he criticized for ignoring the complexities of perceptual mechanisms needed to process information. In a famous article, Swedish psychologist Sverker Runeson (Runeson, 1977) pointed out that stimulus information could be processed directly by 'smart' neural mechanisms that do not require logical operations or internal representations (a classic example is the polar planimeter, an analogue device that can compute the area of arbitrarily complex shapes but uses no rule of geometry). Note that a smart neural process then becomes very similar to a spontaneously organizing one, thereby blending the distinction with at least one form of constructivism. Vision scientist James Cutting, like Gibson a professor at Cornell University, lucidly argued that inference comes in two kinds: deduction, which derives a necessarily true conclusion from information implicit in the premises (like a mathematical demonstration), and induction, which generalizes a possible, but not necessarily true, conclusion from specific instances. If perceptual inferences are deductive, and there are ample reasons to believe that this is what Helmholtz meant (Cutting, 1986), then reasoning-like constructivism is essentially another metaphor for describing how perception may pick up information. To cut a long story short, the debate raged for about a decade, and then it gradually disappeared from the literature and from scholarly meetings.

In one of the most original books about perception written in the past century, Cutting (1986) scrutinized nine theoretical issues that have been advanced as grounds for distinguishing between direct and indirect theories. He came to the conclusion that most are more apparent than real, resting largely on misconceptions or incomplete analysis. He found that only one of these issues promised to provide a useful distinction: the theory's assumptions about *information sufficiency*. This criterion refers to the mapping of information in sensory signals to percepts. In direct theories, information *specifies* percepts as the mapping is one-to-one (Figure 4.1a). Once information in sensory signals has been determined, this suffices to predict what observers will perceive. In indirect theories, conversely, information *underspecifies* percepts as the mapping is many-to-many (Figure 4.1b). Information is not sufficient to predict percepts, and additional computational constraints need to be brought in to disentangle the mapping. However, Cutting's aim in offering this analysis was not to take sides with one of the contenders. He instead argued that a third option needs to be considered, *directed* perception. The key idea of his proposal is that in natural perception the mapping is neither one-to-one nor many-to-many, but many-to-one (Figure 4.1c). In typical natural perception, different sources of information map onto single perceived features. Information *overspecifies* perception, and the job of perceptual systems is to handle this overspecification. For instance, perception may select one source and disregard the rest; it may integrate all the available sources; or it may select a subset and integrate within that set. Whether perception satisfices (by selecting) or optimizes (by integrating) may depend on the task at hand, on environmental or biological constraints, on attentional requirements. Purely direct perception rests at one end of the directed perception continuum, corresponding to situations whereby a single source is selected. Finally, when stimulus information is impoverished (due to special environmental conditions or to deliberate experimental manipulations in the laboratory), internal constraints may be recruited to supplement the available information. Thus, a form of indirect perception may take place. Internal constraints will

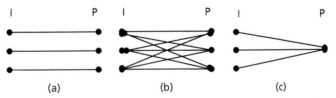

Figure 4.1 Assumed mappings between information and percepts. Mapping varies according to direct (a), indirect (b), and directed (c) perception theories. I: information; P: percepts. After Cutting (1986).

essentially supplement the outcome of directed perception (as the system will still use all the available information), working at the intersection of pure perception and higher-level cognition.

If you have read sections 4.2 and 4.3 of this chapter, you may share with us the impression that optimal multisensory integration models within a Bayesian framework capture many features of directed perception. For instance, they can model situations whereby an object feature, such as its perceived size, is potentially specified by multiple sources of information, such as different visual, tactile, and kinaesthetic signals. As discussed in the aforementioned sections, such modelling successful predicts cases whereby one channel dominates (Cutting's selection) or multiple channels jointly determine (Cutting's optimization) a percept. The analysis of likelihood functions offers a principled tool for understanding sensory information, and the formalization of priors can quantify how internal constraints enter into the equation. The Bayesian approach differs from directed perception mostly in one feature: it assumes a probabilistic mapping of sensory information to percepts. The kind of probabilistic inference implicit in the Bayesian approach, however, is neither deductive nor inductive, as in classical indirect theories, but *abductive*. Abduction (or retroduction, as it is sometimes also called) is a form of logical inference that strives to identify the most supported among candidate conclusions, given a set of premises. Unlike deduction, the premises do not imply a unique and certain conclusion. However, and unlike induction, the conclusion is not mechanically generalized from a set of observations, but is based on probabilistic reasoning and on other constraints that can be formalized. The validity of an abductive conclusion, therefore, can in principle be estimated within a model taking into account the likelihood of the premises, given alternative conclusions, and any other information one may have.

In the Bayesian approach, perception is modelled as a trade-off between information in sensory signals and a priori knowledge about the world. To understand this trade-off, consider the case of the shape of an object's surface. Bayesian models state that perceived shape is chosen from the posterior probabilities of different distal surfaces in the three-dimensional environment, given a sensory signal that consists in a two-dimensional projection on the eye's retina. Assuming that no other information is available, because of projective ambiguity (Figure 4.2) each of the possible distal surfaces is equally likely, that is, the likelihood distribution is uniform. The Bayesian approach, therefore, predicts that perceived shape will be critically dependent on the prior probabilities that enter in the computation. It has long been known that human perception tends to interpret, whenever possible, proximal trapezoids as projections of rectangles. A natural experiment that nicely demonstrates this preference can be performed while visiting New York City. At the corner of 3rd Avenue and 32nd Street in Manhattan lies *The Future*, an apartment building designed by Greek architect Costas Kondylis. A notable feature of the building is its balconies, which are trapezoidal rather than rectangular as almost all balconies in cities. When you look at the building, however, the balconies appear rectangular and, most strikingly, slanted upwards or downwards depending on your position on the street (Halper, 1997; Figure 4.3). The preference for rectangular balconies is so strong that the brain prefers to see architecturally absurd angles relative to the building, rather than more logical right angles but trapezoidal shapes. This happens however only when looking at the balconies from a certain distance. When standing close to the building, the lower balconies appear as they are, that is, at right angles and trapezoidal. Presumably, this happens because other sensory signals enter into the equation, counteracting the influence of a priori expectations. You can see now how this framework lends itself quite naturally to modelling multisensory

2D Projection   Simulation in 3D

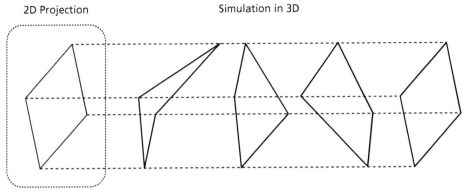

Figure 4.2 Projective ambiguity. Any two-dimensional (2D) projection can be the projection of different surfaces (differing in shape and slant) in three-dimensional (3D) space. For instance, a regular trapezoid in two-dimensions could be the projection of a regular rectangle in three-dimensions, or of infinite other surfaces.

situations, where signals from different sensory channels provide a set of likelihood distributions, and a priori expectations constrain how these contribute to the final percept.

The Bayesian framework can indeed be used to explain many classical puzzles of multisensory perception. One is the so-called *size-weight* illusion: a small object feels heavier than a larger object of equal weight (Charpentier, 1891). You may recall the

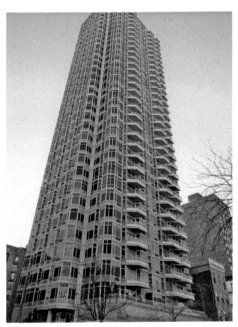
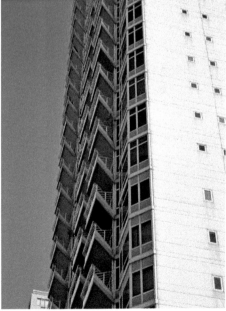

Figure 4.3 Two views of *The Future* apartment building in Manhattan. The balconies are trapezoidal but they appear rectangular and slanted downwards when standing on the right of the building, and upwards when standing on the left.
Photographs courtesy of Paolo Legrenzi.

familiar stumper: 'which is heavier, a pound of lead or a pound of feathers?' The size-weight illusion indicates that the pound of lead is really heavier (perceptually), despite being the same weight (physically). Its first discoverer, the French physiologist Augustine Charpentier (1852–1961), attributed it to the contrast between the visually expected and the haptically experienced effort in lifting differently sized objects. Much debate has arisen on the nature of such expectations and the role of motor and perceptual processes in determining them (see Dijker, 2014; Flanagan & Beltzner, 2000). Whatever one's favourite explanation, the size-weight illusion is puzzling because it seems to contradict the prediction of the Bayesian framework. It stands to reason that priors about the weight of objects should be based on size: visually big might be expected, on the average, to be heavier than visually small. Bayesian models allow that such priors be modified by sensory signals, but in the size-weight illusion the haptically experienced weights for the small and large objects are identical. Thus, whatever change these signals could exert on the prior probabilities, this could not invert actual weight perception relative to the visual expectation. Priors about weight, however, may not depend merely on size—another important factor may be the relationships between size and density. At least for man-made manipulable objects, there is evidence that small objects tend to be denser than large objects (Peters, Balzer, & Shams, 2015). Therefore, density can be inferred probabilistically from size even though it cannot be directly gauged from visual signals. It is only natural at this point to ask if a Bayesian model armed with size-density priors correctly predicts the size-weight illusion. There is recent evidence that it does (Peters, 2016).

In addition, the size-weight illusion is not only a perceptual effect, but also has a sensorimotor side. In an elegant study, Flanagan & Bandomir (2000) found that when comparing two objects, the object that was picked up with a smaller grip, or with a precision grip instead of a power grip (all five fingers), or held such that the contact surface was smaller, was judged to be heavier than a reference object that was visually the same size and had the same weight. Thus, it seems that the size-weight illusion can be induced also when size is perceived via somatosensory channels, or is gauged visually within a sensorimotor process. In another study from the same group (Flanagan & Beltzner, 2000), this motor side of the illusion was examined directly by recording fingertip grip forces along with weight judgements. The results indicated that, upon first lifting equally heavy large and small objects, participants applied more force than needed to the large object, and less than needed to the small one. Over repeated trials, however, participants learned to scale forces to the true weights, although they continued to verbally judge the smaller object as heavier. We can draw several conclusions from these results. First, the sensorimotor size-weight illusion *is* consistent with Bayesian predictions—when attempting to pick up a larger object, one does indeed apply more force than with a smaller object of the same weight, suggesting that force was biased by the visual prior. You may have experienced something of the sort when picking up an empty large suitcase (if not, try—most likely you will pull too much and the suitcase will feel surprisingly light). Second, the sensorimotor and perceptual effects seem to have different time courses. This has been interpreted as evidence that the involved multisensory motor processes are separate and independent (Flanagan & Bletzner, 2000; see also Flanagan, Bittner, & Johansson (2008)). Third, and final, priors seem to be affected by learning. We now turn to this last aspect.

An important question regarding Bayesian priors in perception is whether these are fixed (be them inborn, or formed rapidly in early development) or can be altered by experience. Results from several studies converge in suggesting that experience can change priors. For instance, Flanagan, Bittner, & Johansson (2008) had participants train over several days in a lifting task with blocks having weights that varied inversely with volume. They found that this practice gradually reduced and eventually inverted the size-weight illusion, such that at the end of the experiment participants judged the larger blocks to be lighter. This is consistent with the hypothesis that weight perception priors are based on size-density relationships, not on size alone, and that these priors can be relearned relatively quickly. But perhaps the most convincing demonstration that priors can be relearned comes from a multisensory study of a famous shape-from-shading demonstration (Adams, Graf, & Ernst, 2004). It has long been known that shading gradients affect the perception of surface curvature in accord with the assumption that light will come from above (Figure 4.4).

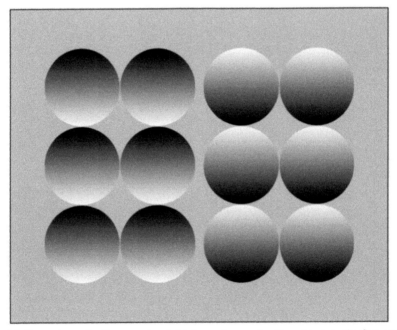

Figure 4.4 Shape-from-shading reveals a light-from-above prior. The objects in the first and second columns appear as concave 'bumps'; those in the third and fourth as convex 'hills'. Turn the page upside down and hills and bumps will exchange positions. Thus, the gradients are interpreted as shading due to illumination coming from the top. Shading information is then used to infer curvature. Computer-generated image drawn by adapting public-domain R code (see http://stackoverflow.com/questions/17333823/plot-gradient-circles).
Courtesy of Tyler Rinker, based on images by Stephen Few and Colin Ware, with thanks to @thelatemail https://stackoverflow.com/questions/17333823/plot-gradient-circles.

To test whether this light-from-above prior can be modified by multisensory experience, Adams and her collaborators established baseline visual preferences for concave or convex interpretations as a function of gradient direction, trained participants with haptic surfaces that were turned upside-down relative to those visually perceived, and then retested them on their visual preferences. The results indicated that at retest the preferences had turned more consistent with the haptically learned new prior. Thus, the light-from-above prior, which is presumably learned among other things from statistical associations between sunlight shading patterns and haptically perceived curvatures, can be rapidly altered by exposing participants to novel associations. This suggests that perceptual priors are remarkably flexible. Relatively brief experience of novel associations can counteract life-long exposure to sunlight coming from above.

In conclusion, there is pretty strong evidence that re-learnable expectations have a role in perception. There is also a growing consensus that Bayesian modelling provides the appropriate framework for understanding the subtle interplay between such prior expectations and current sensory information. The utility of the Bayesian framework, however, is not limited to quantifying the trade-off between likelihoods and priors in determining posteriors. When applied to multisensory interactions, Bayesian modelling can also be used to tackle another delicate problem, the problem of selecting what type of multisensory interaction is appropriate in a given situation. We have already mentioned this problem in the previous section. Given sensory signals A and B, if these are redundant (that is, they come from the same source) then integrating them into a signal estimate is advantageous. For instance, one can better estimate the location of a sound source by integrating visual and auditory signals using a statistically optimal procedure. However, integration will be advantageous only if A and B *do* come from the same source. If they do not, other forms of multisensory interaction may be more appropriate. For instance, the signals may come from the same object but they may be complementary rather than redundant. When I see the front of a cup while feeling with the hand for an handle in the back, visual, and haptic signals about the structure of the object are about different parts and they should be unified in a more complex way than a mere weighted sum. Ernst and Bülthoff (2004) have suggested that this should be called multisensory *combination* rather than integration, precisely because integration would not apply. Finally, often concurrent signals come from different objects altogether and they should be kept separated. If I see a lamb while I hear a growl, locating the sound source where I see the lamb may not only be incorrect but also dangerous—if there is a wolf nearby. Within a Bayesian framework, the problem of selecting the appropriate kind of interaction can be approached by adding an 'interaction' prior, which can be defined in two different ways.

One way to approach the problem of selecting the 'right' kind of multisensory interaction is to construct a model that can infer probabilistically whether different signals come from the same source of from different sources. An influential paper by the group of Ladan Shams at the University of California at Los Angeles (Körding et al., 2007) applied this idea to the problem of perceiving object location from vision and hearing. In the standard Bayesian framework, this is done by integrating likelihoods of visual and auditory information and using these to modify a location prior. In the more complex model of Körding and collaborators, integrated likelihoods modify also an additional interaction prior, which is modelled as the probability of a common as opposed to independent cause for the two sensory signals. To test this model, Körding and collaborators requested participants to judge both the visual and the auditory location (a *dual-report* experiment) for visual and auditory stimuli that could be spatially coincident or disparate. They found that their model including an interaction prior fitted the data of this experiment way better than the standard Bayesian model. In particular, the model correctly predicted most cases whereby visual and auditory judgments were identical (suggesting multisensory fusion of the two signals) and most cases whereby they were different (suggesting that the signals were kept separate). Thus, Körding's model was effectively capable of probabilistically solving not only a perceptual problem (where are current objects located in the environment?) but also a problem of a causal inference (do current sensory signals have a common or independent cause?). If interested in mathematical details, you can find a more technical treatment of this general idea in Shams (2012). At least for this particular situation, this approach provides an elegant solution to the problem of choosing between integration and segregation of signals. Whether, and how, this approach can be extended to signal combination and to other situations remains to be seen.

Another potential way of solving the interaction selection problem is to assume that multisensory interactions are constrained by object recognition and semantic representations in memory. Imagine seeing a kettle that emits a puff of steam while you hear a whistling sound. To decide whether the visual and auditory signals should be integrated for object localization, the brain might exploit semantic knowledge about kettles. More than 60 years ago, Jackson (1953) asked this question in a controlled experiment. He had participants localize sound sources while varying the position of concurrent visual stimuli. In a first study, these were a bell and a light; in a second study, a whistling sound from a compressed air device and an actual puffing kettle. Jackson reported that auditory localization was biased by visual position, but only in the second study. It may speculated that, in the second study, knowledge about kettles dictated that the visual and auditory signals had a common origin, such that multisensory fusion occurred. In the first study, instead, no comparable knowledge could be mustered about bells and lights and the signals were kept separated. Thus, an interaction prior of sorts could be conceived based on object recognition and memory. However, the empirical evidence for such high-level effects on perception should always be interpreted with great caution. In Jackson's studies, the visual and auditory stimuli were very different, and whether this, rather than recognition, caused the different results is very hard to exclude. In a much more recent study, Helbig & Ernst (2007) again proposed that knowledge about a common source for a visual and haptic stimulus promoted multisensory fusion. In their study, knowledge was manipulated by comparing directly viewing a haptically felt object with viewing it in a mirror reflection. Because the two conditions yielded similar multisensory fusion, Helbig and Ernst argued that knowing about mirrors allowed for interaction even if haptic localization (the actual hand position) was different from visual localization (the mirror image position). While this interpretation seems less speculative than Jackson's, it could be argued that the kind of knowledge involved here is not really about object representations but a sort of spatial remapping. In general, it seems to fair to say that the issue of interaction priors needs further theoretical and empirical work.

4.4 Multisensory effects on global unit formation

The multisensory interactions examined so far concern single elementary features of an object, such as its size or weight. Objects, however, do not typically possess only one perceived feature but are rather a unitary representation of grouped elements. This process of global *unit formation* (or *organization,* as baptized by the Gestalt school in psychology, see Tutorial 4.2) is fundamental in determining what we perceive globally from a collection of sensory signals localized in space and time. As exemplified in Figure 4.5, this process

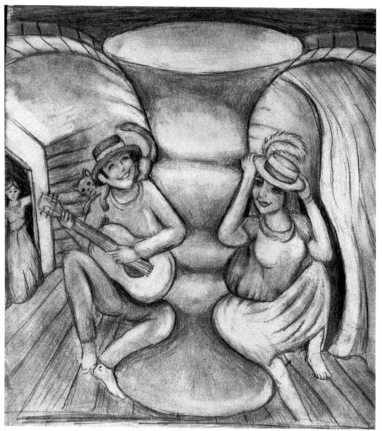

Figure 4.5 Unit formation yields objects segregated from backgrounds. In this variation of a well-known multistable display, three alternative unit formation outcomes compete: a single vase (centre), two full figures (sides), or two facing profiles (sides, extending to the far ends of the frame; if you have a hard time seeing this try looking at the picture from some distance) © Jennelle Brunner.

Tutorial 4.2 Gestalt laws

The notion that objects are the outcome of brain processes of unit formation arises naturally from examining the relationship between distal and proximal stimuli in vision. In the distal environment, variously shaped and sized aggregates of physical materials lie positioned on surfaces of support in multifarious spatial relationships to each other. The job of the visual system is to figure out these distal aggregates—getting to know 'what' is out there—from the sensory signals coded at the level of the retina, i.e. proximal stimuli. However, the relationship of single proximal signals to single distal features is often ambiguous. Consider the spatial structure of proximal stimulation. The optical information impinging on the retinal mosaic can be locally homogeneous or non-homogeneous. Local non-homogeneities correspond to changes (for instance, in light intensity) that possess a spatial structure (e.g. spatially aligned changes in intensity). Such locally aligned non-homogeneities are called *contours* or *edges* whereas homogeneous retinal extents are called *regions* or *uniformly connected regions* (see Palmer & Rock, 1994). Functionally,

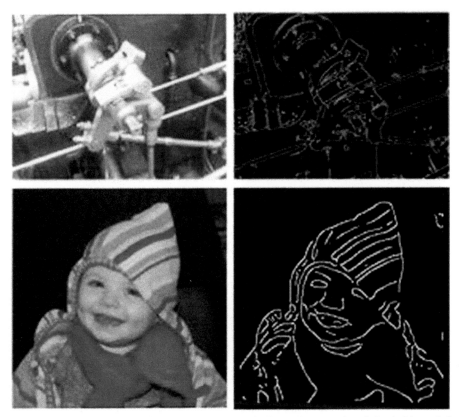

Figure 4.6 Distal boundaries of objects and detected edges. Photographs of distal objects (left column) compared to the outputs of a standard contemporary computer vision algorithm. Note that the relationship between detected edges and the actual object boundaries is not obvious. Although the algorithm does quite well, some of the detected edges do not correspond to boundaries; at the same time, some existing boundaries are not represented by detected edges.

a large part of the initial steps of vision can be interpreted as coding edges within a retinotopic spatial reference frame (Hubel & Wiesel, 1968). Work in psychophysics and artificial vision has devised and tested elegant computational models of edge detection in vision (see Bruce, Green, & Georgeson, 2003). However, this line of work has also clearly revealed that, at least in a single image, detected edges are not easily related to the distal boundaries of objects. This was argued most clearly by computational vision scientists David Marr and Ellen Hildreth (1980) and is neatly illustrated by Figure 4.6. The main lesson to be drawn here is that the relationship of proximal edges to object boundaries is not straightforward: early visual mechanisms may detect edges that do not correspond to actual boundaries (for instance, the short segment below the baby's mouth); at the same time, some boundaries may exist that edge detecting mechanism will miss (for instance, the irises in the baby's eyes).

Despite the non-trivial relationship of contours to boundaries, the human visual system is remarkably good at creating perceptual units corresponding to meaningful material aggregates in the distal environment. Ordinarily, perceived objects prove to be accurate representations of distal entities—at least in the sense that these representations successfully support our internal representations of the outside environment and our bodily interactions with it. A nice example is presented in Figure 4.7. You will agree that a unitary object can be perceived in this picture (a Dalmatian dog), although for some of us this might take some effort, and that this is ultimately a correct way of interpreting this visual input. Close scrutiny of the image, however, reveals that the silhouette of the dog is not specified by proximal contours except in a few places where part of the contours of the black elements happen to be aligned with the perceived silhouette of the dog. Thus this perceived silhouette cannot result merely from contour detection at the local level, it must result from an integrative process of unit formation that somehow 'decides' that some elements belong together, and on the basis of this reconstructs the boundaries of the object, separating this reconstructed figure from the background. This is no obvious feat, for the black elements that pepper the image could in principle be grouped in any number of ways. Taken by itself, there is nothing in each of these elements that connects it with any other element. So how does the brain achieve this?

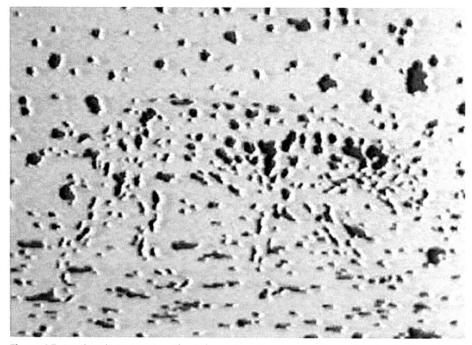

Figure 4.7 Another demonstration of unit formation. Can you see a Dalmatian dog in this picture?

Historically, the merit of having identified functional principles of unit formation in perception is attributed to the Gestalt school, and in particular to Max Wertheimer (1923). Wertheimer was inspired in part by earlier contributions by scholars from European laboratories (reviewed in Vezzani, 2012), but was the first to offer a comprehensive account of factors of organization in perception. According to Wertheimer, unit formation and the concomitant segregation of figures from grounds obey seven general principles (often also called the Gestalt 'factors' or 'laws' of perceptual organization). Wertheimer principles have been listed in countless textbooks of psychology, more often than not in incomplete or incorrect form. As discussed in the original paper (an English translation is available at the extremely useful web resource *Classics in the History of Psychology*, developed by Christopher Green at http://psychclassics.yorku.ca), the seven principles are: *proximity*: other things being equal, closer elements will tend to grouped into a unit; *similarity*: other things being equal, more similar elements will tend to grouped into a unit; *common fate*: other things being equal, elements that move in similar ways will tend to grouped into a unit; *good continuation*: other things being equal, units will tend to be formed yielding contours that minimize changes in curvature; *closure*: other things being equal, units will tend to be formed yielding closed contours; *objective set*: other things being equal, elements that have been organized in some way will tend to maintain that organization; *subjective set*: units will tend to be formed in accord with an individual's past experiences and knowledge. Note that the first five of these principles refer to properties of the stimulus elements (Figure 4.8). Unit formation according to these five first principles is therefore a bottom-up process. The last two principles instead refer to states of the perceiver, implying a top-down component. The Dalmatian dog of Figure 4.7 exemplifies objective and subjective set. The black elements are more easily grouped to form the dog figure if you have already

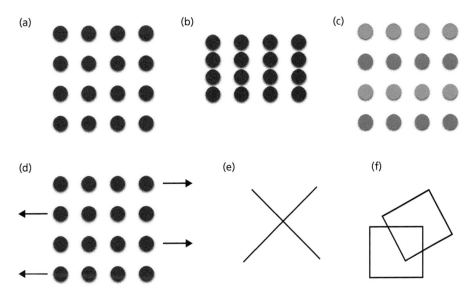

Figure 4.8 Wertheimer's first five principles of unit formation. Wertheimer drew collections of dots or line drawings and observed how they tended to group spontaneously as he looked at them. In a baseline situation, a dot matrix is just as easily seen as rows or columns (a). By reducing vertical distances, the principle of proximity dictates that vertical grouping prevails (b). By making changing colours, the principle of similarity instead favours horizontal grouping (c). Moving alternate rows in opposite directions creates the same units by common fate (d). Good continuation dictates that crossing segments form an 'X' pattern rather than '>' and '<' patterns (e). Closure favours two squares over three irregulars shapes (f).

attained this organization, or if a verbal instruction to look for a dog is given. Another demonstration is provided in Figures 4.9 and 4.10. Although principles of unit formation have been originally investigated within visual perception, similar principles have been shown to predict the formation of auditory units (Bregman, 1990). Auditory unit formation is exploited extensively in polyphonic music, where melodies form identifiable units that are perceptually segregated from other melodies (the 'voices' of classic polyphonic genres like the canon or the fugue) or from accompanying chords. Some studies have also investigated similarities and differences between visual and tactile unit formation (Harrar & Harris, 2007; Serino, Giovagnoli, de Vignemont, & Haggard , 2008).

After the publications of Wertheimer's seminal paper, there have been other attempts to understand the conceptual foundations of his listed laws. For instance, it could be argued that at least the first five laws (as listed here, Wertheimer's order was slightly different) could be considered as manifestations of a generalized principle of proximity in some abstract feature space. Thus, similarity of colour may be considered as proximity in an abstract colour space; common fate as proximity in a space of trajectories or speeds; good continuation as proximity in a space of contour curvature, and so on. There have been also attempts to reduce all of Wertheimer's laws to a general tendency towards simplicity or regularity in perceived forms. This idea is similar to Wertheimer's own suggestion, also discussed in the 1923 paper, that the factors implied a general tendency towards *Prägnanz*, a word often translated as 'good form' or 'good Gestalt' (where 'good' means simpler, more regular, more symmetric).

In addition, there have also attempts to identify other principles of organization, such as for instance synchrony or connectedness. We will not examine all these contributions in full (excellent

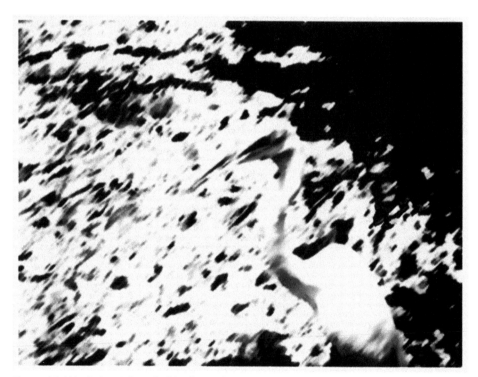

Figure 4.9 Wertheimer's law of *objective set* (part 1). Can you detect a figure in this degraded picture? If you have detected it, would you say that this it was easy or hard to do? (Now look at Figure 4.10).

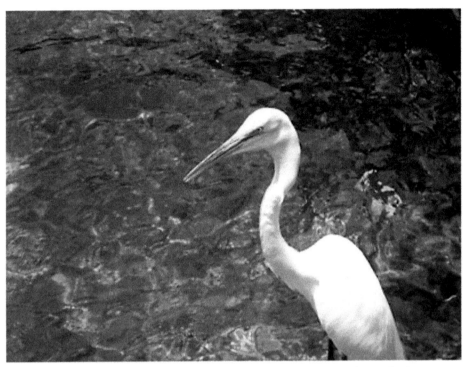

Figure 4.10 Wertheimer's law of *objective set* (part 2). Look at the egret, then go back to Figure 4.9 and you will note that detecting it in the degraded picture has become much easier. Seeing the egret provides anticipatory information that structurally organizes the elements in the degraded image and favours the emergence of the figure.

reviews can be found in Wagemans et al., 2012 and again in Vezzani, Marino, & Giora, 2013). Whatever one's opinion about the correct list of factors, there is now an overwhelming consensus that perceptual organization reflects an adaptive tendency of perception to form units based on heuristics that successfully identify physical objects in the environment (see, e.g. Todorovic, 2011). Indeed, contemporary edge detection algorithms (such as that illustrated in Figure 4.6) actively exploit strategies that are very similar to Gestalt laws to suppress candidate edges that may be due to noise in the image, and enhance candidate edges that are more likely to correspond to true object borders. Biological perceptual systems face a similar challenge when they use information that may be corrupted by low illumination, fog, or partial occlusions within the visual field, or when they attempt to locate animals that make themselves invisible by mimicry. To conclude, a common criticism of the Gestalt approach to perceptual organization is that it is too qualitative and does not lend itself to precise mathematical modelling. Although this was true of the early Gestalt papers (from a century ago), it is certainly no longer true today. Several studies have provided precise measurements of specific instances of Gestalt-like unit formation (the initiators of this trend were Kubovy & Wagemans, 1995; for a comprehensive review see Wagemans et al., 2012a). In addition, Bayesian models have been applied to perceptual unit formation problems with some success (Feldman, 2013; Jäkel, 2016). For instance, Bayesian priors modelling grouping by proximity, similarity, and good continuation have been employed in models of shape perception (Mamassian, 2006).

has several notable consequences. First, note that salient units (objects, in fact) are perceived depending on how individual elements are grouped together. These units possess a size, a shape, a position in space, and so on. Second, these grouped units are distinct from other units, if any, and from parts of the image that are perceived as the background. The background has no 'objecthood'; it has no form, for instance, and is not bounded by a contour—it rather appears to continue behind the contour of the perceived units. Third, when certain units are perceived, they dominate your awareness and it can quite hard to see other candidate units if these compete with those seen. In the case of the figure, a variation on well-known demonstrations of perceptual multistability, there are as many as three different ways that you can group elements into figures: a single vase in the centre, two full figures on the sides, or two facing profiles (this is harder to see, try looking from a certain distance). Thus, unit formation yields objects, and these in turn stand out as figures in front of backgrounds. Playful visual images like this are plentiful, and chances are that you have been entertained by something of the sort on other occasions. Here we will concern ourselves with a more specific issue: is global unit formation affected by multisensory processes, and if so, in what way?

Despite its importance in object perception, empirical studies of multisensory influences on unit formation are surprisingly few (Spence, 2016). Perhaps best documented are situations whereby the formation of units within one perceptual modality, say, a visual object or event, is influenced by localized multisensory signals in another channel, for instance hearing. Studies of these situations have typically exploited multistable stimuli, like that depicted in Figure 4.5, to ask if the insertion of the local signal in the additional channel alters the statistics of spontaneous alternations between outcomes of competing unit formation. A simple but compelling demonstration that this can happen is provided by the *bouncing-streaming* multistable motion display (Metzger, 1934; Figure 4.11). In a typical version of this demonstration, two discs are animated on a computer screen. They are programmed to move on a straight line towards each other, meet at a central point (where for an instant they fuse graphically into a single disc), and then move again on the same straight line until the end of the cycle. Several cycles are usually presented, with

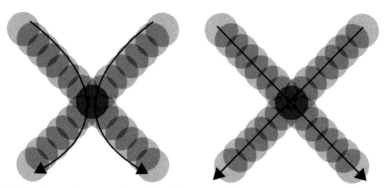

Figure 4.11 The bouncing-streaming effect. The same animation sequence (grey transparent discs) is consistent with two spatiotemporal unit formation outcomes: bouncing (left: two discs collide in the centre and change direction) or streaming (right: two discs cross paths).

the discs going back and forth, and for each cycle participants report whether they had the impression that the discs collided in the centre and bounced back, or rather streamed past each other without changing direction. The two interpretations reflect two alternative unit formations in space-time, and both are fully consistent with the kinematics of the animation. Despite this, however, participants show a reliable bias in favour of streaming (Berthenthal, Banton, & Bradbury, 1993), in accord with the Gestalt factors of good continuation and common fate (see Tutorial 4.2). In a classic paper, Sekuler, Sekuler, & Lau (1997) have shown that merely inserting a click sound when the two discs meet in the centre dramatically increases the probability of a bouncing report, in comparison to the no-click baseline. Thus, the auditory signals modified the visual unit formation process. You can see for yourself by visiting the wonderful website of perceptual demonstrations maintained by Michael Bach at the University of Freiburg (http://www.michaelbach.de/ot/mot-bounce/index.html) and, if you are sceptical that this may be mere suggestion, rest assured that the effect can be replicated with indirect measures that do not require participants to verbally report what they see (Sanabria, Correa, Lupiáñez, & Spence, 2004; we will discuss this phenomenon again in Chapter 8). In fact, interactions of vision and hearing in unit formation have been documented in many other papers in recent years (Bushara et al., 2003; Freeman & Driver, 2008; Grassi & Casco, 2009; Kawachi & Gyoba, 2006; Lyons, 2006; Sanabria, Soto-Faraco, Chan, & Spence, 2005).

Visual unit formation can also be modified by somatosensory signals (Yao, Simons, & Ro, 2009). One good example of this type of multisensory effect is based on a special kind of multisensory stimulus, the three-dimensional Necker cube (Practical 4.1 tells you how you can get a really cheap one and repeat some of these observations). This is simply a wire-frame cube, a solid version of the well-known reversible drawing that almost everyone knows and is reproduced in Figure 4.12. Just like the drawing, the three-dimensional version is also reversible (but only under monocular viewing; with two eyes, binocular disparities precisely specify distances and prevent reversals in depth). Thus, there are visually two competing unit formation outcomes, a regular cube—the 'real' object—or a truncated pyramid (Figure 4.6), such that during prolonged observation most observers tend to alternate between them. A long time ago, Shopland and Gregory (1964) built a small-scale version of the cube that they could hold in their hands; applied fluorescent paint to it, and viewed it in a semi-dark room, such that their hands were scarcely visible. After some

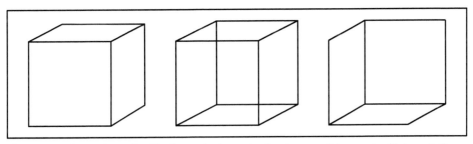

Figure 4.12 The Necker cube. The image in the centre has two possible perceived interpretations (left and right).

experimenting, they noted something unexpected. The cube flipped from the 'real' to the 'inverted' percept not only when it was suspended in mid-air (as one would expect), but also when they held it in their hands. This is surprising because the hands could feel the true shape of the object. Visual dominance? Not really: switching to the pyramid felt harder and seemed to occur less often when they held the cube, in comparison to when they merely looked at it. Thus, it seemed that the somatosensory signals from the hand somehow interfered with the visual process of unit formation, at least to some extent.

In a series of more recent studies of this phenomenon, one of us (Bruno, Jacomuzzi, Bertamini, & Meyer, 2007; Bertamini, Masala, Meyer, & Bruno , 2010) confirmed Gregory's observation and revealed hints as to what might be going on. These studies compared three

---

Practical 4.1 The three-dimensional Necker cube

The Necker cube demonstration is widely known. Try a Google search and you will get thousands of hits, ranging from scientific discussions to popular science, with simple pictures and even animations and applets. Reportedly, the effect was first observed by the Swiss geologist Louis Albert Necker (1832) in drawings of crystals. Necker's drawings were not of regular cubes, but the effect is now typically illustrated as in Figure 4.12 (centre) which can be perceived in two alternative arrangements of a cube. Both percepts are compatible with the proximal stimulus as provided by the drawing, but the cube resting on a horizontal support surface (left in the figure) is perceived more readily, perhaps because of priors about typical viewpoints and support surfaces (Troje & McAdam, 2010). Under prolonged observation, most observers experience spontaneous reversals, although this may require some patience (up to 1 to 3 min according to one estimate; Girgus, Rock, & Egatz, 1977). Shortly after Necker's publication, Wheatstone (1838) reported similar reversals in three-dimensional wireframes (see Wade, Campbell, Ross, & Linglbach, 2010).

The aim of this practical is to let you experience reversals with a three-dimensional wireframe object (not quite a cube, as you shall shortly see, but this is not important). Assuming you don't want to spend time or money to build one, we suggest you go buy a bottle of sparkling wine. The cork of sparkling wines, such as champagne, and of some beers, are reinforced by a steel wire hood, known as a *muselet*. The purpose of muselets is to prevent the cork from popping due to the pressure of carbonates in the wine, but we will use them to learn something about the perception of form and depth. We start by pulling the cork. To do this, you need to loosen and then remove the muselet—if you are careful not to deform it too much this will not affect the practical. You can also drink the wine at this point—this will make the demonstration more fun but it is not strictly necessary. The other thing you have to do is to remove the flat metal cap on top of the muselet. At this point, you will have a wireframe 'cuboid' that looks more or less as that in Figure 4.13. Note that the muselet is equipped with a small handle. Gently bend it downwards. Hold the muselet by the handle, and look at it with one eye. Take care not to move your head. Wait. After a while, you will experience a reversal: the wires will invert their position in depth and a different three-dimensional shape will appear. Try not to move at this point as this might cause the percept to reverse back to its true shape. Remember that binocular and motion cues signal the true shape to your brain: by viewing the muselet with one eye and keeping your head stationary, you suppress these cues. After experiencing a few reversals, some learning will take place and switching from one shape to the other will become easier. This is already quite interesting, but it is not the most interesting thing you can do with a three-dimensional Necker cube. So try this now. Look at the muselet (again, one eye and don't budge!) and wait until you get the illusory reversal. Now, very gently, oscillate your head sideways while trying to maintain the inversion. You may lose it the first time you try, but don't despair, be patient and try again. Sooner or later (for most of us, it really isn't that difficult) you will see something unexpected. Try it, the key is to stay relaxed, maintain fixation, and move gradually.

Did it work? Did the inverted wireframe appear to move, as if it rotated in depth following your sideways movement? We are not talking here about inferring that things have changed position relative to your eye, we are talking about motion that looks real, as if the wireframe actually rotated relative to

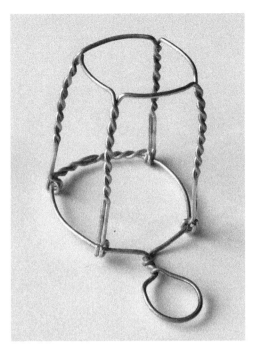

Figure 4.13 The wirehood, or muselet, from a champagne bottle. This is essentially a three-dimensional Necker 'cuboid' once you remove the cap.
Joriola/Wikimedia Commons (CC BY-SA 3.0)

the handle. Once you see it, you will know what we mean. This spectacular illusion is due to perceptual mechanisms that stabilize the perceived world during active vision. As we move, object projections on our retinas are subjected to changes that depend on distance, fixation, and type of movement. Yet the perceived world is stable: Somehow the brain 'knows' how we move and somehow manages to discount the optical changes that can be attributed to these movements. This stabilizes the cube when seen in the true arrangement, as the retinal motions can be interpreted as due to the changes in three-dimensional positions that would be expected given the movement of the observer. When the cube is seen in the reversed illusory arrangement, however, the interpreted changes in relative three-dimensional position cannot be due to the movement of the observer, and this tricks the brain into interpreting the retinal motions as movement of the object. If you are curious, more details about this can be found in Bruno (2017).

Unfortunately, a muselet is too small to hold in the hands. This makes it a bit difficult to demonstrate what happens when reversals occur for a hand-held three-dimensional Necker cube. Although you won't be able to reproduce the stimuli of the studies described in the chapter, you can, however, approximate the experience in this way. Forget about the handle and try balancing the muselet with your index fingers on opposite corners of the frame, one up and one down. Keep your hands on the sides to have a full view, and wait for a reversal. At this point, move the head. The cuboid will move, but now the fingers are touching it. So the fingers will move with it, as if they had broken or become elastic. As we have seen in Chapter 2, the brain is quite willing to modify its representation of the body to account for certain combinations of multisensory signals. Even more fun, wait for a reversal and now move your fingers slightly instead of moving your head. The wireframe will start to deform, looking almost rubbery, and it will *feel* rubbery in a strange, paradoxical way. It is almost as if this peculiar combination of visual signals could induce a completely illusory haptic sensation. But if you have read the book so far, this conclusion will perhaps surprise you only up to a point.

ways of holding the wireframe cube: with a two-finger pincer grip (fingertip contact with the wireframe and no shape information); with the palms of the hands cupped over opposed corners (static tactile shape information); or with the hands actively performing a short-range slide of the palms across a limited region around the corners (active haptic shape information). The results showed that, in comparison to the pincer grip baseline, reversals occurred less often and the pyramid percept was briefer in the static touch condition, and of even shorter duration in the haptic touch active condition. Importantly, Bruno and collaborators identified a signature of these haptic effects by analysing how the cumulative probability of reversals changed as a function of the changes from static to active touch. Specifically, they observed that switches to the illusory reversals never occurred in a well-defined time window: this 'vetoing' of reversals occurred about two seconds after the switch from stationary to haptic touch, and lasted about two further seconds. This seems to indicate that somatosensory signals affected unit formation by promoting the 'real' solution over its reversal. This effect, however, was critically dependent on the nature of the somatosensory information. Static touch did not completely prevent reversals, only active touch did. This makes sense, if you assume that haptic touch is presumably much more informative about shape than static touch. That sensing this information would take some time (about two seconds) is also understandable, as haptics implies exploratory behaviour within a perception-action cycle, a process that happens at a longer time scale. Less obvious is why the vetoing effect of haptics lasted only for an additional two seconds, and then reversals started again to become possible. If we have piqued your curiosity, you can read some speculations on why this might be case in the original paper (Bruno, Jacomuzzi, Bertamini, & Meyer, 2007).

These studies indicate that, when different unit formation outcomes are possible from the same visual stimulus, a local signal in another sensory channel can bias the outcome in favour of one of the possible solutions. This mechanism may correspond to a general disambiguating function of multisensory perception. When stimulus conditions are partly ambiguous in one channel, such that different global unit formations are possible, then signals from other channels can reduce the ambiguity. Note, however, that this implies that competing units are still formed within a single multisensory channel (in the examples that we have described, a visual one), and the multisensory interaction affects the decision process that chooses a perceived alternative. As pointed out by Spence (2016), however, this is not the only question on could ask about multisensory unit formation. A deeper question is whether multisensory interactions can form a single multimodal unit, namely, if perceptual organization can take place between elements that are, in fact, coded by different sensory channels, and perceived in separate perceptual modalities. Spence (2016) called this the problem of *intersensory Gestalten* (a Gestalt is, in the classic terminology of the Gestalt school, a perceptual unit).

To understand how a multimodal perceptual unit might be created from multisensory elements, imagine the following situation: you are sitting in front of an opaque screen with two vertically aligned LEDs in front and two small horizontally aligned speakers in the back, mounted as shown in Figure 4.14. Note that LEDs (visual stimuli) and speakers

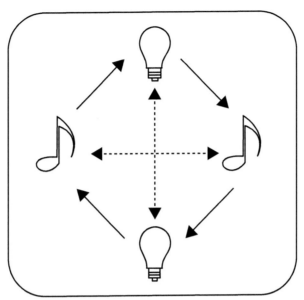

Figure 4.14 Spatial arrangement of the audiovisual stimuli used by Huddleston et al. (2008). Dotted lines show unimodal motion paths (horizontal for sounds and vertical for lights). Solid lines show the hypothetical multimodal motion path, which was never perceived by participants.

(auditory stimuli) are positioned at the vertices of a diamond. Lights and sounds can be controlled independently. We start by alternating the lights: top, then bottom, then top again, and so on. You can change the timing of the alternation (or, more precisely, the *interstimulus interval* or ISI), and we ask you to experiment until you perceive *apparent motion* of a single object moving vertically up, down, up, down, and so on. This is visual unit formation: the two LEDs are grouped into a single moving unit given the appropriate spatiotemporal proximities. Now we turn off the lights and turn on the sounds. We alternate clicks from the speakers: right, left, then right again, and so on. Again, you can change the timing of the alternation until you perceive horizontal apparent motion of a single entity. This is auditory unit formation—nothing new so far. But now we do something more complicated; we alternate both light and sound. Specifically, we turn on the top LED, then sound the right speaker, the turn on the bottom LED, then sound the left speaker, and so on. Again you can change the temporal parameters. Will you be able to perceive apparent motion along the perimeter of the diamond (or perhaps along a circular trajectory)? This would entail the perception of a multimodal unit, one emerging from visual and auditory perceived elements. Is this possible?

At present, the answer to this question seems to be more 'no' than 'yes'. Evidence for this conclusion comes from studies that have compared unisensory visual and auditory unit formation with a combined condition that in principle could be grouped into a multimodal unit. Huddleston, Lewis, Phinney, & DeYoe (2008) used exactly the display described in the previous paragraph (Figure 4.14) to demonstrate visual apparent motion of the LEDs and auditory apparent motion of the sounds. They then combined the two stimuli to ask whether participants could perceive bimodal motion along a circular trajectory. They tested seven participants, and none was able to perceived bimodal motion. They reported that they could track the order of appearance of the visual and auditory stimuli when the ISIs were sufficiently long, such that they could *infer* that the stimuli were positioned at the vertices of a diamond. However, they never perceived a single bimodal unit moving along a diamond-shape trajectory.

In another study, Watanabe and Shomojo (2001) introduced an interesting variation on the bouncing-streaming effect that we described earlier. They assessed the frequency of bouncing reports in three main conditions: a no-sound baseline, a single sound presented when the paths of the two discs crossed, and a sequence of three sounds presented 300 ms before the time of visual coincidence, exactly at visual coincidence, and 300 ms after visual coincidence. In the no-sound conditions, they observed that bouncing was reported in about 20 percent of the tests. This is in line with previous descriptions of the bouncing-streaming effect: the streaming interpretation is favoured over bouncing in accord with visual laws of unit formation. In the single sound condition, bouncing reports instead occurred in more than 80 percent of the tests. Thus, in accord with the observation of Sekuler, Sekuler, & Lau (1997), the single auditory signals strongly affected unit formation of the visual elements. Now recall that the three-sounds sequence contained exactly the same sound that was presented in the single-sound condition. In the three-sounds condition, however, participants reported bouncing in only about 40 percent of the tests. This suggests that a global multimodal unit encompassing the visual and the auditory elements was not perceived. Instead, two units, one visual and one auditory, were separately formed and this prevented the element embedded in the auditory unit from interacting with the formation of the visual unit. In support of this interpretation, Watanabe and Shimojo (2001) performed two control experiments. They reduced the strength of auditory grouping by using sequences of sounds with different frequencies or different intensities. In these conditions, reports of the bouncing interpretation raised again to the level of the baseline no-sound condition.

These observations provide compelling examples whereby multimodal perceptual units could not be formed. Whether this is true in general (as argued by Spence, 2016) is, at present, hard to say. Relevant studies are few, and it might be that these studies looked at the wrong stimulus conditions. For instance, it could be that audiovisual multisensory combinations are not the best choice for identifying multimodal units (Allen & Kolers, 1981). In a study comparing unit formation between pairs of visual, tactile, and visuo-tactile signals, Harrar, Winter, and Harris (2008) attached small stimulators to the index fingers of participants. The stimulators consisted of small wooden cups containing an electrical device that applied pressure to the finger when powered, and an LED. The participants were asked to keep their fingers 5 cm apart and to keep fixation on the point between their hands. The stimulators were turned on in sequence using a wide range of ISIs, in three randomly interleaved conditions: visual–visual using only the

LEDs, tactile–tactile using only the pressure devices, or visual–tactile (LED and then – pressure). After each presentation, participants rated the quality of perceived apparent motion (an indirect indicator of unit formation) from one finger to the other finger locations. They found that participants almost never reported no motion at all (that is, ratings of 0 in a 0 to 5 scale); that at shorter ISIs they tended to report better quality of perceived motion in the visual–visual condition, intermediate quality in the tactile–tactile condition, and somewhat worse quality in the bimodal condition; but also that in all three conditions participants reported medium-quality perceived motion (an average rating of about 3) at longer ISIs. They therefore concluded that visuo-tactile bimodal unit formation can occur, that its saliency is comparable to that of unimodal unit formation at longer ISIs, and that its temporal dynamics are different from those of the unimodal cases.

These results may be taken to suggest that, unlike the audio-visual case, visuo-tactile unit formation is possible given sufficient time. Given the nature of the task, however, it is not easy to rule out that participants were rating inferred rather than actually perceived motion (as in the study by Huddleston and colleagues). In addition, because the three conditions were intermixed within the same experimental session by the same participant, it is also possible that bimodal motion perception resulted from carry-over effects from previous unisensory trials. In conclusion, it seems to us that the available evidence still points more in the direction of a negative answer to the question of multimodal unit formation, although further studies may of course modify this conclusion.

4.5 **Crossmodal object recognition**

Human perception is generally very good at what it does. And of the things that perception does, object recognition is clearly one of those that it does best. When we look at objects, we just know what they are. This is so fast that it feels instantaneous, and so accurate that we are rarely mistaken. For instance, we can reliably report whether a previously unseen photograph contained an animal even if the photograph is flashed on a computer screen for as little as one-fiftieth of a second (20 ms). This is an incredibly short time for transducing a complex visual signal. Our eyes have barely time for a single fixation. But even more impressive is the speed of the whole process, from the initial transduction up to the recognition of the object category. It has been shown that the EEG signature of an animal/not animal decision can be measured just 150 ms after stimulus onset, and a key-press response can be observed after about twice this time in humans (Thorpe, Ftize, & Marlot, 1996; vanRullen & Thorpe, 2001) and even earlier in monkeys (Fabre-Thorpe, Richard, & Thorpe, 1998). These times suggest that recognition of entry-level categories, such as animal (or, in other of these studies, means of transport or food), can happen immediately after the initial sweep of incoming visual signals arrives at the brain—no additional operations are needed. Recognition of subordinate categories, such as bird or airplane or fruit, can take longer than this, depending on several factors. But it remains, in general, extremely efficient. For instance, object recognition remains accurate even when objects are seen from different viewpoints, under different illuminations, and in different contexts. Even moderate amounts of occlusion by other objects usually have very little effect on our ability to recognize. To account for the remarkable efficiency of recognition processes, two types of theories have been proposed.

According to *viewpoint-independent* theories, each object is stored in memory by a single, general representation regardless of size, position, or orientation. This is type of representation usually referred to as a *structural* description (Marr & Nishihara, 1978), that is, a full three-dimensional model of the spatial relationships between an object's parts. (We will neglect here another possible, but implausible, viewpoint-independent approach—that based on symbolic lists of features.) In viewpoint-independent theories, recognition consists in constructing a structural description of the object from current visual input, and then matching the current description with those in memory (Biederman, 1987). Viewpoint-independent structural descriptions fare well on two scores. They successfully predict accurate and fast recognition over a range of changes in viewpoint, and they offer a parsimonious strategy for object representation. These theories, however, have a problem. They predict that recognition should be even more efficient than it has been shown to be. Biederman & Gerhardstein (1993) detailed conditions whereby structural description theory predicts viewpoint independence in object recognition. This prediction has been repeatedly falsified even in experiments that satisfied these conditions (Hayward & Tarr, 1997; Tarr, 1995; Tarr & Bülthoff, 1995).

According to the alternative *viewpoint-dependent* theories, objects are represented as single views in viewer-centred coordinates, that is, as seen from the perspective of the viewer. You can think of single-view representations as equivalent to two-dimensional snapshots of objects, as opposed to the three-dimensional descriptions of structure assumed by viewpoint-independent theories. In a nutshell, viewpoint-dependent theories propose that recognition consists in matching stored views with current input views, with no need to build higher-level structural descriptions. This approach, however, also entails a problem. To account for successful recognition of objects seen from diverse viewpoints, viewpoint-dependent theories have to assume that a very large number of views are stored in memory. It could even be argued that, logically, infinite different views need to be stored, as potential viewpoints for seeing objects are indeed infinite. To address this problem, and to account for the empirical data that do suggest at least a degree of viewpoint dependence, three classes of solutions are possible (Tarr & Pinker, 1989). In *single-view* models, object views are stored only once in a 'canonical' orientation. Recognition is then achieved by means of an internal transformation that 'rotates' or otherwise modifies the current view to fit the canonical stored view. In *multiple-view* models, object representations include a small set of familiar views and recognition happens if the current view fits one of these familiar views. In *hybrid* models, finally, a small set of views is stored, including canonical views (Palmer, Rosch, & Chase, 1981). Recognition, however, is attained as in single-view models by transforming current views to the nearest or more similar stored view.

The debate between proponents of viewpoint-independent and viewpoint-dependent models has been especially lively during the last decade of the past century. Although many issues remain relevant, not only for theories of human perception, but also for computational and robotic vision, the literature seems to have reached a consensus that hybrid viewpoint-dependent models fit the specific observed patterns of viewpoint dependence best (see also Bülthoff, Edelman, & Tarr, 1995). These models can account for very efficient recognition of canonical or very familiar views (these are assumed to be the stored views, which can be matched directly to the input signal), and correctly predict that recognition efficiency will depend on the 'distance' between a given unfamiliar view and the 'nearest' stored view. At the same time, it could be argued that the internal transformations needed to match novel inputs to the nearest stored views imply some degree of representation of the object's structure, although this needs not be a full three-dimensional model. In this way, this feature of hybrid models could be said to blur the distinction between structural description and view-based models. In addition, it could be argued that the two approaches need not be mutually exclusive. Structural descriptions could be used in some conditions or tasks, while view-based recognition may occur in others. This has been called the *multiple routes* hypothesis (Vanrie, Willems, & Wagemans, 2001; see also Humphreys & Riddoch, 1984; Lawson, 1999). This possibility is especially relevant for the problem of crossmodal object recognition. As we shall now see, studies of crossmodal recognition have also provided some evidence for matching based on structural descriptions, but also some intriguing evidence for a multisensory form of viewpoint dependence.

The problem of crossmodal recognition is conceptually different from unisensory object recognition as introduced so far. Standard unisensory recognition is, by definition, a process of matching sensory input to representations stored in memory. Its final goal is to access semantic and verbal memorized information about the object, such that we know 'what is out there' (Marr, 1982). In crossmodal recognition, the goal is somewhat simpler: an object is presented within one perceptual modality, for instance vision, and then presented again in another, for instance haptic. The brain's task is to determine if the sensory signals from the second presentation match those from the first, across the two modalities. We are often extremely good at doing this. In Gibson's (1962) famous cookie-cutter study, for instance, participants were essentially perfect in matching seen cookie-cutters to previously studied cookie-cutters when the study was based on haptics (you may recall our extensive discussion of this work in Chapter 1). This ability could be based on two separate, unisensory recognition processes, leading to semantic representations of the object and a final match between these two representations. Alternatively, however, matching could take place within a multisensory process that precedes semantic-level processing. For instance, matching could result from the activation of a shared, multisensory representation of object structure by the visual and haptic signals. Gibson's results are consistent with both possibilities, because he used an explicit naming task with familiar shapes. Gibson's student Caviness (1964) showed that equal levels of performance can be attained with unfamiliar three-dimensional shapes, but again using an explicit task so even in this case the two interpretations cannot be distinguished.

More recently, Reales and Ballesteros (1999) studied crossmodal matching using a classic paradigm of experimental psychology known as *priming*. In priming, processing of a test stimulus is facilitated (for instance, reaction time is lower) when the stimulus is preceded by a related 'prime'. The prime can be any other stimulus, and the relation can be along any given dimension. For instance, in a word/non-word classification task, responses to 'bread' are faster when 'bread' is preceded by 'butter' than when it is preceded by a no-prime baseline; in contrast, they are slower than baseline when 'bread' is preceded by 'hammer'. In the crossmodal priming experiment performed by Reales and Ballesteros, primes and tests were everyday manipulable objects (such as a spoon, a glove, or a pipe). However, the priming stimulus was irrelevant for the task, so any observed facilitation or cost could be attributed to an automatic, obligatory process. The experiment involved two phases. In the study phase, participants were presented a sequence of objects and for each were required to either generate a meaningful sentence including the object's name (semantic study) or to rate the object's volume on a five-point scale (physical study). In the test phase, participants were presented with the objects and had to name each as quickly as possible. This was done in two unimodal conditions (visual study and visual test, or haptic study and haptic test), and in two crossmodal conditions (visual study and haptic test, or haptic study and visual test). The results were clear. In both crossmodal conditions, response times were as fast as in the equivalent unimodal conditions. This suggests that the sensory signal presented in the priming modality was automatically matched to the test and could not be ignored, even though it was irrelevant for the naming task. In addition, there was no difference whatsoever between the semantic and physical study conditions. In explicit memory tasks, the level of processing of the encoded material (semantic, or 'deep', vs physical or 'shallow') has usually a large impact: we remember best information encoded at the semantic level (Schacter, 1994). That no level of processing effect was found is therefore consistent with the conclusion that matching occurred not only automatically but also pre-semantically. Reales and Ballesteros suggested that visual and haptic encoding of an object elicit a single, multisensory structural description, and that crossmodal recognition is mediated by this shared pre-semantic representation.

Other studies have largely confirmed Reales and Ballestero's conclusion. For instance, priming effects comparable to those reported by Reales and Ballesteros have been described by Easton, Greene, and Srinivas (1997). In addition, direct evidence for shared visual and haptic representations of object shape comes from neuroimaging data. Using fMRI, James et al. (2002) documented that haptic exploration of novel objects activates not only the primary somatosensory cortex, but also areas of the occipital lobe that are associated with visual processing. Critically, these same areas were shown to be activated by visual exploration of the same objects, and the activation was found to increase when the objects were primed, both in the same modality or in the other modality. Finally, if multisensory structural descriptions are elicited by signals in different perceptual modalities, one would expect that perceptual learning in one modality would improve perceptual discriminations in another modality tapping into the same multisensory process. Using a crossmodal three-dimensional shape discrimination task, Norman, Clayton, Norman, and

Crabtree (2008) have documented significant learning across experimental trials for both haptic-to-visual and visual-to-haptic discriminations. Importantly, Norman and collaborators used non-familiar shapes that belonged to the same entry level category (they produced casts of eight similarly sized, but differently shaped bell peppers) and gave no feedback to participants during the experiment. Thus, their results indicate that implicit haptic learning of the shapes occurred over trials, and that learning refined visual discriminations despite the fact that participants had no verbal labels corresponding to the distinctions.

If structural information learned through haptic exploration can benefit visual perception, what is the nature of the interaction between the two systems in crossmodal recognition? Recent studies indicate that this interaction is sensitive to the orientation of the object relative to the effector that performs the exploration, yielding a sort of 'viewpoint' dependence in crossmodal recognition from haptics to vision. This counterintuitive result was reported for the first time by Newell, Ernst, Tjan, and Bülthoff (2001) using a variant of the standard crossmodal recognition paradigm that we have already described. In each trial, participants studied four custom 'objects' made from Lego blocks either haptically or visually. Study was unconstrained: participants were left free to move both hands around the objects or to move their head and, of course, their eyes. (The only constraint was that participants could not move the objects or walk around them.) Immediately after study, another set of four objects was presented and participants had to decide if any of the objects in the new set were present in the study set, or not (this is often called an *old–new* task). The test set was presented in the same modality as the study set (thus, visual–visual or haptic–haptic) or in the other modality (visual–haptic or haptic–visual), and in the same orientation or after a 180 degree rotation about the vertical axis (such that the backs of test objects now faced the participant). Recognition accuracy was strongly influenced by the change in orientation, but, surprisingly, in completely different ways in the unimodal and crossmodal trials. Both in visual–visual and haptic–haptic conditions, changing the orientation at test caused a drop in recognition accuracy. In haptic–visual and to some extent also in visual–haptic conditions, conversely, changing the orientation caused an *increase* in recognition accuracy. In fact, rotated haptic–visual trials yielded the highest mean accuracy in comparison to all other conditions. Thus, a haptic analogue of 'viewpoint' dependency was found, but with an important difference. While the eye's viewpoint is determined by the line of sight, allowing exploration of the front part of objects, the hand's natural posture during exploration is such that we get information preferentially about the back. Thus, the hand 'feels' the back of the object while the eye 'sees' its front. Due to this complementarity of exploratory behaviour by eye and hand, transfer of information across the two sensory channels is most efficient after the front and back of the object have been swapped. To test their hypothesis, Newell and collaborators performed two additional control experiments. In one, they rotated study and test objects around the horizontal axis, such that front and back were again swapped (together with top and bottom). In the other, they rotated around the depth axis, such that only top and bottom were rotated but not front and back. Critically, they found again better accuracy in the crossmodal trials in the first control, but not in the second. When they swapped top and bottom, accuracy was always worse in all four conditions.

4.6 **Sensory substitution**

Studying multisensory interactions in object perception naturally leads to a practical question. When different sensory signals are available to separate channels about a distal object, in what respect can these signals be said to be *equivalent*? In terms of perceptual theory, this question can be approached in different ways. One answer, of course, is that sensory signals are equivalent when they are about the same object. This, however, is not particularly useful, for the brain has no way of knowing a priori that signals in different channels are about the same object. Other possibilities are more interesting (Marks, 1983). Multisensory equivalence can be defined in relation to interactions between different sensory signals about objects, as in the cases of multisensory integration and combination that we have discussed in this chapter. Alternatively, it could be defined in terms of analogies between perceptual attributes, such as perceived light intensity and perceived sound intensity, which have structural similarities in their psychophysical behaviour when the underlying physical quantities are varied, or of similarities in the information contained in different signals. Yet other criteria for equivalence could be sought in shared neural substrates. All these become a practical problem when one considers the possibility of compensating for a missing sensory channel using signals from another, intact channel. This is the problem of *sensory substitution.* We are all familiar with the white cane used by blind people to acquire information about objects outside the range of reachability, or with the Braille alphabet. The research program that characterizes sensory substitution work is, however, more ambitious. Is it possible to provide a blind individual with information that is equivalent to what is available to sighted people, such that she will be able to perform 'visual' tasks? Would that be a new form of 'seeing' (most work on sensory substitution has concentrated on developing visual aids for blind people, but the concept can be extended to any kind of sensory deafferentation; see Amedi et al., 2007; Maidenbaum, Abboud, & Amedi, 2014)?

The early work on sensory substitution was done by the American neuroscientist Paul Bach-y-Rita (1934–2006). At the end of the 1960s, Bach-y-Rita initiated a research programme based on the concept of processing images captured by a video camera to transform them into patterns of vibro-tactile stimulation (Bach-y-Rita, 1967). The ultimate aim of the programme was to develop systems that could serve as visual substitutes for blind people to use. The original device delivered the tactile patterns to the back of participants, but Bach-y-Rita later moved to smaller applications that could be applied to the fingertips or that delivered electrical signals to the tongue. Perceptual learning with tactile visual substitution has been studied extensively (for reviews see Bach-y-Rita, 2004; Bach-y-Rita & Kercel, 2003), and there is one published first-person report of the training involved (Box 4.2). In general, tactile visual substitution has shown some degree of

Box 4.2 A first-person account of 'seeing' with one's skin

In 1974, Gerard Guarniero was a PhD student in the Department of Philosophy at New York University. His planned doctoral thesis was on the relation between visual and tactile space. This is not an unusual interest for a philosopher of science, as you may have gathered from reading the initial chapters of this book and especially Box 4.1. What made it special in his case was that Guarniero is congenitally blind, and had therefore never experienced visual space, although he had a repertoire of conceptual notions about it from reading philosophical and scientific literature. He therefore decided to seek a way to achieve some perceptual understanding of visual space, or at least 'something resembling it sufficiently ... to gain some notion of it.' He obtained a grant from ATT to undergo a three-week training programme with a tactile vision-substitution system (TVSS) at the University of the Pacific in San Francisco. His experience during training is described in a paper published in the journal *Perception* (Guarniero, 1974). This paper remains, to the best of our knowledge, the only detailed first-person account of perceptual learning with a sensory substitution device. The TVSS consisted in a device that converted images acquired by a camera into vibratory tactile patterns applied to the user's back (Bach-y-Rita, 1972).

The paper describes a rather fast development of a series of perceptual abilities. In the beginning, Guarniero was only able to determine if something out there was moving or still. This entailed learning the distinction between changes in tactile stimulation due to camera movement and changes due to object movement. After two days, he became capable of doing this and started to train his ability to recognize objects. Later on, he experimented also with judgments of relative distance, hand-eye coordination, and object orientations. Overall, he achieved some degree of success in solving these challenging perceptual problems, although he never became fully proficient. For instance, he wrote: 'I had always been given a side view ... when [the object] was displayed head-on ... I had difficulty in identifying it. This difficulty decreased but was never entirely overcome.' In describing his training in recognition, which involved associating names and haptic exploration to the sensory-substitution input, he wrote: 'I never discovered any correlation between how something 'looked' and how it felt ... Since I could not recognize the objects which I 'saw' as the same as those I felt ... it took some time ... to associate their names and their appearances.' Nonetheless, he reported that after learning, tactile sensory signals no longer resulted in percepts located on his back, and awareness of the vibrating pins contacting the skin faded away. At this point 'objects had come to have a top and bottom; a right side and a left'. However, he also stated that these objects had no depth, that is, they did not appear to be located in a three-dimensional environment. They were perceived 'in an ordered two-dimensional space, the precise location of which has not yet been determined.'

Guarniero's account is fascinating precisely because it attempts to convey the phenomenal character of perception through sensory substitution. This fascinating feature

Box 4.2 Continued

is, however, also the main weakness of the account. It is very difficult to fully grasp from his words the nature of his experience, as Guarniero himself acknowledged: 'I can relate only what I did and how I did it—I cannot convey the qualitative aspect of the experience ... The difficulty is not merely one of vocabulary; rather, it is a conceptual one.' Perhaps the most interesting aspect of this difficulty is his remark about percept locations: no longer on his back, but in an unspecified external two-dimensional space. It is tempting to interpret this report as evidence of the primitive manifestation of a defining feature of true perception (as opposed to cognitive judgment). Perceived objects appear to be located outside our body, not on the locus of proximal stimulation. When we look, objects appear out there, not on the eye. When we touch, we perceive the external object not the pattern of mechanical stimulation on the hand. Even when we perceive the flavour of an edible object, we perceive it as a property of something external that happens to be in our mouth, not as a complex constellation of gustatory, mechanical, noxious, and especially olfactory sensory signals in different parts of the oral cavity and in the nose (we discuss this in detail in Chapter 5 on the multisensory perception of food). This feature is often called *distal referral*. Guarniero's account may taken as evidence that a degree of distal referral is possible after extensive training with sensory substitution. At least in Guarniero's account, however, it seems that this was never complete or at least comparable to distal referral in ordinary perception. Objects never gained perceived positions in three-dimensional space. Whether this would have happened eventually, had he undergone longer training—perhaps over several months—is impossible to tell. As discussed in section 4.6 on sensory substitution of this chapter, it is quite possible that tactile visual substitution can never become a true form of 'seeing' through the skin, for theoretical rather than practical reasons. Our impression is that this possibility needs to be taken seriously.

success in allowing blind individuals to perform some 'visual' tasks such as object detection, form discrimination, and especially spatial orientation (Segond, Weiss, & Sampaio, 2005). Reportedly, the most successful clinical application, however, has been in the treatment of balance disorders (Danilov, Tyler, Skinner, & Bach-y-Rita, 2006; Vuillerme et al., 2007). Bach-y-Rita worked on these towards the end of his career. His tactile vestibular substitution system consists of a set of accelerometers mounted on the patient's body. Signals captured by the accelerometers are processed by software and transformed into weak electrical signals that are delivered to an array of electrodes on the tongue of the patient. Different regions of the tongue are stimulated as a function of the accelerometer inputs, establishing a mapping between tongue stimuli and the body's orientation relative to gravity. Treatment with this device has been reported to improve balance in patients with vestibular diseases more than conventional physiotherapy (Ghulyan-Bedikian, Paolino, & Paolino, 2013).

In the last decade of the past century, much work has been done with an alternative approach based on auditory visual substitution. In these systems, video frames are converted into 'sound landscapes' (*sonification*) according to different rules, that must be learned through extensive training. For instance, the *vOICe* system (Meijer, 1992) codes frames as a two-dimensional array of pointwise light intensities (akin to the pixels of a computer monitor), and then represents each point using frequency for the vertical dimension (low frequencies for the bottom row of the image, high frequencies for the top) and time for the horizontal dimension (each auditory 'frame' becomes a complex sound that lasts about a second; at the beginning of the sound are frequencies for the left columns of the image, as the sound unfolds frequencies for successive columns are then presented). Light intensities are represented with sound intensity (soft sounds for dark pixels, loud sounds for light ones). Examples of sonified images and even downloadable apps can be found at https://www.seeingwithsound.com. The *PSVA* system (Prosthesis for the Substitution of Vision by Audition; Capelle, Trullemans, Arno, & Veraart , 1998) is even more complex. The image is processed based on a model of the retina, which takes into account the higher resolution at the fovea in comparison to the periphery, and converted based on a model of the cochlea. Other systems have also been developed (Cronly-Dillon, Persaud, & Gregory, 1999; Fontana et al., 2002; Hanneton, Auvray, & Durette 2010). There is evidence that well-trained users of these systems can to some extent navigate the environment, point to objects, and categorize them (Arno et al., 1999; Cronly-Dillon, Persaud, & Gregory, 1999; Proulx et al., 2008).

As you can easily verify with a quick search on the world-wide-web, sensory substitution systems have been often the object of enthusiastic reports by the press. Magazine articles describing the wonders of seeing with one's tongue, or with the ears, are no doubt fascinating and they do raise scientifically interesting issues. Despite the media hype, however, it is clear that sensory substitution devices have yet to become viable visual aids for blind people. For one, after more than 50 years of research, none of these systems is used routinely in clinical settings and very few blind individuals use them (and when they do, it is more for experimentation than for regular everyday use). Given the great advances in miniaturization and in computer science over this period, this situation is unlikely to depend merely on technical problems. One begins to suspect that the problems are not only technical but also theoretical. In addition, although trained users can perform some spatial tasks using a sensory substitution, the scope of these tasks is limited. Even more critically, those that seem most capable of learning these systems are blindfolded sighted individuals (usually, as control participants in experiments) or late blind users. For instance, there is evidence that visual effects such as the Ponzo and vertical-horizontal illusions (Figure 4.15) can be perceived through an auditory visual substitution device, but only by sighted controls and not by individuals who are blind from birth (Renier et al., 2005; Renier, Bruyer, & De Volder, 2006). It remains possible that these limitations can be overcome if training is begun at birth or soon thereafter (Aitken & Bower, 1983), but this of course would raise delicate ethical problems.

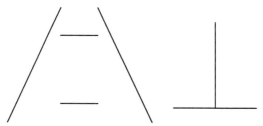

Figure 4.15 The Ponzo (left) and vertical-horizontal (right) illusions. The two horizontal segments on the left have the same length, but the top one appears wider. The two segments on the right also have the same length, but the vertical one appears longer. Blindfolded sighted controls report the illusions when they 'see' the patterns via auditory substitution, suggesting an analogy between their visual and auditory substituted experiences. Congenitally blind participants, however, do not (Renier, Bruyer, & De Volder, 2006).

In an interesting review, Lenay and collaborators (2003) suggested that the very notion of sensory substitution suffers from two key conceptual flaws. According to these authors, these devices do not *substitute* a missing perceptual modality and do not work at the *sensory* level. There is no real substitution, they argue, because perception through the device is never in the 'substituted' perceptual modality. Percepts remain tactile, or auditory, even though with training their character changes in interesting ways (see Box 4.2). This is not merely because some key features of the visual modality cannot be conveyed (colour, for instance, is not coded by these devices), but also for a deeper reason. The kind of spatial information that can be represented in a tactile or auditory signal remains unavoidably different from that available in visual signals. Thus, it is more appropriate to talk about sensory *augmentation* than substitution. Said otherwise, these systems are better understood as technologically advanced white canes that can work at longer distances than the familiar aid almost all blind individuals use. The augmentation, moreover, is not just a sensory process. To become proficient in the use of these systems, participants need to engage in active exploration and to learn new couplings between the substituting sensory signals and their own movements. Therefore, what is augmented is in fact a *sensorimotor* process. The devices create new lawful co-variations of sensory signals and exploratory movements, and learning these is the key component of training (Auvray, Hanneton, & O'Reagan, 2007).

Recently, these ideas have been further developed in a lucid theory article by Deroy and Auvray (2012). Sensory substitution theorizing, they argued, has been performed under a *perceptual* assumption, the assumption that these systems produce percepts that are equivalent to the substituted ones. Deroy and Auvray convincingly suggest that this is not the case, and propose an interesting alternative model. They propose that learning sensory substitution should, instead, be defined as something similar to the acquisition of reading skills, a culturally implemented extension of natural perception. Just as in reading, sensory substitution training involves recoding information already available in a pre-existing route (visual pattern recognition in vision, auditory, or tactile processing in sensory substitution) and attaining a level of proficiency such that the process becomes automatic up to the recognition of novel meaningful units (words, or sensorily substituted objects). In reading, this results in the establishment of a second processing route, whereby visual patterns are directly experienced as meaningful words instead of coloured shapes. In sensory substitution, whether an equivalent qualitative change in experience can be obtained remains at present doubtful. The analogy, however, remains useful, if anything because it provides a novel framework for the development of sensory substitution devices and designing training programmes, and for understanding the theoretical implications of sensory substitution for multisensory perception in general.

Chapter 5

Perceiving Food

5.1 Why does food taste as it does?

Human perception has evolved to deal with many different types of objects. Among these, a special place is occupied by *edible* objects. As we interact with our environment, we come into contact with things that are potential sources of nourishment. Being able to detect, discriminate, and recognize such things is indispensable for survival. In addition, food consumption represents an important form of reward behaviour which underlies many forms of socially shared experience in rituals, ceremonies, and celebrations in all cultures. For these reasons, it is perhaps not surprising that eating is amongst the most multifaceted aspects of human psychology (see Meule & Vögele, 2013) and that food perception and recognition involve numerous complex multisensory interactions. The appreciation of a dish during a meal is not based only on sensory signals coded by receptors in the oral cavity (the 'taste sense' in the naïve definition), but depends critically also on signals coded in the nose ('olfaction sense') and on somatosensory signals from the mouth as well as the hand that brings food to the mouth. In addition, food appreciation is influenced by anticipatory information from visual and even auditory signals. Indeed, eating and drinking are multisensory experiences par excellence (Stillman, 2002) and the active processing of so many sources of sensory information may be considered as perhaps the best example of a perceptual system as defined at the beginning of this book (see also Green, 2002; Auvray & Spence, 2008; Bruno, Pavani, & Zampini, 2010).

The multisensory nature of food perception underlies the well-established distinction between primary tastes, that can be perceived in the mouth even when multisensory contributions are prevented, and *flavour* (Prescott, 1999; Stevenson, 2009), the integrated experience of food in normal multisensory conditions (see Practical 5.1). Most of us intuitively understand that the nose is important for flavour perception, as testified by the deprived perception resulting from a stuffed nose due to a cold, and many culinary traditions pay intense attention to visual and tactile features such as the colour, shape, and size of ingredients and to the relationships between these features when the ingredients are assembled on the plate. Cooks and food critics are increasingly aware that food perception is heavily influenced by more global environmental factors, such as room illumination, furniture, or ambient music (see Box 5.1). Thus, that food tastes as it does due to multisensory interactions is increasingly becoming part of common knowledge. The scope and variety of these interactions, however, often escapes us, and the natural tendency to take perception for granted can obscure features of food perception that need to be explained.

Practical 5.1 Of cheese and men

To fully enjoy this practical, first go to the shop and buy a portion of *Parmigiano-Reggiano* cheese. We recommend that you check the origin of the product: true Parmigiano-Reggiano is only made in Italy in the provinces of Parma, Reggio-Emilia, and Modena, and in part of the provinces of Bologna and Mantua. It should have a denomination-of-origin mark branded on the crust. For best results, we also suggest going for cheese that has been aged for at least 24 months. The cheese should look more or less like the example in Figure 5.1. The seller should best divide it by inserting a special almond-shaped knife and forcing a chunk of cheese to detach from the bigger part, such that the borders of the portion remain irregular and grainy. Try to avoid neat slices made with a sharp cut. The colour should be an even straw-yellow (if you have the software and want to try, RGB values for your computer monitor are approximately 250, 248, 227) and you should see tiny white crystals on the cheese paste. These are due to the release of the amino acid tyrosine during the process of protein breakdown and are a sure sign of the maturation of the cheese.

Our aim in this practical is to expose readers to the intricacies of *sensory analysis* as done in the food industry. From the standpoint of this book, sensory analysis can be considered as an application of research and methodologies in multisensory perception and psychophysics. Sensory analysis is usually performed to define the perceived dimensions of a given food product, that is, what sensory analysis experts call the product's *sensory profile*. This profile is useful for several purposes. For instance, an industry might be interested in determining why customers prefer one food product over another, or in finding novel ways of differentiating their product from those of competitors. By quantifying perceptual similarities and differences between different products within the respective profiles, data can be collected that can contribute to addressing these issues. Another important use of sensory profiles is standardization of the product's perceptual characteristics, to issue production guidelines, to perform quality control, or

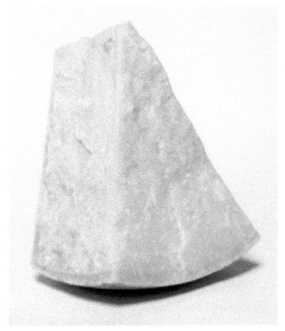

Figure 5.1 It may help to get a piece of Parmigiano-Reggiano like this for this practical.

to identify characteristics that are required to label the product with specific territorial origin denomin-ations. As you may have guessed, we will focus on sensory analysis for Parmesan cheese, a product which is relatively easy to acquire, highly consistent in its perceptual characteristics, and, of course, very good. The present description is based on the methods described in Garavaldi, Pacchioli, and Vecchia (2009), who outline the results of standardization efforts by several research laboratories funded by the Emilia-Romagna region in Italy. Similar methods are used for the sensory analysis of most other food products, including cooked meat and sausages, wines, and oils.

In the preliminary part of the procedure, a panel of judges is trained in detecting, discriminating, and verbally labelling specific flavour components. Training sessions typically include discrimination tasks, scaling tasks, and qualitative descriptions. An example of a discrimination task is the so-called *triangular test*. Judges are presented with three samples of a product. Two samples are identical and the third one is different for some flavour characteristic. Judges try to identify the odd one out. By contrast, an ex-ample of a scaling task is the *ordering test*. Judges are presented with different samples of the product and they are asked to order them based on the intensity of certain perceptual characteristics, such as its colour, flavour, or texture, often with reference to a known standard that serves as anchor for the judg-ment. Qualitative descriptions, finally, aim at identifying relevant perceptual dimensions and at defining

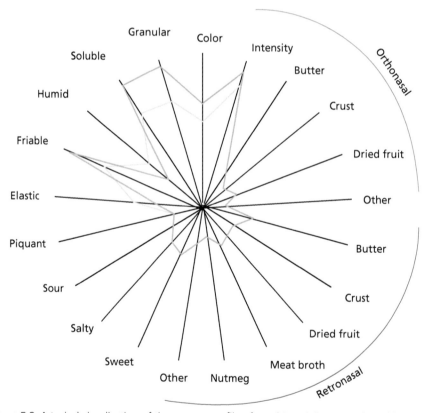

Figure 5.2 A typical visualization of the sensory profile of aged Parmigiano-Reggiano (dark yellow-green). The slightly different profile for fresher cheese is also provided for comparison (light yellow).

Adapted from di A. Garavaldi, M.T. Pacchioli, and P. Vecchia, *L'analisi sensoriale per caratterizzare il parmigiano reggiano*, p. 6 © Opuscolo C.R.P.A, 2009.

standardized verbal descriptions. Training sessions are also aimed at familiarizing judges with the standardized terminology that must be used by all in the same way to promote consistency within and between the panel judges.

Based on the results of the preliminary tests, the consortium of laboratories has agreed on a set of verbal descriptors for the cheese odour and flavour dimensions, and on a standardized tasting procedure which consists of several successive steps: visual examination of the cheese's colour, visual texture, and tyrosine crystals; haptic examination by hand to evaluate consistency, granularity, and elasticity of the paste; orthonasal olfactory examination, first of the overall intensity of the cheese odour and then of specific odour components; haptic examination by mouth to confirm evaluations performed by touching with the hand and to evaluate the cheese's solubility (how easily it dissolves in saliva while chewing); examination of primary tastes and of spicy, astringent, and piquant notes (these three are sometimes called *trigeminal sensations*); examination of the flavour in the mouth while chewing and expiring air from the nose to enhance retronasal olfaction. At this final step, the checklist of verbal descriptors is key in defining all potential flavour dimensions that need to be considered. A sensory profile is typically obtained by averaging across several judging sessions on different days and is visualized by a chart like the example in Figure 5.2. Aged Parmigiano-Reggiano is granular and soluble in the mouth, tastes slightly salty and sweet with an umami component (usually described by comparison to meat broth and cheese crust); has additional flavour notes of fresh milk, yoghurt, melted butter, nutmeg, pepper, and tends to include also a discrete piquant note.

You may want to take a piece of your cheese and follow these steps to taste it. We believe the experience will nicely recapitulate most concepts that have been discussed in this chapter about the multisensory perception of food. In particular, pay special attention to the anticipatory effects from viewing, smelling, and touching the cheese morsel with the hand and the mouth, as well as to the difference between the tastes that you perceive during the initial contact of the morsel with the tongue and oral cavity, and the rich, long-lasting flavours that become apparent while chewing and expiring from the nose. And most importantly enjoy your cheese!

One such feature is the very fact that food is experienced in the gustatory modality. Given that food-related perception is so heavily multisensory, it is not obvious that stimulation of multiple sensory channels should eventually result in unimodal experiences. Yet, flavour is experienced as having the modal character of taste and that character only. Naturally, when eating we also have corollary percepts in other modalities, such as olfaction or vision. Think about the recommended procedure for wine tasting, which begins with the observation of the colour of the liquid in the glass, followed by sniffing the wine *bouquet*. No doubt, such anticipatory percepts are part of the overall appreciation of food. However, they are different from the multisensory interactions that occur when food is in the mouth and we experience its flavour. When we do so, there is a form of *unimodal referral* of multiple concomitant sensory signals. Signals come from many channels, but result in percepts in one modality only. This is not uncommon whenever multiple sensory signals are bound into a unified percept: when listening to speech, we are not aware of lip movements even though viewing them influences what we hear. This binding process itself requires an explanation. How does the brain bind multiple sensory signals from the nose, the mouth, the eyes, and the ears into a unified flavour percept? Several physiological and neuroimaging results are now beginning to shed light on this problem, as we will see in section 5.2.

Box 5.1 Dinner at the Futurist table

Futurism was a European artistic and social movement of the early twentieth century. It originated in Italy after poet Filippo Tommaso Marinetti launched his Futurist Manifesto in 1909, soon to be joined by a large group of painters, composers, architects, and other artists, and by parallel initiatives in other countries and especially in Russia. The futurists had surprisingly modern—and multisensory— ideas about cooking. In 1913, French cook Jules Maincave converted to Futurism and published a *Manifeste de la cuisine futuriste,* where he stressed the importance of harmonizing food taste with food colours and with the dining context, including the choice of cutlery, glassware, and tablecloths. The idea was later developed in the article 'Futurist cooking' (Culinaria futurista) in the Italian magazine *Roma Futurista* of 1920. The author, a Futurist woman poet writing under a pseudonym, advocated harmonizing food with contextual colours and paying special attention to the 'architecture' of the servings—how foodstuff were arranged on the plate to form plastic complexes. After other magazine articles, a full-length book, *La cucina futurista*, appeared in Italy in the early thirties co-authored by Marinetti himself and a less known Futurist artist writing under the pseudonym of Fillìa (Marinetti & Fillìa, 1932, Figure 5.3).

Among other things, Marinetti and Fillìa proposed a ban on pasta (this bit obviously did not catch on) and described a few 'formulas,' the Futurist word for recipe, such as Fillies' *carneplastico* (roughly, 'meat diorama') which consisted of minced veal mixed with 11 different cooked greens, shaped as a vertical cylinder and adorned by an encircling sausage, all this resting on three disks of roasted chicken and topped by honey (we have never tried this but it sounds a bit on the heavy side). Marinetti and Fillia's book was read and translated into several foreign languages but, in the conservative Italian society of the times, their unusual ideas did not have much influence on cooking styles. However, futurist ideas about cooking and serving meals are today widely regarded as precursors of the modern movements of nouvelle, deconstructivist, and multisensory cuisines. Especially interesting in this respect are the Futurists' ideas about eating as a multimodal experience and the use of multisensory interactions to enhance flavours. For instance, Marinetti and Fillìa suggested that cutlery, glassware, and table clothing should harmonize with food flavours and colours; that foods should be shaped into plastic complexes that can be mouthed without forks or spoons, favouring an anticipatory tactile experience before actual tasting; that appropriately chosen perfumes should precede each dish and be later dispersed by ventilators to prepare for the next one; that appropriately chosen music should be played between courses or during eating. More than one avant-garde restaurant is currently pursuing similar ideas to update the dining experience and enrich the flavour of the food served.

Although they were based solely on artistic and hedonic considerations, much recent research on the multisensory perception, appreciation, and consumption of

Box 5.1 Continued

food has confirmed many of the Futurists' intuitions. Contextual factors are now widely recognized to affect food choice, intake, and evaluation (Clydesdale, 1993; Spence, Harrar, & Piqueras-Fiszman, 2012; Wadhera & Capaldi-Philips, 2014; Wansink, 2004), including the size of the plate (van Ittersum & Wansink, 2012), its colour (Bruno, Martani, Corsini, & Oleari, 2013; Genschow, Reutner, & Wänke, 2012; Harrar, Piqueras-Fiszman, & Spence, 2011; Piqueras-Fiszman, Alcaide, Roura, & Spence, 2012), and the material composition of the cutlery (Piqueras-Fiszman, Laughlin, Miodwnik, & Spence, 2012). The general ambience of the tasting room has been shown to affect ratings of whisky (Velasco, Jones, King, & Spence, 2013), and

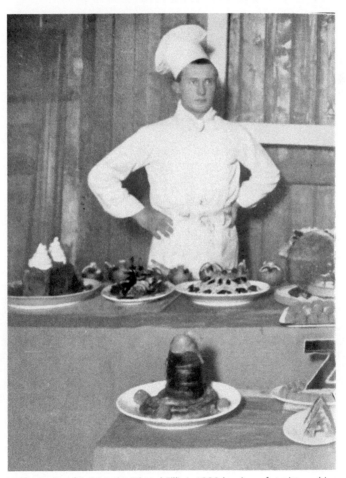

Figure 5.3 An illustration from Marinetti and Fillìa's 1932 book on futurist cooking.
The Bodleian Library, University of Oxford (Arch. 80.IT.1932).

Box 5.1 Continued

the colour of ambient illumination has been shown to alter the wine drinking experience, modifying participant's ratings on several sensory dimensions (Spence, Velasco, & Knoeferle, 2014). These environmental effects are very much in line with the Futurists' suggestions. Finally, a recent paper by Michel, Velasco, Gatti, and Spence (2014) compared ratings of three versions of the same salad: a traditional presentation, a 'neat' presentation with all ingredients forming a quasi-regular grid on the plate, and an 'artistic' presentation that mimicked Vassily Kandinsky's *Panel for Edwin R. Campbell No. 4* (Figure 5.4). Results revealed higher tastiness ratings and higher general appreciation for the Kandinsky salad, despite the fact that exactly the same ingredients in the same proportions were present in all three versions. No doubt, Marinetti and Fillìa would have loved this finding.

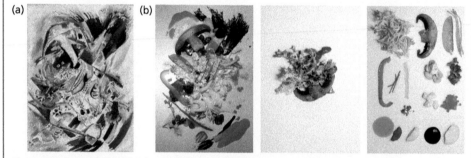

Figure 5.4 Example of the stimuli used by Michel et al. (2014). Kandinsky's *Panel for Edwin R. Campbell No. 4,* 1914, a salad presentation inspired by this abstract painting, and two control presentations.

Figure 5.4a: (Kandinsky) Digital image, The Museum of Modern Art, New York/Scala, Florence.

Figure 5.4b: Reproduced from Charles Michel, Carlos Velasco, Elia Gatti, and Charles Spence, A taste of Kandinsky: assessing the influence of the artistic visual presentation of food on the dining experience, *Flavour,* 3 (7), Figure 1, doi:10.1186/2044-7248-3-7 © Michel et al.; licensee BioMed Central Ltd. 2014. This work is licensed under the Creative Commons Attribution License (CC BY 2.0). It is attributed to the authors Charles Michel, Carlos Velasco, Elia Gatti, and Charles Spence. Photos by Charles Michel.

A second, related general feature of multisensory food perception is that tastes have a definite spatial location: in the mouth. This also implies a multisensory process, as the taste and somatosensory components of the flavour experience do originate in the mouth, but the olfactory ones do not. Odorants must first reach the nose via the retronasal route and stimulate the olfactory epithelium. However, these sensory signals are not experienced as odours coming from the outside environment. Instead, they are bound with the signals originating from receptors in the mouth and the resulting multisensory integration yields a unified flavour percept located where the food actually is, a phenomenon known as 'oral referral.'

Much has been said about the oral referral of olfactory sensory signals. Prescott (1999), for example, deemed it an illusion and Marks (1991) suggested an analogy with ventriloquism: just as in the ventriloquist effect the auditory signals are referred to the viewed mouth of the puppet, so are the olfactory signals referred to the food in the mouth. Upon further reflection, however, we realize that the oral referral of sensory signals from the nose is really no different from what happens with all percepts. Visual percepts, for instance, appear to be located out there, not at the receptor surface. We perceive objects and events in the environment, not neural events in the eye's retina. Early on, we have called this general property of perception *distal* referral. When we perceive food, distal referral takes place for an object inside the oral cavity, but the object is still an external object, at least until one initiates the process of digestion by chewing. In fact, even the analogy with ventriloquism is not completely appropriate, as in the ventriloquist effect visual and auditory signals come from different locations and therefore it makes sense to talk about vision capturing hearing. In oral referral, the taste and olfactory signals have instead a common origin, the food bite in the mouth. Thus, there is no capture to speak of, and oral referral could well be regarded as a multisensory interaction that produces a correct, and veridical, perceptual representation of the object in the environment. This is perhaps not surprising, given that the moment when food is in our mouth represents the last chance to spit it out, avoiding harmful consequences if perception suggests that the substance is not edible. From the standpoint of evolutionary psychology, food flavours are what they are precisely because they serve basic adaptive functions: encouraging consumption of high-energy, carbohydrate-rich substances, and avoiding the ingestion of potentially harmful ones.

5.2 **Sensory coding of basic tastes: myths and facts**

If food flavours result from multisensory interactions, what exactly is the role of 'taste' proper, that is, of the sensory channel that originates with the chemoreceptors in the oral cavity? A quick look at the neural bases of sensory coding in the taste channel provides some answers. Chemoreceptors in the oral cavity lie within the so-called taste buds, minuscule onion-shaped structures mostly located on the soft palate and on the tongue. Tongue taste buds are located within papillae (the small bumps on the tongue's surface) and these come in four kinds. The *fungiform* or mushroom-like papillae are located on the front part of the tongue. The *circumvallate* or wall-like are located in the back of the tongue and the *foliate* or leaf-like lie on the rear side. The *filiform* or thread-like papillae, which are the most numerous, actually do not contain taste buds and are involved only in somatosensory processing. Within the buds are the taste cells, which have tiny hairs, or microvilli, protruding from the top of the bud. Through these, chemicals dissolved in saliva can make contact with taste cells. The interaction results in an electrical change, that in turn triggers the taste cells to send chemicals signals that ultimately cause neural impulses to be sent to brain centres. Interactions happen in different ways, depending on what type of chemical is involved: salts, acids, sweet substances, or bitter substances. This provides some grounds for the popular notion that there are four basic tastes. However, how sweet, sour, salty, and bitter percepts map on chemical classes is not completely clear-cut. Taste cells respond to tastants but also to temperature and mechanical changes. Many carbohydrates, such as sugar, are sweet but some are not. Chemicals that taste salty or sour can be very similar. Conversely, widely different chemical structures can have similar tastes, such as for instance chloroform, the artificial sweetener aspartame, and sugar. In addition, it has been proposed that there exist a fifth basic taste, *umami* (roughly, 'delicious taste' in Japanese), which is associated with savoury or meaty substances (Karamura & Kari, 1987). Thus, although advances in molecular biology and genetics have greatly advanced our understanding of sensory coding by oral chemoreceptors, many details are still not completely understood (for recent reviews see Gravina, Yep, & Khan, 2013; Liman, Zhang, & Montell, 2014; Roper, 2013).

What is clearly understood today is that basic tastes *do not* map to locations on the tongue. Although your grade school teacher might have told you that we taste sweet on the tip of the tongue, salty and sour on the sides, and bitter in the back, this factoid has no empirical basis. It apparently originated from misreading an early psychophysics paper in German (Hanig, 1901). Hanig measured detection thresholds for sweet, sour, acid, and bitter substances. Although he noted that some regions tended to respond most to certain classes of substances, overall he found relatively little variation across the tongue surface. The diagram summarizing his findings is reproduced in Figure 5.5, where greater dot density represents better sensitivity. In a more recent paper, Collings (1974) has confirmed that differences as a function of localization on the tongue are so small as to be devoid of any practical significance. For instance, people missing the anterior part of the tongue continue to experience sweet tastes. However, the myth of a taste map on the

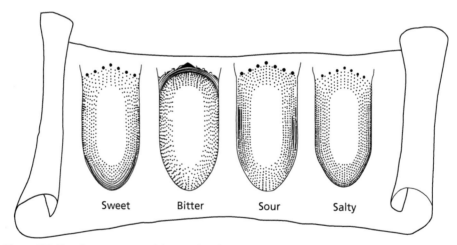

Figure 5.5 The diagram summarizing Hanig's findings. Sensitivity in detecting four kinds of edible substances as a function of location on the tongue, as described in a classic paper by Hanig. Note that there is somewhat greater clustering on the tip for sweet and in the back for bitter, but that generally the whole surface is responsive to all categories.

Adapted from David P. Hänig, Zur psychophysik des geschmacksinnes, *Philosophische Studien*, 17, pp. 576–623, Figures 2, 4, 6, and 7, 1901.

tongue surface has made its way in to many biology textbooks, especially for elementary and secondary schools, and has proved hard to eradicate.

Much debate has taken place on the scheme used by taste neurons to code tastes. In general, these neurons tend to respond to a variety of different substances, but respond most vigorously to certain groups. This was originally interpreted as evidence that each basic taste is coded by the activity of particular cell type, that is, by 'labelled lines.' The idea was that cells that respond best to salt code for saltiness, cells that respond best to sweet code for sweetness, and so on. This proposal, however, fails to explain the broad sensitivity to different substances, and is generally inconsistent with schemes that are observed in other sensory channels. In vision, for instance, there are no neural labels for specific colours. Rather, each cone class is broadly tuned to a range of wavelengths within the visible spectrum. As a consequence, neural responses from individual cones do not contain information about wavelength per se, and colours are coded by relative amounts of activity in each cone class. Analogously, it is known that olfactory neurons code odorants by relative response patterns (Buck, 1996). By the early 1980s, evidence that this scheme may be relevant also to taste became available. Smith, Buskirk, Travers, and Bieber (1983a, 1983b) studied neural response patterns of taste neurons in the hamster brain stem. Using multivariate statistical techniques, they observed three patterns of response profiles, corresponding to sweet-tasting substances, salts containing sodium, or acids and non-sodium salts. Within these patterns, analysis of the profiles suggested that certain neurons were critical for coding specific tastes, as one would expect with labelled lines. However, these neurons coded similarities and differences in across-neuron patterns, such that the neural classification of tastants, in fact, depended on the 'across-fibre pattern' of activity. Thus, these findings suggest that both approaches capture some feature of the data. However, the resolution of the debate is not completely clear and is further complicated by species differences (see e.g. Liman, Zhang, & Montell, 2014).

Whatever the solution, what remains clear is that neural coding within the taste sensory channel can account only for certain simplified sensations, loosely, the five 'primary' tastes. To experience food flavours, additional contributions from other channels, most notably olfaction, are indispensable. Projections from taste cells project to the medulla and the thalamus and from there they reach the insular cortex. The anterior insular cortex is generally regarded as the primary taste cortical area. However, the insula is also an important region for multisensory integration responding to signals from the tongue, the nose, interoceptive somatosensation, as well as signals from emotional and cognitive regions (see Frank, Kullmann, & Veit, 2013). From the insula, the taste pathway reaches the orbitofrontal cortex, which is also heavily multisensory. In a milestone study on the orbitofrontal cortex of the macaque, Rolls and Baylis (1994) documented neurons that responded to tastants, odours, and visual stimuli. These multisensory neurons lay intermingled with unisensory ones on the cortical surface, suggesting that the orbitofrontal cortex implements multisensory interactions involved in flavour perception. This suggestion has been supported by studies that used fMRI to study the functional properties of orbitofrontal cortex (Osterbauer, Matthews, Jenkinson, Beckmann, Hansen, & Calvert,

2005). These studies have demonstrated that activity in caudal regions of orbitofrontal cortex was modulated by the congruency of colours and odours. For instance, they observed an increase in orbitofrontal activation after presenting yellow with lemon odour (congruent) but a decrease after presenting blue with strawberry odour (incongruent), in comparison to the unisensory presentation of odours without colours.

5.3 Somatosensory signals and food perception

The mouth does not contain only chemoreceptors. Receptors that respond to tactile stimuli, thermal stimuli, and pain are also abundantly present not only in the filiform papillae, but also in fungiform and circumvallate papillae. There is even evidence that somatosensory innervations of fungiform papillae may outnumber gustatory ones (for a review, see Green, 2002). Electrophysiological evidence indicates that many 'taste' cells respond also to temperature and mechanical stimulation (Zotterman, 1935; Oakley, 1985), and multisensory neurons that respond to tastants as well as to somatic stimulation are common in the primary gustatory areas (see Green, 2002). Behavioural observations confirm that the perception of substances in the mouth can be altered by somatic stimulation. For instance, warming the anterior edge of the tongue is associated with perceived sweetness, and cooling the same part can elicit sourness or saltiness (Cruz & Green, 2000). If you have the patience to wait a few seconds, and can stand the chill, you will notice that an ice cube applied to the side of your tongue begins to taste slightly salty. Ingredients such as chilli or pepper contain capsaicin, a substance that stimulates oral nociceptors (for a review, see Green & Lawless, 1991). Tannins are chemicals that cause actual tactile stimulation within the mouth, such as general dryness, roughness on the tongue and palate, and feeling of outer tension of the cheek muscles. The interaction of nociceptor or mechanoreceptor signals with signals from taste receptors adds the spicy note to your curry and the astringent note to your red barriqued wine. Based on the abundance of tactile, thermal, and pain-related receptors in the mouth and their obvious contribution to flavour, it has been suggested that taste is as much a cutaneous sense as it is a gustatory one (Green, 2002).

The contribution of somatosensation to the perceptual experience of food, however, is not limited to adding characteristic notes to its flavour. A defining feature of how we experience food is that the flavour 'feels' located in the mouth and fills it in a characteristic way. These aspects of how we perceive food depend critically on interactions of the chemosensory signals with somatosensation. For instance, if a taste target is presented within the mouth among tasteless distractors, it is immediately identified. However, if the tasteless target is presented among distractors that have a taste, identifying the tasteless target becomes quite difficult (Delwiche, Lera, & Breslin, 2000). This asymmetry suggests that the target can 'inherit' the taste of the distractors, in accord with somatosensory signals that place it at the same or nearby location. Similarly, when they have to rate a tasteless swab surrounded by two neighbouring swabs imbued in a tastant (such as sugar or common salt), participants often mislocalize the taste to the tasteless swab (Green, 2002).

When a tastant is slid on the tongue from a taste-sensitive region to a region containing no taste receptors, we have a continuous experience of taste on all locations touched by the applicator. However, the spreading of taste to taste-insensitive areas of the tongue does not occur after anaesthesia preventing somatosensory afferents from the tongue. These phenomena are grouped under the label *tactile capture of taste* (Stillman, 2002). Tactile capture of taste is presumably one of the factors that contribute to the oral referral of chemosensory signals (Todrank & Bartoshuk, 1991).

Finally, for those of us who are into cooking, a most obvious somatosensory contribution to the food experience stems from tactile signals that specify food texture. Mushy, overcooked pasta does not taste as good as the firm, *al dente* dish. Most of us like tender meat and don't appreciate the fibrous, hard feel of an overcooked steak, and there is something definitely wrong with a lumpy, gritty custard cream. It is not clear, at present, to what extent these tactile signals actually modify food flavour within a process of multisensory integration, or rather combine with flavour, adding another perceptual dimension to the perception of food although this dimension remains perceptually separate from flavour proper. In a recent paper, Slocombe, Carmichael, and Simner (2016) compared taste evaluations of foodstuffs having a rough or a smooth surface and found that the rough stimuli were judged to be more sour. Elegantly, they included a control condition with rough or smooth plates rather than foods, and there they found no effect. This rules out task demands, but the fact remains that participants were providing introspective evaluations. So the jury is still out on the question whether these aspects of the food experience influence actual perceptual mechanisms of flavour perception (say, by modifying thresholds), or rather change a post-perceptual evaluation of the dish as a whole. We will return to this issue in the final section (6.5) of this chapter.

5.4 Perceiving food with the mouth and the nose

Let's try a simple experiment. Ask a friend to buy some fruit juice and have him pour it in a glass, without letting you know what fruit flavour it contains. Don a blindfold and apply a laundry clip to your nose. Now try drinking the juice, but do it in two steps. First, hold the liquid in the mouth without swallowing and concentrate on taste percepts coming from the mouth. You will notice that the experience is not particularly rewarding. Suppose for instance, that the glass contained lemon juice. Most likely, you will have experienced this as combination of sweetness, sourness, and acidity. However, the juice will not have the characteristic flavour of lemon. Most people do not recognize lemon juice with the nostrils closed. Now remove the clip, expire to open up the nostrils, and swallow the juice. Within a few seconds your experience will become much richer, you will become aware of the juice flavour, and most likely you will recognize it. The characteristic flavour of lemon depends on terpenes, volatile biomolecules that are found in the essential oils of many plants and most notably in those of citrus. Normally, terpenes will reach the olfactory mucosae through the so-called retronasal passage which connects the oral cavity with the nose. The olfactory signals that arise from sensory coding of terpenes would then be fused with the taste signals to create the flavours that we perceive. The laundry clip however prevents this by keeping the nostril tightly closed, and this is the reason for the altered flavour of the lemon.

As shown by our little experiment, the experience of flavour depends critically on stimulation of olfactory receptors (Murphy, Cain, & Bartoshuck, 1977). Support for this general conclusion is so overwhelming that a few selected facts will suffice to prove the point. For instance, many individuals have trouble distinguishing between a boiled potato, an apple, and a pear when tested for recognition with a blindfold and a clip to block the nose. Or consider reports of loss of taste by patients, a common complaint following head trauma. True loss of the taste channel, or *ageusia*, is in reality quite rare. Most often, a report of taste loss depends on malfunctioning of the olfactory channel, or *anosmia*. Partial loss of taste signals from the mouth often, in fact, remains completely unnoticed. For instance, anesthetizing the chorda tympani branch of nerve VII on one side of the cranium will block afferents from the front of the tongue ipsilaterally. Despite this, food flavour is still experienced as coming from the whole mouth and the effects of anaesthesia can remain completely unnoticed (Östrum, Catalannotto, Gent, & Bartoshuk, 1985). Conversely, anosmia has significant effects on one's quality of life, as depriving an individual of the experience of flavour can have negative effects on dietary habits and on a score of emotional, motivational, and social factors. Or consider the effect of adding odours to taste stimuli. Stevenson, Prescott, and Boakes (1999) obtained sweetness, sourness, liking, and intensity rating from participants who were presented with 20 odours. They then obtained taste ratings for solutions with these odours added as flavourants, and compared these with ratings without the added odours. They found that certain odours strongly modified perceived taste: for instance, caramel odour enhanced sweetness ratings in sucrose solutions and suppressed sourness ratings in citric acid solutions.

These observations suggest that sensory signals from the tongue and the nose undergo a complete fusion when we perceive food flavours, such that physically different combinations of odorants and tastants can result in identical percepts, that is, in multisensory metamers. This strongly suggests that the interaction of taste and smell signals is a form of multisensory integration. Dalton, Doolittle, Nagata, and Breslin (2000) have conducted a series of elegant experiments to test this idea. They presented participants with different concentrations of the odorant benzaldehyde (the characteristic odour of almonds), of the tastant saccharin (sugar), or of monosodium glutamate (umami taste). They used psychophysical techniques to determine the smallest concentrations of the odorant and of the tastants that could be reliably detected by each participant, that is, the *nasal detection threshold* for benzaldehyde and the *oral detection thresholds* for saccharin and glutamate. Next, they measured benzaldehyde thresholds again, but this time the odorant was accompanied also by subthreshold concentrations of the tastants. They found that the nasal threshold was decreased (that is, sensitivity was increased) when participants received the subthreshold concentrations of saccharin, relative to control conditions whereby the odorant was presented without a tastant, with odourless water. Given that the saccharin concentration was below the detection threshold, participants did not consciously perceive it. Therefore, this result rules out higher-order, strategic, or attentional effects. The taste stimulus was actually fused with the smell stimulus, and the multisensory taste— smell interactions resulted in improved sensitivity, in comparison to taste or smell alone.

Given that taste and smell signals were integrated, an interesting question arises. How does the brain decide that the signals must, in fact, be integrated? In other words, how does it solve the binding problem in this particular situation? Another feature of the study of Dalton and collaborators provides a preliminary answer. When studying changes in sensitivity for the odorant stimulus, they observed that an increase in sensitivity occurred with a simultaneous presentation of saccharin, but not with that of glutamate. Pairing the odorant with subthreshold concentrations of glutamate had the same null effect of pairing it with water. Given that sweet tastes are often associated with almond door in Western culture (think of cookies) but not with glutamate, this suggests that multisensory integration takes places specifically for previously encountered pairings of tastants and odorants, and not in general for any pairing. This final point is quite consistent with studies of the phenomena of sweetness enhancement–suppression which we have discussed in the previous paragraph (for review see Auvray & Spence, 2008). For instance, sweetness can be enhanced by caramel or strawberry odour, but not by peanut butter. Repeated experience with odor-taste mixtures can produce conditioned change in perceived odours (Stevenson, Boakes, & Wilson, 2000). Thus, one's exposure to the statistical co-occurrence of multisensory stimulus pairs appears to be a critical factor in determining how the brain tackles the binding problem. This is consistent with other observations that we have discussed previously regarding the role of experience in binding in multisensory object perception. In the epilogue to this book, we suggest that this may, in fact, be a general principle regulating multisensory interactions.

The scope of multisensory processes involved in food perception, however, extends well beyond the multisensory integration of taste and smell. As we see in the next section, sensory signals from the nose interact with the coding of flavour in another important way, along with and visual signals and, surprisingly, even somatosensory signals from the hand as well as auditory signals. Studies of this other kind of multisensory interaction provide new qualifications on the popular notion that 'one eats with eyes first' (Delwiche, 2012), and suggest that anticipatory effects are not limited to vision. We eat with our eyes first, but in some cases we eat first also with the nose, the hands, and even the ears.

5.5 Anticipatory multisensory interactions in the perception of food

So far, we have described multisensory interactions that take place while food is in the mouth. As food is chewed, sensory signals from taste, somatosensory, and smell receptors are merged into a unified perception of the food flavour. This process itself can extend in time, as different features of the flavour can be revealed, for instance, at the initial contact of the tongue with a solid morsel or a liquid, in comparison to the successive chewing and swallowing. However, multisensory interactions affecting the perception of flavour are not limited to what happens as food is in the mouth, but begin even before. Sensory information which is made available by sniffing, viewing, or touching an edible object, or by hearing sounds associated with, for instance, biting it, can also affect how we perceive food. Whether these anticipatory multisensory interactions actually modulate food perception at the sensory level, by modifying sensory thresholds for the intensity of a particular flavour or flavour feature, or rather modulate higher-order processes of categorization and identification of flavour features remains the object of debate. That anticipatory olfactory, visual, somatosensory, or auditory signals can modulate hedonic responses to food as well as categorization and identification processes is now generally accepted. Conversely, evidence regarding the possibility that anticipatory signals can alter the intensity of perceived dimensions of flavour remains ambiguous (Spence, Levitan, & Zampini, 2010). Here we will review the main findings supporting the first of these two outcomes, as well as some evidence that suggests that the second may also occur at least in some conditions.

Before placing food in our mouth, we usually perceive its odor. In fact, sensory analysis protocols usually recommend doing this deliberately and paying intense attention to the smell. Wine tasters, for instance, actually insert the nose in the glass and repeatedly sniff to evaluate the wine's *bouquet* before they bring the liquid to the mouth. When we sniff doors in this way, odorants from the external environment reach the olfactory mucosa through the nasal passages, that is, via *orthonasal* olfaction. When smell signals reach the nose from the oral cavity during actual eating, we are instead using *retronasal* olfaction. Thus olfaction is a dual system, and you may note that this provides additional grounds for our critical approach to the notion of 'the senses'—there is no unitary 'smell' sense; rather, the coding of olfactory signals serves two different perceptual functions (Rozin, 1982). The first is that of integrating signals originating in the mouth in the actual perception of flavour, the process described in the previous section of this chapter. There is, however, a second and equally important function, which is geared to detect the presence of specific substances or objects by exploiting volatile chemicals that objects release. Sensory signals from this orthonasal process can then interact with later perceptual processes, as in the anticipatory effects of smell on flavour, or, to mention just another example, the effects of smell on hand shaping when grasping seen objects (see Chapter 3). Anticipatory orthonasal signals may also be interpreted in relation to the well-known phenomenon that odours are often verbally described as having taste qualities. For instance, the odours of vanillin or caramel are spontaneously described as sweet. Presumably, sniffing vanillin prompts us to access memories of sweet foods, and activation of a semantic network in turn links the odour to sweetness (discussed in Prescott, 1999). Additional clues about the anticipatory role of visual signals on flavour perception also come from studies that have investigated the neural basis of the so-called *tip-of-the-nose* phenomenon, the quite common feeling of knowing what a certain odour is, but of being unable to retrieve the verbal label for it (Qureshy, et al., 2000). Interestingly, these studies have observed that when participants attempt to identify odour stimuli, in addition to olfactory areas there is also activation of the primary visual area.

In addition to its smell, it is generally accepted among experts of gastronomy that the visual appearance of food is also extremely important. Food that is presented in atypical formats, or has unusual colours, can look less appetizing and therefore have a lower probability of being consumed or liked. In a famous study, Weathley (1973) asked participants to sit at a dinner table and consume dishes that were served under conditions of illumination that masked the colours of the food. Participants started to eat and initially reported enjoying the dishes. At one point during the dinner, however, researchers brought illumination conditions back to normality revealing a blue steak, green potato chips, and red peas (Figure 5.6). Weathley reported that merely seeing these 'wrong' colours induced nausea in many participants, and that some felt sick and had to run to the toilet. In general, consumers report that food ingredients such as margarine, orange juice, bacon, or cheese are seem to have better quality and more pleasant flavours when they have normal colours in comparison to when they are given unusual colours (Christensen, 1983). When margarine was first introduced in Australia and the US, consumers showed little appreciation. Reportedly, the initial flop of the new product depended on a shade of white that made it resemble the colour of lard. Although producers of butter opposed this, eventually the colour was modified to make it more yellowish and closer to the colour of butter, and this is what we now find on supermarket shelves (discussed in Packard, 1957).

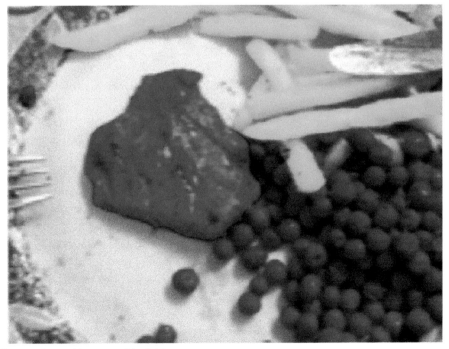

Figure 5.6 Would you eat this dish?
Reproduced from J. Wheatley, Putting Colour into Marketing, *Marketing*, 67, pp. 24–29, 1973.

The effects described in the previous paragraph suggest that anticipatory information from colour can have a strong influence on how we respond to food. But is this response confined to hedonics, that is, whether we like or dislike the flavour, or is the actual perception of the flavour altered? For instance, is the multisensory flavour of a drink modified if we change its colour? At present, the best answer to this question seems to be: it depends on which feature of the flavour you want modified. Consider flavour *intensity*. The food industry has assumed for a long time that the right amount of colorant will increase the perceived intensity of a flavour. Add green colorant to a mint-flavoured drink, and tasters will report that the mint flavour is now stronger. Increase the amount of red colorant to strawberry yogurt and even food quality experts will report a more intense strawberry flavour (Teerling, 1992). However, the empirical evidence from controlled studies of the effect of vision on flavour intensity is rather mixed. In a recent influential review, Spence, Levitan, Shankar, and Zampini (2010) discussed 24 studies testing changes of perceived flavour intensity after manipulations of food colour. They classified twelve of these as reporting a statistically significant effect of colour, five as reporting a non-significant effect, and seven as reporting a complex mixture of significant and non-significant effects. Thus, as many as half of the studies included negative evidence, and Spence and colleagues concluded that support for a modulation of flavour intensity by colour is really rather weak. On the other hand, it may be noted that these studies measured changes in basic taste features, such as sweetness, saltiness, or sourness. Although these are relevant dimension of food flavour, it may be that anticipatory effects of colour work their magic only on more complex dimensions of flavour, such as those that cannot be detected by taste alone but require actual multisensory interactions.

Evidence supporting the latter hypothesis comes from studies of flavour *identification*, our ability to categorize flavours and label them verbally. In a widely cited study, DuBose, Cardello, and Maller (1980) asked participants to sample drinks with colours that could be either consistent or inconsistent with the drink ingredients (for instance, a red-coloured vs. a green-coloured cherry drink), and compared flavour identifications to those of drinks presented in colourless solutions. In many of the tested drinks, they found that flavour identification depended much more on the colorant than on the flavorant, that is, sensory signals from the eyes were more important than the combined effect of the mouth and nose signals. In particular, when they sampled a cherry drink all participants identified it correctly when the drink was red, but most also identified it as lime when it was green, and about 20 percent of participants identified it as orange when the drink had an orange colour. Numerous other studies have consistently reported similar effects of colour on flavour identification (see, e.g., Zampini, Sanabria, Philips, & Spence, 2007). An important question regarding these effects is whether they occur at the interface between perception and memory, altering processes involved in recognition, or if they instead modulate the criteria adopted by participants when formulating verbal categorization responses. Distinguishing between these two possibilities is not easy, and more research is called for on this issue (Spence, Levitan, Shankar, & Zampini, 2010).

One potential explanation for anticipatory effects of colour on flavour is that colour engenders expectations about the sensory signals that will become available once the food is in the mouth. These expectations may structurally coordinate information in different sensory signals (Booth, 2013), such that certain ways of solving the binding problem or even of grouping specific elements across sensory channels are favoured over others. We speculate that this process is analogous to what happens in vision with Wertheimer's law of objective set (see Chapter 4): once local stimulus signals have grouped in a certain perceptual unit, they tend to preserve that specific organization. At the functional level, one processing route for such an anticipatory process may involve the mediation of olfaction. Consider the case of wine. If you have had some exposure to wine, you probably know that the flavour of white wines is often described by referring to fruit such as lemon, grapefruit, banana, melon, mango, peach, apple, apricot, or pineapple; conversely, the flavour of red wines is often referred to fruit such as prune, raspberry, bilberry, cherry, red currant, or black currant. Although there is some overlap in the use of some of these terms, there is little doubt that our ability to detect olfactory 'notes' in the wine bouquet is affected by colour. When wearing a blindfold, novice and intermediate wine tasters perform poorly (although still better than chance) in comparison to true experts when they have to guess the colour of a wine from its bouquet (Sauvageot & Chapon, 1983) and even experts have difficulty distinguishing white and red wines from rosé wines (Ballester, et al., 2009).

In a study that received much attention from the press, Morrot, Brochet, and Dubourdieu (2001) compared the terms used by enology students to describe the bouquets of a white Bordeaux, a red Bordeaux, and the same white Bordeaux after adding an odourless red colorant. Unsurprisingly, they observed that typical white wine descriptors were used for the bouquet of the white wine, and typical red wine descriptors for the bouquet of the red. However, and much less predictably, they also found that almost the same proportion of red wine descriptors were used for the red and for the red-coloured white. These results suggest that colour has a strong effect on the processing of orthonasal signals when we try to identify odours. This might reorganize multisensory interactions between olfactory and taste signals, leading us to miscategorize the flavour and perhaps even to experience a change in its perceived quality or intensity.

If visual cues have an anticipatory effect on food perception, it seems only reasonable that other signals that may become available before we bring edibles to the mouth may have similar effects. In a recent report, Barnett-Cowan (2010) studied the perception of pretzels that participants had to grasp and bring to the mouth while blindfolded. To this end, Barnett-Cowan used three types of pretzels: ordinary fresh pretzels, treated pretzels that were fully immersed in water for 20 seconds and then dried, and partly treated pretzels having one half that had been immersed in water and another half that was kept fresh. Participants received one end of each pretzel on their index and thumb, made a single bite using their front teeth, spat out, and rated the pretzel on fresh–stale and crisp–soft response scales. The results indicated that both freshness and crispness ratings were highest when both the hand and the mouth received a fresh pretzel, and lowest when they both received a treated pretzel. Conversely, when the hand received a treated pretzel and the mouth a fresh one, or vice versa, freshness and crispness were somewhere in between these two extremes. Thus, when the hand felt a treated pretzel, participants tended to report less crispness and freshness even if the sensory signal from the biting action was that of a fresh pretzel; when the hand felt a fresh pretzel, they reported more crispness and freshness even though they bit a treated one. This is quite consistent with an anticipatory effect of the hand signals on the evaluation of food in the mouth.

Similarly, one might expect anticipatory effect from the sounds that are produced when biting, and that are known to vary systematically in amplitude, frequency, and phase depending on the type of food. In an elegant study that won the authors the infamous *IgNobel* prize for improbable (but serious) research, Zampini and Spence (2004) reported strong evidence that these acoustic changes also modulate the multisensory perception of food. For their study, Zampini and Spence used commercially available potato chips that all look, smell, and taste the same, and manipulated the sounds produced when biting them using a custom-made apparatus. This consisted of a microphone that fed the sound into a device that selectively amplified or attenuated either the whole spectrum or only high frequencies, and returned the modified sound to earphones worn by participants. The results indicated that crispness and freshness were rated higher when hearing the amplified versions, both with the whole-spectrum and in the high-pass filtered sounds, in comparison to the attenuated versions. Given that the chips were otherwise identical, this shows that sounds affected the response to food. When debriefed, out of the 20 participants as many as 15 refused to believe that they had been sampling from the very same batch of chips!

Chapter 6

Synaesthesia

6.1 An unusual, intriguing condition

The term *synaesthesia*, from the ancient Greek *syn* (union) and *aisthesis* (perception or sensory-based experience), refers to a curious anomaly of multisensory perception. For a true synaesthete, stimulation of one sensory channel evokes, in addition to percepts in the perceptual modality associated to that channel, an additional percept in the modality that is usually associated to a different channel. The evoking stimulus is called *inducer* whereas the associated percept is called *concurrent*. For instance, synaesthesia researcher Richard Cytowic has described the amazing case of MW, an individual that experiences the 'shapes' of the foods he tastes. For MW, tasting foods includes a set of tactile perceptions, as if 'things were rubbed against the face or were sitting on the hands' (Cytowic, 2002, p. 4). When he cooks, MW therefore strives to create not only pleasant tastes, but also interesting shapes: He uses sugar to make the taste 'more round'; citrus to add 'points' (p. 66). Thus, for MW tasting is a multimodal experience. The multisensory interactions that underlie the perception of food flavours in most of us, and that for us result in a unified percept in the taste modality, for MW result in a double percept in the taste and somatosensory modalities. Moreover, MW's experiences of the shape of foods are not imagined or conceived, they are actually perceived—they are 'there'—and he cannot help perceiving them. In true synaesthetes, such as MW, multisensory perceptual processes seem to be genuinely different from those of the rest of us.

Although synaesthesia is sometimes described as a neurological anomaly, the condition is not cited in psychiatry or psychopathology textbooks. It usually does not have negative effects on the quality of life of synaesthetes, except, perhaps, for the feeling of being different, 'not right,' that some report especially when recalling their childhood realization that their synaesthetic experiences were not shared by others. In regard to this, scientific investigations of synaesthesia have had a valuable side effect. By making the condition more generally known, they have helped synaesthetes to understand that nothing is wrong. The specific differences in their perception in comparison to that of non-synaesthetes is notable, but within the range of normal group variation. In this, we suspect that synaesthesia might be compared to other unusual variants of perceptual experience such as absolute pitch (see Takeuchii & Hulse, 1993) or superior odour identification by perfume or wine experts.

Synaesthesia is relatively rare. Estimates of the prevalence of the condition range from about 1 in 100,000 (Cytowic, 2002) or 1 in 2000 (Baron-Cohen, Burt, Smith-Lattain, &

Bolton, 1996) to about 1 in 200 (Ramachandran & Hubbard, 2001). These large differences presumably depend on which generic definition one adopts (see section 6.3 and Box 6.1). In addition, although relatively few of us are synaesthetes, specific manifestations of the condition vary widely (see Day, 2005). Estimates differ on exactly how many inducer-concurrent associations have been found, with those involving colour concurrents being the most frequent. For instance, the following inducer stimuli have been described in relation to colour concurrents: musical pitch, chords, or timbre; other auditory stimuli, such as the human voice or sounds in general; tactile or thermal stimulation; letters or numbers; pain; odour; and even emotional or somatosensory experiences such as, for instance, the experience of female orgasm. Taste or odour concurrents have been described in relation to visual and auditory inducers. Yet other peculiar cases are well known, such as the case of MW who has tactile concurrents from taste inducers. This combination of rarity of occurrence with diversity of manifestation represents an especially difficult challenge for attempts to draw valid generalizations.

Synaesthesia is linked to sex, runs in families, and has been related to superior memory. Female synaesthetes are about six times more frequent than male synaesthetes (Galton, 1883) and children of synaesthetes are more likely to have the condition than children of non-synaesthetes (Baron-Cohen et al., 1996). These characteristics of synaesthesia suggest a genetic basis (Gregersen et al., 2013), although the mode of transmission remains unclear (see Brang & Ramachandran, 2011), and different criteria for estimating prevalence may lead to different results (Simner & Hubbard, 2006). Superior memory performance by many synaesthetes is presumably related to additional cues for recall that are not available to non-synaesthetes. Suppose that hearing certain names caused you to experience colours, such that, for instance, 'Judith' is pink but 'Helena' is orange. You meet a young lady but can't recall her name. But wait a minute—you remember she had a pink name ... oh, yes, it's Judith. The process is analogous to what happens to all of us with non-synaesthetic cues. (What's her name ... I remember it started with J ... oh yes, it's Judith.) Individuals endowed with prodigious memories are often synaesthetes. For example, the famous S described in neuropsychology's classic *The Mind of a Mnemonist* (Luria, 1968) reported actively exploiting his automatic synaesthetic associations both when encoding and when retrieving information to perform complex memory tasks. Enhancement of memory might be one of the selective advantages of the synaesthesia trait, although it is also possible that it is merely a by-product of some other useful adaptation.

6.2 Synaesthetic metaphor

The term synaesthesia is used in literary circles to refer to a figure of speech whereby words that apply to a perceptual modality are used to qualify experiences that come in a different modality. This is sometimes called a *synaesthetic metaphor* (Takada, 2013). Consider, for instance, Eugenio Montale's 1920s masterpiece *I limoni*—in our favourite translation (Montale, 1993) titled *The lemon trees*. In the final part of the poem, the yellow

---

Box 6.1 Is flavour a universal form of synaesthesia?

As we have seen in detail in Chapter 5, chemosensory signals from the tongue and the nose interact when we perceive food flavours. In fact, flavour perception depends on sensory signals picked up retronasally by olfactory receptors much more than on signal picked up by receptors in the oral cavity. As a consequence, presenting odours to the nose in conjunction with tastants to the mouth can substantially alter perceived flavour. It has been suggested that this phenomenon, perception of taste induced by odours, could be considered a form of synaesthesia that is experienced by everyone (Stevenson & Boakes, 2004). There is, however, a crucial difference between synaesthesia as defined in this chapter and the perception of flavour. In synaesthetic experiences, perceivers report two percepts: the percept that is normally associated with the inducer plus the additional synaesthetic concurrent. The two percepts are distinct and often experienced in different locations. For instance, MW reports experiencing the flavour of foods he is cooking, and having an additional somatosensory experience of solid shapes. In the perception of flavour, instead, a single percept is experienced and referred to the substance in the oral cavity. For this reason, we believe that defining flavour as a universal form of synaesthesia would be misleading. Flavour is better understood as a form of multisensory interaction between tongue- and nose-related signals, which under certain conditions are bound and result in a single unified percept (Auvray & Spence, 2008).

---

colour of lemons evokes the sound of songs and trumpets, which in turn are felt peppering one's breast:

> And, one day, through a gate ajar,
> among the trees in a courtyard,
> we see the yellows of the lemon trees;
> and the heart's ice thaws,
> and songs pelt
> into the breast
> and trumpets of gold pour forth
> epiphanies of Light!

Although this often remains unnoticed, synaesthetic metaphor is not confined to the verses of Nobel laureates. In fact, language teems with synaesthetic metaphor (Marks, 1978). Expressions like *warm colour, sweet smell,* or *bitter cold* are so commonplace that we hardly notice their synaesthetic nature. The fact that all of us understand them, however, suggests that they rely on similarities that are universal. This poses the problem of the perceptual and cognitive basis of these universally understood associations, an issue that we address in the fourth section of this chapter. On the other hand, the universal nature of these associations indicates that synaesthetic metaphor is a different phenomenon from true perceptual synaesthesia, although the two might be related. As suggested by Marks (1978), the ability to expand the limits of how we think of and conceptualize events is fundamental to cognition. By disclosing novel analogies and resemblances, metaphor plays an important role in weaving these into a coherent fabric, creating a new manner of organizing a set of concepts. Metaphor is key in promoting creativity, and synaesthetes may possess a special sensitivity for metaphor.

The possibility of a link between synaesthesia and creativity is perhaps one of the most-cited features of the condition. Many famous artists are reputed to have been synaesthetes, including, for instance, the composer Olivier Messiaen, the painter Vassily Kandinsky, and the writer Vladimir Nabokov. Ramachandran and Hubbard (2001) cited a study by Domino (1989) reporting that, in a sample of 358 fine-arts students, 84 or 23 percent were synaesthetes and that these scored better on measures of artistic creativity compared to controls. To the extent that a synaesthete's brain more readily and comprehensively produces associations between percepts and concepts, it is not unlikely that this might produce a greater propensity for mapping across unrelated ideas in a creative fashion (Ramachandran & Hubbard, 2001). This idea is seductive. If synaesthesia is related to creativity, this would provide interesting insights for both art psychology and for the already-mentioned issue of understanding the adaptive value of synaesthesia, if any. Despite its considerable interest, however, evidence for a causal link between synaesthesia and creativity remains inconclusive (Brang & Ramachandran, 2011). We will therefore set the issue aside, and concentrate on synaesthesia as a phenomenon of multisensory perception. The first step in this direction is mapping the territory of synaesthetic phenomena. What forms of synaesthesia have been observed? How do they differ? And what did we exactly mean when we referred to 'true' synaesthetes early on in the chapter?

6.3 Defining synaesthesia

Several generic forms of synaesthesia have been described, and there have been difficulties in providing a comprehensive definition and terminology. However, some conceptual dimensions have proven useful in identifying variants that are most relevant for multisensory research. Here we will address the distinctions between synaesthetic perception and synaesthetic conception; between developmental, acquired, and pharmacological synaesthesia; between unimodal and multimodal synaesthesia; and between projector and associator synaesthetes.

The distinction between *synaesthetic perception* and *synaesthetic conception* (Grossenbacher & Lovelace, 2001) refers to the nature of the inducer. In synaesthetic perception, concurrents are induced by actual sensory signals coded by a sensory channel that is not usually associated with the modality of the concurrent. The case of MW, the man who tastes shapes, is an example of synaesthetic perception. In synaesthetic conception, conversely, concurrents are induced by thoughts or mental images. Individuals that experience coloured flashes (photisms) when thinking about the days of the week or the months of the year have synaesthetic conception. Synaesthetic conception has also been called *ideaesthesia* (Nikolic, 2009). In some cases, both kinds of synaesthesia coexist in the same person. In a most unusual report, Nikolic, et al. (2011) recently described the case of two experienced swimmers for which each swimming style evokes a different colour concurrent. For instance, breaststroke is red-brown, whereas front crawl is yellow. The concurrents reportedly occur from somatosensory and motor signals during actual swimming, but also from seeing illustrations of each style and thinking about the style.

The distinction between *developmental, acquired,* and *pharmacological* synaesthesia refers to the onset of the synaesthetic experiences. Developmental synaesthetes routinely experience automatic and stable synaesthetic perception or conception. They report having had synaesthesia at least for as long as they can remember, and typically remain synaesthetes till old age. Acquired synaesthetes, on the other hand, start to experience synaesthesia after an incident such as a brain lesion or sensory deafferentation. For instance, in a recent paper Goller, Richards, Novak, and Ward (2013) observed that some amputees reported tactile percepts on their phantom limbs (see Tutorial 2.1) when watching someone else being touched. Acquired synaesthesia may be limited to synaesthetic perception—to the best of our knowledge, there have been no reported cases of synaesthetic conception after neurological insult. Pharmacological synaesthesia, finally, refers to synaesthetic hallucinations from taking psychedelic substances such as LSD or mescaline. Although these hallucinations do consist of percepts induced by stimulation of other sensory channels, the nature of these percepts appears to be quite different from that of developmental or acquired synaesthetes. For one, the hallucinations are often rather complex, including people, imaginary animals, monsters, or complex coloured patterns. Concurrents experienced by the other two types of synaesthete, instead, consist of simple features such as colours, shapes, texture, or light touch. In addition, the manifestations of pharmacological synaesthesia are variable. In one drugged trip, music might induce the perception of beautiful landscapes; in another, of fearful monsters. The inducer-concurrent associations of developmental synaesthetes are instead relatively stable over their entire existence.

An additional important distinction is that between *multimodal* and *unimodal* synaesthesia. In multimodal synaesthesia, a signal coded within one sensory channel (the inducer) engenders a percept in the modality usually associated with that channel. In conjunction with this 'normal' percept, however, a second percept (the concurrent) is experienced in a different perceptual modality. A common form is tone-colour synaesthesia, a condition that may be associated to absolute pitch (Gregersen et al., 2013) and that may account in part for the superior memory for tones of possessors of absolute pitch. The case of MW discussed at the beginning of this chapter is also a case of multimodal synaesthesia. In unimodal synaesthesia, conversely, both the percept associated with the inducer signal and the concurrent percept occur within the same perceptual modality. A common form is grapheme-colour synaesthesia, whereby visual forms evoke visual colours. Note that unimodal synaesthesia seems to run counter to the idea that synaesthesia is a 'union of the senses.' Upon further reflection, however, you might realize that this seeming contradiction is merely a consequence of a confusion between perceptual modalities—a concept that belongs to the domain of subjective experience and phenomenology—and sensory channels—which refer to mechanisms of neural encoding.

Box 6.2 Acquiring synaesthesia from refrigerator magnets?

Is it possible that the inducer-concurrent associations of an individual synaesthete somehow depend on his or her idiosyncratic childhood experiences? Plausible as it seems, this hypothesis is hard to test. One would need to trace an adult's specific synaesthesia back to specific environmental features during the childhood of the synaesthete, a task that requires considerable detective work and good luck. To the best of our

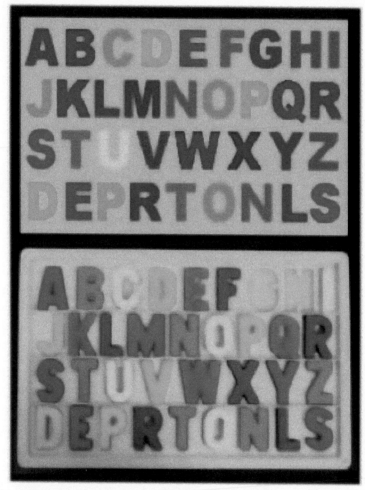

Figure 6.1 Acquiring synaesthesia from refrigerator magnets? A.E.D.'s synaesthetic associations between letters and colours (top) compared with a photograph of her magnetic letter set as provided by her parents (bottom).

Reprinted from *Cortex*, 42 (2), Nathan Witthoft and Jonathan Winawer, Synesthetic Colors Determined by Having Colored Refrigerator Magnets in Childhood, pp. 175-83, doi: 10.1016/S0010-9452(08)70342-3 © 2006 Elsevier Masson Srl., with permission from Elsevier.

Box 6.2 Continued

knowledge, there has been only one documented case of synaesthesia that could be reliably related to childhood environment. Witthof and Winaver (2006) stumbled across AED, a grapheme-colour projector synaesthete. AED actually recalled having had a set of coloured magnetic letters as a toy, and her parents were able to retrieve most of the set at the family home. Compare AED's adult colour concurrents, as measured objectively with a colour-matching procedure, to the toy set (Figure 6.1). Although there are some notable differences, for the large majority of the letters the colour is essentially the same. Perhaps not surprisingly, this report has received a lot of attention within recent attempts to re-evaluate the role of learning in synaesthesia (Yon & Press, 2014; Watson et al., 2014). Still, evidence for childhood environmental effects remains hard to accrue. Even in the case of AED, it has proved impossible to extend testing to concurrents of numbers, which also were part of the toy set but were lost. And for more esoteric forms, such as MW's taste-shape synaesthesia, we find it very hard to imagine what childhood experience might ultimately explain it.

In instances of unimodal synaesthesia, such as the grapheme-colour variety, sensory signals encoded by the retina-parvocellular channel produce the 'normal' percept of a visual form; at the same time, they somehow evoke an additional percept of visual colour, which is normally produced by signals encoded by the retina-magnocellular channel. Thus, the distinction is more apparent than real, and rests only on a misguided definition of the supposed 'sensory modalities'. If you compare their manifestations to the definition given at the beginning of this chapter, you will easily convince yourself that both multimodal and unimodal synaesthesia in fact obey the same logical scheme—although of course they involve different neural pathways.

Finally, the distinction between *projector* and *associator* synaesthetes (Dixon, Smilek, & Merikle, 2004) refers to the nature of the concurrent experienced after stimulation by the inducer. In some cases described in the literature, and in all the examples that we have mentioned so far, the concurrent is indeed a percept with an apparent location outside of the body. For instance, in the case of MW, who has taste-shape synaesthesia, the experienced shapes are felt on the hand or the face. In grapheme-colour synaesthesia, synaesthetes report coloured photisms that seem to fill the printed letters, or that appear as if there was a transparency bearing a coloured letter on top of the page, or as if they were placed on an invisible screen within arm's reach (see also Grossenbacher & Lovelace, 2001). Individuals reporting such percepts are called projectors. In other cases, synaesthetes report that concurrents are 'in the mind's eye', that is, the inducers evoke a perception-like internal experience rather than a true percept. These experiences are presumably akin to imagery, whereby we can readily bring to consciousness a visual image of a colour, or an auditory image of a sound. These images, however, are experienced internally and not projected onto the outside world. Individuals experiencing internal concurrents are associator synaesthetes. As we see in the next section, the distinction is not merely based on the synaesthetes' reports, but finds strong support also from quantitative laboratory results (Dixon, Smilek, & Merikle, 2004).

Armed with this set of conceptual distinctions, we can now delimit the object of this chapter with greater precision. We will define a true synaesthete as an individual having projective or associator synaesthetic perception of the developmental or the acquired varieties. We believe that pharmacological synaesthesia, although interesting in itself, belongs more to the domains of psychopharmacology and neurology than perception science. And we will not address the distinction between multimodal and unimodal synaesthesia as we believe that this distinction is misleading, as we have argued. Thus, we have now defined a conceptual space based on two binary distinctions: the developmental-acquired distinction and the projector-associator distinction. The first obviously corresponds to two qualitatively different categories of individuals. The second is more likely, in our opinion, to define the polarities of a continuum. We suspect that projectors and associators may not be different in kind, but merely stronger and less strong manifestations of the same general phenomenon. This, however, remains a speculation, and more research and theoretical work is needed before we can reach a firm conclusion.

An especially thorny issue here is that synaesthesia is a first-person experience. Unless she is a synaesthete herself, a synaesthesia researcher is in a situation similar to that of the famous thought experiment of Mary, the blind colour scientist (Jackson, 1982). Mary has trained to become an expert about the physics, physiology, and psychology of colour. Yet, she has never experienced colour directly for she is congenitally blind. Can she truly understand what colour is? Is there a way that she can relate her conceptual knowledge about colour to the object of her science, which remains a subjective experience? These are deep epistemological problems, and a thorough discussion would require writing a second and very different book. Despite this, psychophysical methods exist that can be used to address specific aspects of a synaesthete's subjective experience. We turn to these in the following section.

6.4 Synaesthesia beyond subjective reports

If synaesthesia is a first-person experience, one might be justly sceptical that the reported concurrents are actually perceived. One argument against the idea that synaesthetes are somehow making up surprising stories is the perceived quality of the concurrents, which invariably consist of features such as colours, textures, or simple shapes. If synaesthetes were fabricating these reports, one would not expect such consistency across widely different forms of synaesthesia. In addition, although mapping of concurrents to inducers is highly idiosyncratic, inducer-concurrent associations are remarkably stable within each individual. Baron-Cohen, Harrison, Goldstein, and Wyke (1993) assessed the coloured concurrents evoked by hearing more than 100 words in a group of nine sound-colour synaesthetes. After one year, in a second assessment more than 90 percent of the reported inducer-concurrent associations were identical to those of the original assessment. This finding is particularly striking when considering that participants where not informed that a retest was planned. And a control group of non-synaesthetes retested after only a week yielded 38 percent consistency, a much poorer performance especially if considering that controls *were* informed of the planned retest before taking the measurements.

Clever phenomenological and psychophysical studies also provide evidence of actual perception of the concurrents. Consider Figure 6.2. On the left top panel, you see a matrix of black letters. If you are like the authors of this book, you will tend to see that the lines form separate horizontal rows. This is an instance of visual grouping by proximity, which we have already described in Chapter 4. But if you have digit-colour synaesthesia, things might be different. Suppose that for you, threes and sevens are green, and eights and zeros red. You will see the matrix as we have drawn it on the right top panel, not as we have drawn it on the left. And its organization will no longer depend only on proximity, but also on similarity which supports vertical columns rather than horizontal rows. Ramachandran and Hubbard (2001) have shown that in two grapheme-colour synaesthetes the perceived organization of letter matrices was modified, relative to controls, in the direction predicted by the similarities of their idiosyncratic colour concurrents. And not only this. These authors have shown that one of the two synaesthetes could perform an even more remarkable feat. Consider the bottom left panel of Figure 6.2. Here a triangular pattern formed by H letters is embedded in a field of distractor letters F and P. For non-synaesthetes, these letters are quite hard to distinguish in these conditions as H, F, and P share a prominent vertical edge. As a consequence, the triangular pattern is masked and detecting it requires considerable effort. If you have grapheme-colour projector synaesthesia, however, the Hs might have a different colour from the Fs and Ps, and the configuration might resemble the right bottom panel. The triangular pattern would pop out

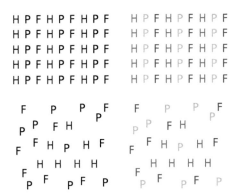

Figure 6.2 Stimuli as in Ramachandran and Hubbard (2001). Top left: A matrix of black letters organizes visually into separate rows. Top right: To a grapheme-colour synaesthete, the letters might organize into columns due to the similarity of the concurrents. Bottom left: Spotting the triangle formed by the Hs is hard due to perceptual similarity to the Fs and Ps. Bottom right: To the synaesthete, the triangle might pop out.

Data from V. S. Ramachandran and E. M. Hubbard, Psychophysical investigations into the neural basis of synaesthesia, *Proceedings of the Royal Society B: Biological Sciences*, 268 (1470), pp. 979-983, DOI: 10.1098/rspb.2000.1576, 2001.

right away, and this will show in quantitative measures of your detection performance, such as percent correct responses and reaction time. This is precisely what Ramachandran and Hubbard report for their synaesthete, suggesting that he really does see something akin to a coloured letter.

Applying the same general principle, in a later paper Ramachandran and Azoulai (2006) have also demonstrated that synaesthetic colour concurrents can, in digit-colour synaesthetes, engender the perception of apparent motion. In this study, the authors have shown a pair of images containing groups of the digits 2 and 5 in black on a white background. The 2s were placed at random positions, whereas the 5s were arranged in a horizontal line. In the first image, the row of 5s was on the left of the image, whereas in the second image it was on the right. The two images were shown in rapid sequence one after the other. When non-synaesthetic controls viewed the sequence, they reported seeing a chaotic ensemble of short movements in all directions. The 2 and 5 digits are almost mirror-reversals of the same shape, and they are hard to distinguish (more or less like the H, F, and P of the previous example). For this reason, controls failed to segregate the lines and simply perceived individual elements displacing from one presentation to the other in random directions. For the synaesthetes, however, the 2s were green and the 5s were red. Thus, a horizontal red line popped-out in two different positions in the first and second image, producing left-to-right apparent motion.

Synaesthetes also report that their unusual experiences are automatic and obligatory, that is, they 'just happen' and cannot be avoided. To investigate this feature of synaesthetic experience experimentally, the paradigm of choice has been the Stroop task (Stroop, 1935). In the Stroop task, participants have to name the colours used to write words. Suppose, for instance, that you see the word 'house' written in red. Your task is to say 'red.' Presumably, you agree that this seems easy to do. But now suppose that the names were themselves names of colours. Then you could have words such as 'blue' that can be written using colours that are either congruent (blue) or incongruent (e.g., yellow) with the name. This situation generates the so-called Stroop effect, that is, naming the colours is easy when the word is congruent with the colour, but much harder when it is incongruent. To convince yourself of this, just take a look at Figure 6.3. Naming the colour of the first letter string (red) is straightforward; something funny instead happens when one tries to name the colour of the second string (blue). The Stroop effect is evidence that reading is automatic and obligatory. When presented with a word, we cannot help accessing the entry in our mental lexicon for that word. This speeds up linking to the name of the ink colour when it is congruent with the word, but slows it down in the other case. The facilitation and corresponding interference can be readily quantified by measuring reaction times and error rates.

Capitalizing on this idea, several studies have created modified Stroop tests to investigate the automaticity of the perception of synaesthetic concurrents. For instance, Dixon, Smilek, Cudahy, and Merikler (2000) studied C., a digit-colour synaesthete. When C. views a black 2, she experiences red; when she views a 7, she experiences yellow, and so on. Dixon and collaborators first mapped C.'s idiosyncratic digit-colour associations. Then they presented her with coloured digits that were either congruent or incongruent with

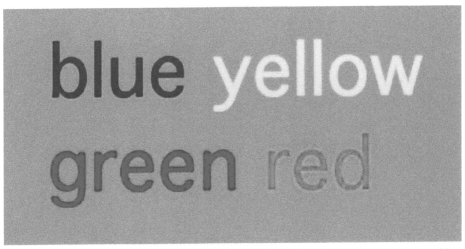

Figure 6.3 The Stroop effect. Try naming the colour used to write the top words; compare with naming the colour used to write the bottom words.

the colours elicited by the written digits. When tested in this manner, C. showed robust Stroop interference. For instance, she was slower when she had to name the colour of a yellow 2, but faster when she had to name the colour of a red 2. This suggests that she could not ignore the coloured photisms even though they were irrelevant to the task, as one would expect if the photism were elicited automatically and in an obligatory fashion. In a later paper, Dixon, Smilek, and Merikle (2004) introduced an additional elegant manipulation to differentiate between projector and associator synaesthetes. They studied 12 digit-colour synaesthetes that were first classified as projectors or associators based on their subjective reports. Each participant performed two modified Stroop tasks. In one task, their job was to name the colour of the ink used to write the digits. In this task, therefore, Stroop interference could be expected when the concurrent photism was incongruent with the actual colour. In the other task, they were asked to name the colour of the coloured photism elicited by the digit. In this second task, therefore, interference could be expected when the actual colour was incongruent with the photism. Their results are summarized in Figure 6.4. Both groups of synaesthetes showed Stroop interference in both tasks, as you can see for yourself in the graph: Congruent trials are faster than incongruent trials in all conditions. However, the interference effect was stronger in the colour naming task for the projectors, and in the photism naming task for the associators. In other words, projectors had a harder time ignoring their photisms, as one would expect if the synesthetic experience of the photisms was stronger, or at least as strong, as the experience than the perception of the actual colours. This is what one would expect if the photisms were actually perceived, and if their spatial location coincided or was near that of the actual colour (spatial interference). Associators, conversely, had a harder time ignoring the colours, suggesting that the synaesthetic experience of the concurrents was

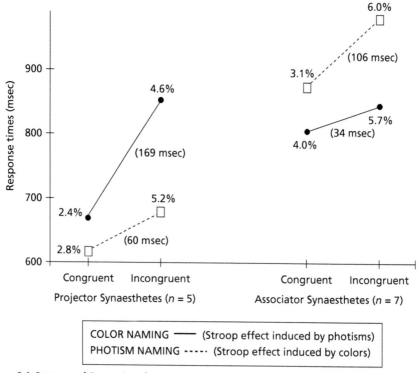

Figure 6.4 Patterns of Stroop interference in projector and associator grapheme-colour synaesthetes.

Adapted from *Cognitive, Affective, and Behavioral Neuroscience*, Not all synaesthetes are created equal: Projector versus associator synaesthetes, 4 (3), Mike Dixon, Daniel Smilek, and Philip M. Merikle, p. 338, Figure 1, doi: 10.3758/CABN.4.3.335, Copyright © 2004, Psychonomic Society, Inc. With permission of Springer.

somehow weaker than the perception of the actual colours, and presumably not spatially coincident.

In conclusion, it is well established that true synaesthetes are not making up their subjective reports. Quite convincing evidence for this conclusion comes from several studies that employed phenomenological, psychophysical, or cognitive-psychological methods. Even stronger evidence, however, comes from studies addressing the neural basis of synaesthesia, as we now see.

6.5 The neural basis of synaesthesia

A major breakthrough in the study of the brain basis of synaesthesia occurred when Paulesu and collaborators (1995) used PET to compare regional blood flow, a measure of brain activation, in a group of speech-colour synaesthetes and controls. Unsurprisingly, they found that in both groups spoken words activated regions classically implied in language processing, such as the superior and middle temporal gyri and the left inferior frontal gyrus. In the synaesthetes, however, they also observed specific activations in several other areas. Critically, they observed activations in the left posterior inferior temporal cortex, an area that has been related to the processing of object colours and in verbal tasks referring to visual features of objects, but not in the primary visual area V1. This study provided the first evidence of actual differences in the pattern of cortical activity of synaesthetes, and located it in higher-level vision centres as well as in other areas, but not in primary sensory cortices. Note further that these results are consistent with a notion of synaesthesia as centrally synthetized perception and argues against interpretations in terms of mental imagery or metaphorical thought.

Other studies have replicated and extended the findings of Paulesu and collaborators. These studies have typically used fMRI or electro-encephalography (EEG) to more precisely locate brain areas related to synaesthesia. For instance, Nunn, Gregory, Brammer, and Williams (2002) observed that colour area V4, but not the primary area V1, was activated by speech in speech-colour synaesthetes. In contrast, no V4 activation was present in controls when hearing speech or when imagining colours in response to spoken words, despite extensive training on the associations reported by the synaesthetes. In a compelling recent report, Holle, Banissy, and Ward (2013) presented movies of faces being touched to individuals with mirror-touch synaesthesia, a condition whereby watching another person being touched evokes touch concurrents. Their data showed two notable effects. First, both synaesthetes and controls exhibited activations in regions SI and SII, the primary and secondary somatosensory areas, when feeling touch but also when watching another person being touched. This striking result is presumably related to the multisensory coding of peripersonal space (see section 7.5) and to mirror systems (see Tutorial 3.1). Second, synaesthetes but not controls exhibited activations of a posterior SII region (in addition to SI and to posterior temporal lobe) when watching touch. Notably, activation of this synaesthesia-specific region correlated with subjective reports of the mirror-touch synaesthesia.

Similar findings have been reported by several other laboratories (Beeli, Esslen, & Jäncke, 2008; Hubbard, Arman, Ramachandran, & Boynton, 2005; Sperling et al., 2006; van Leeuwen, Petersson, & Hagoort, 2010). In addition, evidence for cortical involvement has come from behavioural studies. Palmeri and collaborators (Palmeri et al., 2002) used a clever psychophysical technique to present letters to a letter-colour synaesthete. Using this technique, they were able to provide information about the letters only by binocular or motion cues which are known to be processed after binocular or temporal integration. Even in these conditions, the inducers continued to elicit colour. This is what one would expect if the locus of multisensory interactions involved in synaesthesia was at the level of higher-order cortical visual centres. A later study using transcranial magnetic stimulation (TMS) demonstrated that TMS applied to a right parieto-occipital region disrupted performance in a synaesthetic Stroop task in a group of grapheme-colour synaesthetes (Muggleton et al., 2007). As a whole, therefore, these studies provide evidence for two main conclusions. First, cortical areas appropriate for the modality of the concurrents are activated in synaesthesia. Second, additional areas, including motor areas and other areas in the parietal lobe, are likely to be part of the network that constitutes the neural basis of synaesthesia (Rouw, Scholte, & Colizoli, 2011). As knowledge about the brain of synaesthetes improves, it is hoped that a satisfactory model of the neural causes of the condition will emerge. At present, two main classes of hypotheses have been advanced: those assuming an altered balance of inhibition and disinhibition between different brain centres, and those assuming anomalous cross activation of brain centres.

One of the earliest attempts to model the brain basis in terms of inhibition was the *limbic mediation* hypothesis (Cytowic & Wood, 1982). According to this hypothesis, synaesthesia results from anomalous multisensory integration at the level of the limbic system, and especially in the hippocampus. The hypothesis proposes that critical to synaesthesia is inhibition of the neocortex, which alters the balance between limbic and cortical activation and in turn enhances the awareness of multisensory associations. In support of the hypothesis, measurements of cerebral blood flow (CBF), by means of a non-tomographic xenon inhalation technique, revealed a widespread decrease of CBF at the level of the neocortex during synaesthesia in patient MW (the taste-shape projector which we have already mentioned; Cytowic, 1989). However, due to the technical limitations of the xenon inhalation technique, no direct measurements of limbic activations could be obtained at the time. As discussed earlier, later studies employing more modern techniques, such as PET and fMRI, have revealed that several cortical centres are active during synaesthesia. These observations seem to run counter cortical disengagement.

A quite different proposal is the *disinhibited feedback* hypothesis (Grossenbacher & Lovelace, 2001). In this proposal, synaesthesia stems from disinhibition of feedback from higher-level cortical areas. It is well known that feed-forward neural signals from different sensory channels often converge at the level of higher-level cortical areas, and that these bottom-up projections are reciprocated by top-down signals carried by feedback projections. The hypothesis assumes that, normally, these signals are inhibited in the absence of the bottom-up sensory signals that are normally associated with percepts in the concurrent modality. In synaesthetes, conversely, disinhibition allows these top-down signals to activate centres that are involved in the production of the concurrent percept. As in limbic mediation, therefore, the hypothesis assumes normal connectivity in the synaesthete brain and emphasizes differences in the balance of inhibition across brain centres. In contrast to limbic mediation, however, the disinhibited feedback hypothesis proposes that the difference occur at the level of cortico-cortical connections rather than between the limbic system and the neocortex. As supporting evidence, proponents of the hypothesis cited an early study using event-related potentials (ERPs) to compare the evoked electrical brain activity in grapheme-colour synaesthetes and controls (Schiltz et al., 1999). In this study, significant differences between the two groups could be detected only after 200ms from the presentation of visual graphemes, which was interpreted as evidence that the generation of synaesthetic concurrents depends on feedback signal at a later stage than the initial feed-forward neural signals. However, later studies have found evidence that synaesthesia-related activations can be recorded at much earlier times as we discuss in the next paragraph. Proponents of the hypothesis have also suggested that the ability of some drugs to induce synaesthetic hallucinations in non-synaesthetes might arise precisely due to disinhibition of normally present feedback connections. This proposal, however, is also not free of problems as the phenomenology of pharmacological synaesthesia is quite different from that of developmental synaesthesia.

According to the *cross activation* hypothesis, finally, synaesthesia results from an abnormal excess of anatomical connections between the brain areas responsible for the inducer and the concurrent. The cross-activation hypothesis has been first introduced by Ramachandran and Hubbard (2001) as an account of grapheme-colour synaesthesia. These authors were struck by the fact that the brain region responsible for processing graphemes and digits (often called the 'visual word form area,' or VWFA) is adjacent to the colour processing area V4. In analogy to the *neonatal synaesthesia* hypothesis (Maurer, 1993; see also Baron-Cohen, 1996), they assumed that these areas are densely interconnected at birth, that pruning occurs in normal development, and that such normal pruning does not occur in synaesthetes. Therefore, they suggested that in synaesthetes activation can pass directly from neural mechanisms that code the inducer to brain centres that generated concurrents. Although originally developed for grapheme-colour synaesthesia, the logic of the hypothesis can be extended to other forms (Hubbard, Brang, & Ramachandran, 2011). The cross-activation hypothesis has received substantial empirical support from studies of the functional connectivity in synaesthesia-related brain regions. These studies (Hanggi, Wotrube, & Jancke, 2011; Jäncke & Langer, 2011; Rouw & Scholte, 2007) applied sophisticated statistical techniques to resting-state EEG or MRI data in synaesthetes and controls. Results revealed several important differences in the degree of connectedness between the two groups at relevant cortical centres, as one would expect if abnormal connections were indeed present. In addition, the predictions of the cross-activation theory have been confirmed by magnetoencephalography (MEG), a technique that allows joint measurements of the time course and the cortical location of evoked activity. Using magnetoencephalography, Brang et al., (2010) have been able to demonstrate that colour area V4 becomes active as early as 110ms after presentation of a letter or digit in grapheme-colour synaesthetes. Such early activation in colour-related areas is consistent with the notion that synaesthetic experiences arise through a bottom-up processing stream as proposed by cross activation.

6.6 **Crossmodal correspondences**

Crossmodal correspondences underlie the automatic, spontaneous, and near-universal experience that certain percepts within different perceptual modalities are associated, that is they 'go together.' A striking example is the Maluma-Takete phenomenon (see Tutorial 6.1), a form of spontaneously perceived phonosymbolic association between a linguistic element and a visual shape. However, many other examples have been described. For instance, high-pitched sounds are spontaneously experienced as associated to small and bright objects in higher spatial locations; low-pitched sounds to big dark objects in lower locations (for a review see Spence, 2011). In his classic paper *Die Einheit der Sinne* (The Unity of the Senses), von Hornbostel (1927) described many other such

Tutorial 6.1 The Maluma–Takete phenomenon

When asked to match the nonsense names 'Takete' and 'Maluma' with the two patterns shown in Figure 6.5, most of us have little hesitation. Takete is spiky, Maluma is curvy. Reported about 90 years ago by Wolfgang Köhler, one of the leading figures of the Gestaltist movement, the Takete-Maluma phenomenon is extremely robust. It can be readily observed in informal demonstrations using Köhler's names or variants such as 'Bouba' and 'Kiki' or 'Momo' and 'Zizi.' It is observed in prelinguistic toddlers (Maurer, Pathman, & Mondloch, 2006; Spector & Maurer, 2013), has been replicated in different cultures (Rogers & Ross, 1975; Bremner, et al., 2013), and has been observed not only with explicit choices of names but also with implicit tasks based on reaction times (Westbury, 2005). These results suggest that the multisensory interactions underlying the Takete-Maluma phenomenon occur prior to semantic processing, a conclusion that has attracted enormous interest by linguists and philosophers of language. Non-arbitrary, pre-semantic mappings of sounds to visual percepts potentially ground linguistic symbols to external objects (Harnad, 1990). This may provide a crucial first step in the evolution of language in humans, 'jumpstarting' an iterative process that could then gradually include more arbitrary sound-object pairings (Ramachandran & Hubbard, 2001).

What is the brain basis of the Maluma-Takete phenomenon? It has been reported that name-sound associations are not observable, or greatly reduced, in aphasics—patients with impaired speech production

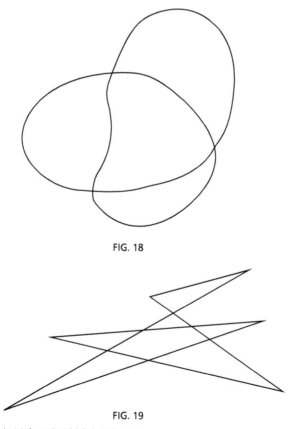

FIG. 18

FIG. 19

Figure 6.5 Which is *Maluma*? Which is *Takete*?
Reproduced from Wolfgang Köhler, *Gestalt Psychology*, Figures 18 and 19, (London, 1929).

due to a brain lesion (Ammon, Moerman, & Guleac, 1977) and in individuals with autism-spectrum disorders (Oberman & Ramachandran, 2008). These reports are consistent with an explanation based on analogies between the arm movements that draw the shapes and the oral movements required to articulate the sounds. The curvy shape requires a continuous round movement of the arm; this has analogues in the presence of consonants that are articulated by a relatively prolonged touching of the lips as well as of vowels, such as 'ou' and 'oh,' that are articulated by forming a circle with the lips. The spiky shape, conversely, requires several abrupt changes of direction and straight lines; this has analogues in the presence of consonants that require the tongue to sharply strike the palate as well as of vowels, such as 'ah,' 'ee,' 'eh,' which are articulated by spreading the lips sideways. To the extent that similar bodily movements underlie the production of visual shapes and auditory sounds, shapes and sound may be associated by *common embodiment* (Kubovy & Minhong, 2014). Common embodiment is consistent with the recent observation that visual shape and luminance affect phonatory behaviour in a task that required participants to utter the vowel 'ah' in response to visual stimuli (Parise & Pavani, 2011). It has been suggested that mirror systems (see Chapter 3) are an obvious candidate neural basis for a common embodiment of auditory speech and visual shapes resembling articulatory gestures (Ramachandran & Hubbard, 2001). The proposal is more than mere speculation: mirror systems have been observed in the monkey analogue of Broca's area, one of the primary lesion sites for aphasia (di Pellegrino, et al., 1992) and are thought to be impaired in autism (Rizzolatti & Fabbri-Destro, 2010).

Plausible as it seems, however, the common embodiment hypothesis is not free of problems. Perhaps the most serious one is that the Maluma-Takete phenomenon readily extends to other sensory channels. For one, there is a robust tendency to associate 'Bouba' and 'Kiki' to unseen curved and spiky three-dimensional shapes that are felt with the hands (Fryer, Freeman, & Pring, 2014). Based on what is known about hand exploratory procedures (Lederman & Klatzky, 2009; see Chapter 4), it is not at all obvious how finger movements in three-dimensions during haptic perception could be considered analogous to visual shapes. In addition, complex food flavours also spontaneously and reliably associate with names such as Maluma and Takete (Gallace, Boschin, & Spence, 2011). For instance, potato chips are more easily paired with Takete whereas brie cheese is more easily paired with Maluma. In this case, there is no obvious movement associated with tasting the foods that could be considered analogous to the articulatory movements for pronouncing the words. Finally, odours reliably associate to visual shapes (Hanson-Vaux, Crisinel, & Spence, 2013). For instance, lemon and pepper scents associate with spiky shapes, whereas raspberry and vanilla associate with curvy shapes. There is simply no way that these associations could be mediated by common motor representations. We might conclude that these findings imply some bad news but also some good news. The bad news is that the Maluma-Takete phenomenon, despite its salience and considerable interest, clearly is still not well understood. More research is needed! The good news, however, is that the phenomenon may prove remarkably useful as a tool for understanding our preferences for foods, drinks, and other products in terms of spontaneous associations, as well as for choosing appropriate names, labels, and packaging—a well-known practical problem in marketing science (Krishna, , Cian & Aydınoğlu, 2017; Irmak, Vallen, & Robinson, 2011).

---

spontaneously perceived associations. In the last 40 years, several studies have documented the perceptual reality of crossmodal correspondences measuring reaction times in information processing tasks with crossmodally corresponding and non-corresponding stimulus pairs (Bernstein & Edelstein, 1971; Evans & Treisman, 2010; Ferrari, Mastria, & Bruno, 2014; Gallace & Spence, 2006; Marks, 2004). These studies generally show that although participants have to classify stimuli in one channel (e.g. small vs large shapes), they fail to ignore the task-irrelevant paired stimuli in the other (e.g. high or low tones). As a consequence, they respond more quickly to crossmodally corresponding pairs and more slowly to non-corresponding pairs, relative to a unimodal baseline. This body of phenomenological observations and quantitative findings underscores the salience and wide practical relevance of crossmodal correspondences, a theme that we will discuss in greater detail in Chapter 10.

Crossmodal correspondences have been used successfully as a tool to study multisensory binding. In an elegant study, Parise and Spence (2009) paired small and large figures with high- or low-pitched sounds, generating pairs that form crossmodal correspondences as well as pairs that do not. They then presented these pairs at slightly different times or slightly different positions in space, and asked participants to give judgments of temporal order or relative position. They found that the precision of discriminative judgments was worse for crossmodally corresponding pairs than for non-corresponding pairs. For instance, participants were less certain of their responses when they had to decide which of a small figure or a high-pitched sound had been presented first, or presented to the left, in comparison to when they had to discriminate between a small figure and a low-pitched sound. This suggests that crossmodally corresponding stimuli were harder to discriminate than crossmodally non-corresponding ones, as one would expect if multisensory binding somehow causes multisensory processes to form perceptual units despite discrepancies in time or space. Using a simplified version of Parise and Spence's paradigm, Bien et al., (2012) have been able to show that TMS applied to the right intraparietal sulcus temporarily eliminated the behavioural effect of crossmodal correspondences. In addition, having observed that crossmodal correspondences correlated with a characteristic increase in a right parietal ERP component, they showed that this EEG marker was also eliminated by TMS at the right intraparietal sulcus. These results suggest that crossmodal correspondences may play a role in the solution to the binding problem, and that a critical brain site for this might be in the right parieto-occipital cortex.

Practical 6.1 Are you a synaesthete?

Although true synaesthesia is relatively rare, most of us have experiences related to synaesthesia, such as certain crossmodal correspondences or phonosymbolic spontaneous associations. Thus, synaesthetic phenomena may be regarded as a continuum rather than all-or-none. If you are at one of the ends of the continuum, chances are you already know the answer to the question in the title. Let's say you are a genuine synaesthete. Then you experience consistent, vivid concurrents whenever you are exposed to the appropriate inducers. Presumably you had already begun to realize that your concurrents are not experienced by everyone in your childhood, and by now you are well aware of your peculiar condition. At some point, perhaps, you might have even wondered whether 'there is something wrong.' If you are a genuine non-synaesthete, conversely, you simply have no first-person experience of any of the phenomena described here. But if you fall somewhere in the middle of the continuum, as does for instance the writer of this chapter, perhaps some of the phenomena described here have felt vaguely familiar. Perhaps you recall having experienced something similar at some point, perhaps something that happens only in very specific, peculiar conditions, or something that you have learned to disregard. Does this make you a synaesthete? Is there a way of assessing where you fall in the hypothetical continuum of synaesthetic phenomena?

Answering the aforementioned questions requires an objective measure of synaesthesia, a goal that is far from trivial for at least two reasons. First, as detailed in this chapter, synaesthesia comes in many kinds. Measures that work for, say, grapheme-colour synaesthesia may not work with other forms. And, of course, two possessors of grapheme-colour synaesthesia may show completely different inducer-concurrent mappings. Second, synaesthesia is subjective and highly unusual. Awareness of synaesthetic percepts varies widely across individuals, synaesthetic percepts are often difficult to describe precisely with words, and these words are bound to remain ambiguous for non-synaesthetes who have never experienced anything of the sort. However, an important step in solving this problem has been made by Eagleman, Kagan, Nelson, and Sagaram (2007). These synaesthesia researchers have created an on-line test battery that attempts to pin down what kind of synaesthesia one might have, and provides an objective, quantitative measure for the most common forms using a clever experimental paradigm. The synaesthesia battery can be viewed on the world-wide-web at http://www.synesthete.org and is freely available in many languages. The results remain anonymous but, for purposes of research, registered synaesthetes can specify the email of a researcher to have the results sent to that address. We will not reproduce all items here—we encourage interested readers to visit the website—but we will try to give a general idea of how the battery works.

The battery takes you through three basic steps. Before taking the tests, a questionnaire will present a set of questions to determine whether you are likely to be a synaesthete, and what kind of synaesthesia you might have. You will asked whether: i) numbers or letters cause you to have a colour experience; ii) weekdays or months have specific colours; iii) weekdays, months, or years have a specific location in space around you; iv) hearing a sound causes you to perceive a colour; v) words trigger tastes; vi) smells trigger tactile sensations. These are believed to be the most common forms of synaesthesia. In addition, many more forms have been reported, such hearing a sound when seeing a movement, sensing a shape when tasting something, or experiencing colour when feeling pain. The questionnaire therefore offers the possibility of reporting other forms that the test taker might have. This preliminary step can be skipped if you are already clear as to what kind or kinds of synaesthetic experiences you have. However, we find it of particular interest for those who are less well versed in the topic. The second step (first if you skipped the initial questionnaire) actually begins the battery. You will be offered a checklist to indicate what kind of synaesthetic associations you experience. Based on which boxes you checked, the program will then select different sections of a questionnaire and different versions of the programs that will test your synaesthesia. After going through the checklist, therefore, you are ready to begin the actual battery.

The initial part of the battery consists of a longer, more detailed questionnaire. The questionnaire has up to 80 questions but only those that are relevant to the taker's form of synaesthesia are actually presented. Thus, the time to complete the questionnaire varies somewhat across takers but in general it can be completed within a few minutes. Questions are meant to identify traits that may be common across synaesthetes, and to gather information about the presence of neuropsychological conditions such as autism, head trauma, or tumours. Text fields for additional comments are also offered to encourage test takers to share their personal experiences. It is hoped that these might provide novel clues about what it is like to be a synaesthete and what might cause the condition. Once the questionnaire has been completed, the program will administer two experimental tests.

The first is an inducer-concurrent consistency test. At the time of the writing of this book, only programs testing colour concurrents are available. This restricts the scope of the battery somewhat. However, it still covers several forms of synaesthesia, such as the grapheme-colour, number-colour, sound-colour, note-colour, timbre-colour varieties. All these are based on the same general idea. The inducing stimulus is presented while takers are offered a computer-controlled colour palette that can be navigated with the mouse. Test takers use the palette to indicate which colour they experience in the presence of the inducer. Over many trials, as well as over successive sessions, data can be collected about the consistency of the responses. A natural metric for the consistency of the responses is the variability in colour space of the selected colours for each inducer. True synaesthetes are expected to choose approximately the same colour every time they see, say, a given letter or sound. Thus, the distances in colour space between their responses will be small. Conversely, weaker synaesthetes are expected to be much more variable.

The second experimental test is a speeded congruency test. Test takers are presented inducers, such as letters, in their previously specified concurrent colours (congruent trials) or in another colour chosen among those they used for other inducers (incongruent). They are asked to respond, as quickly as they can, whether the physically presented colour matched their synaesthetic concurrents. Their response times are recorded as well as their accuracy (a correct response being defined as one that matches the concurrents chosen in the inducer-concurrent congruency test). This test provides an even clearer distinction between true synaesthetes and weaker ones. True synaesthetes are almost perfect, with accuracies well above 95 percent, and relatively fast. Weaker synaesthetes are much less accurate and relatively slower.

Finally, crossmodal correspondences have also attracted considerable attention for their theoretical implications in studies of synaesthesia and of multisensory interactions in general. According to some researchers (Hubbard, 1996; Martino & Marks, 2001; Marks, 2013), crossmodal correspondences are in fact a 'weak' form of synaesthesia. In this view, strong and weak synaesthesia lie at opposite ends of a continuum and share a similar brain mechanism. However, this idea is problematic. For one, the phenomenology of crossmodal correspondences differs from that of true synaesthesia on several scores. True synaesthesia involves a double percept where there should have been only one. Crossmodal correspondences involve two percepts where it is perfectly appropriate that the percepts are two; what is surprising is that the percepts are perceived as associated when there is no obvious reason why they should be. True synaesthesia is, in most cases, unidirectional: Sounds induce colours but colours do not induce sounds. Crossmodal correspondences are instead bidirectional: After hearing high-pitched sounds, one spontaneously pairs them with small objects; after seeing small objects, one spontaneously pairs them with high-pitched sounds. In addition, as argued by Spence (2011), Spence and Deroy (2012), and Deroy and Spence (2013), the most important difference between synaesthesia and crossmodal correspondences is found in their respective relations to learning. Convincing evidence that true synaesthesia is due to learning remains very difficult to obtain (see Box 6.2). At least for some crossmodal correspondences, instead, it seems quite plausible that perceived associations reflect internalized statistical associations in the environment or in the structure of objects and events. For instance, larger objects tend produce lower sounds when bumped into than smaller objects, and small objects are more easily found in higher places as they are lighter to lift. These statistical associations are bound to be far from perfect, but they may well be sufficient to cause implicit learning either over an individual's development or even across the evolutionary history of our species. If this is correct, they may also represent a powerful form of prior knowledge that could be used to solve the binding problem in multisensory perception (see Chapter 4).

Chapter 7

Spaces

7.1 **Multisensory spaces in the mind**

A fly just landed on your left arm. You heard it buzz; then you saw it near your forearm; and then you saw it land and you felt its light weight on your skin. While you were feeling all this, you knew *where* in space all these sensations were happening. The fly was approaching you in the room, then was near your arm and, finally, it was on a definite position on your skin. You can use all of these multisensory stimulations for planning an action—for instance chasing the fly away—because for each of them you know *where* they have occurred. If you are familiar with Euclidian geometry you might even think that your mind gave the fly a set of coordinates—*x, y,* and *z*—in a three-dimensional, continuous space, instantaneously merging the multisensory inputs that contributed to your perception of the insect while it made its way towards your arm. In this space, there are no boundaries: the space near you gradually turns into the space several metres away, without discontinuities. To your introspection, space appears *unitary, continuous,* and *uniform.* What's more, you perceive space in itself, as the medium in which all the sensory events concerning the fly took place; the *empty* container in which all objects lay. This is how most us think of *space.*

In our intuitive notions about space, we are in good company. Many scientists, philosophers, and psychologists of the past shared similar views. George Berkeley (1685–1753), in his celebrated *Essay on a new theory of vision* (1709) argued for a three-dimensional, empty, continuous space. In this medium, distances are simply lines from points in space to points on the fundus of the eye, and as such they are lost in the projection. Isaac Newton (1642–1727) also suggested that space is like a container, that exists independently of objects. Immanuel Kant (1724–1804) proposed that space is something that makes acquisition of all perceptual experiences possible, and yet we do not directly perceive it. While these ideas resonate with our intuitive notion of space, when applied to the perception of space they are mostly wrong. In this chapter, we will show how empirical observations in psychology, cognitive neuroscience, animal behaviour, and neuropsychology converge in challenging these introspective notions. Rather than a unitary and continuous perceptual representation of space, the mind holds a collection of *multiple* spatial representations, each tied to specific multisensory and motor processes.

This chapter lies at the very heart of the notion of multisensory perception that we are proposing in this book. It aims to show that even a concept that may appear as a prerequisite of perception is, in fact, built and structured on the basis of multisensory and motor processes. We will begin with a description of the different ways to obtain information about locations within specific sensory channels. As we shall see, available spatial information differs depending on the form of energy (electromagnetic, mechanical, or chemical) that carries it to receptor arrays. Early unisensory processing of space is therefore also different for the various sensory systems. Next we will re-examine the notion of sensory-motor transformation (already introduced in Chapter 3), to reveal the baffling problem that the brain has to solve when coordinating multiple spatial maps (e.g. eye-centred, hand-centred) to plan and execute an action in space, such as chasing away a fly. Finally, we will examine multisensory integration in three different portions of space: the space occupied by the body, sometimes called *body space* or *personal space*; the space immediately surrounding the body and the space where we can use our hands, termed respectively *peri-personal space* and *reaching space*; and the space located further away from us, termed *extra-personal space*.

7.2 Coding space in different sensory channels

In most real-life situations, multisensory stimulations originate from distinct spatial locations. This book is seen and felt in your hands, the lamp is somewhere else in the room, the ticking clock hangs from the wall, and perhaps the distinct aroma of coffee comes from the mug on the table. Becoming aware of the spatial locations of these objects and events seems a single, effortless mental act. However, the structure of the information available to each of the relevant sensory channels is quite different, as is the type of processing that is needed to represent space. Let us briefly review some of these differences.

In vision, information is carried by patterns of electromagnetic energy (i.e. light in the visible range). The great theorist of perception James J. Gibson, whose work we discussed in Chapter 1, argued that such patterns are best described by the notion of the *ambient optic array*: the set of solid angles formed by surfaces in the environment to a given viewpoint (Gibson, 1979). Gibson's key idea was that the spatio-temporal structure of the optic array is not arbitrary, but depends in specific ways on the structure of the world. Figure 7.1 illustrates an example of ambient optical array for an observer sitting in the centre of a room. From this specific viewpoint, the observer's eye (here magnified for explanation purposes) 'sees' various portions of the surrounding environment: some parts of the floor, walls, and ceiling, some parts of the table and lamp, and some parts of a bush and a lorry through the open window. Figure 7.1 also highlights four solid angles (A, B, C, and D), together with their corresponding visible surfaces (A', B', C', and D') and their projection onto the retina (A″, B″, C″, and D″). The fact that A is higher in the optical array relative to B, specifies a possible vertical relationship between surface A' (the wall above the window) and surface B' (the wall below the window). Note, however, that the optical array is potentially ambiguous, as exemplified by the surfaces resting on the flat ground (C' and D'). Here, the vertical arrangement of solid angles C and D should be interpreted as a difference in distance, not elevation. Nonetheless, it is clear that some aspects of the structure of the environment are preserved in the optic array.

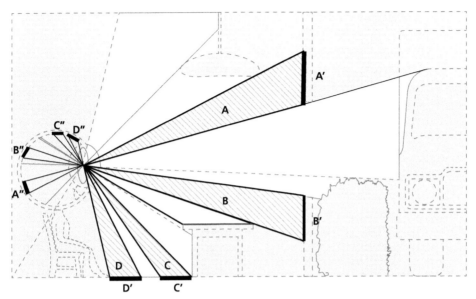

Figure 7.1 Gibson's ambient optic array as sampled by an eye placed at a viewpoint. Uninterrupted lines and white regions indicate visible surfaces and ground regions; dashed lines and shaded areas indicate the portions of the array that are not visible. For explanation purposes, four visible 'solid angles' (A, B, C, and D) are also emphasized, with the corresponding surfaces in the environment (A', B', C', and D'), and projections on the retinal surface (A″, B″, C″, and D″). Adapted from James J. Gibson, *The ecological approach to visual perception*, 1979.

Furthermore, if the viewpoint moves (e.g. the observer stands up), the optic array will dynamically change over time, providing further information about the relative position of surfaces. Traditionally, perception textbooks refer to these as instances of static and motion-related spatial information as *monocular depth cues*. The most important aspect to appreciate here is that spatial information about visual directions, and to some extent even about relative distances, can be coded by the pattern of neuronal activations at the level of the retina (in the example: A″, B″, C″, and D″). Thus, spatial information in the optic array will be represented by a spatial map in retinal coordinates—a *retinotopic map*.

In tactile signals, information is carried by patterns of mechanical energy (forces acting on locations on the skin), not by light. In addition, these patterns originate from objects that are in direct contact with the skin, such that there is no need of a medium carrying information through the environment. (Incidentally, this is the reason for the traditional distinction between vision as a 'distal' sense and touch as a 'proximal' sense.) With regard to spatial information, however, there are strong analogies with the visual case as some information about locations of external objects is preserved in the spatio-temporal pattern of mechanical events on the skin. For instance, suppose that two crabs pinch you on two different toes while you are walking on the beach. If pinched toe A is left of pinched toe B, then you can also infer that crab A' was left of crab B' in the sand. In some respect, we can say that the spatial layout of the stimulated regions of skin is informative about the spatial layout of the environment. Yet, as already explained for the case of vision, spatial information on the skin may not be sufficient to reconstruct the spatial layout of objects in the environment. In the case of touch, an important source of confusion is the fact that the body can adopt many different postures, altering spatial relations between different skin regions. Imagine, for instance, that you were picking up a shell next to your foot when one crab pinched you on one finger and the other pinched you on one toe. Although the receptors on your fingers and your toes are almost two metres away in terms of skin surface, you might still perceive the sources of pain as hidden next to each other under the sand. The reason why you perceived the veridical spatial relationship between the crabs has to do with your ability to integrate 'skin space' (a *somatotopic map*) with representation of spatial positions of your body parts relative to the environment—that is, your brain knows that your right hand moved next to your right foot (we will return to this topic in section 7.3).

But consider now the case of information carried by chemical energy, the 'olfaction' sense. Here the situation changes radically. Although the chemical particles that convey the coffee aroma originate from a defined location in the environment (the mug on the table), they diffuse in all directions under the action of air currents. In this diffusion process no spatial information is preserved. When odorant molecules travel up the nostrils to reach the olfactory epithelium, activation of the receptors will not reflect a spatial map. Indeed, we know that maps of neuronal activation in olfactory ganglion cells change as a function of odour type, not odour location.

Finally, let us consider spatial encoding for hearing. Auditory information is again carried by mechanical energy, but in contrast to somatosensation, sound-emitting objects need not be in contact with your body: information is carried by pressure waves propagating through an elastic medium (typically, air). Sound waves, like odours, diffuse in all directions in the medium and therefore they contain no information about the direction of the source relative to the receiver. The signal arriving at the tympanic membrane is completely described by temporal modulations of pressure, with no spatial dimension retained. Indeed, when we look into the cochlea we discover that the layout of the receptors is by no means related to the position of the sound source in the environment, and reflects instead the temporal changes of the pressure wave as a function of time (i.e. the temporal frequency of the sound). Sounds with similar temporal frequencies, for instance the C and D notes played on the same octave of the piano keyboard (corresponding approximately to frequencies of 262 Hz and 294 Hz, respectively) will be encoded by nearby populations of receptors. In contrast, sounds that are farther apart in terms of temporal frequencies, for instance a C in the central octave and the same note in the upper octave (corresponding to 262 Hz and 523 Hz, respectively), will be encoded by cochlear receptors that are farther apart. Researchers call this a *tonotopic map* to imply that the spatial arrangement of receptors on the cochlea reflects tonal differences—not the layout of sound sources in the environment.

Yet we can perceive auditory space and we can very roughly know the origin of an odour. How does the brain achieve these spatial representations whose construction does not start in the sensory epithelium? We answer this question by presenting the case of hearing. When it comes to reconstructing the location of sound sources the brain extracts spatial information from *cues* that originate from the interaction between the sound source, the head and the external ears (Blauert, 1997; King, Schnupp, & Doubell, 2001). An important first cue results from the spatial separation between the two ears, which determines different times of arrival of the sounds at each ear as a function of auditory source position. A sound on the right side of the head, for instance, reaches the right ear before the left one, whereas a sound directly in front of us reaches the two ears approximately at the same time. Although this temporal difference at the two ears is in the order of fractions of milliseconds, the brain uses this tiny temporal gap to estimate sound source location. Another important cue depends on the fact that the ears are separated by a physical barrier: the head. A sound on the right side of the head is louder at the right than the left ear. Again, the brain takes advantage of this intensity difference at the two ears to estimate sound location. Finally, the constituent frequencies of the incoming sound are intensity-modulated as a function of their direction of arrival on the external ear. These three sources of spatial information are known as 'interaural temporal difference cues', 'interaural intensity difference cues', and 'spectral cues', respectively. What is very important to appreciate here is that all these auditory cues change whenever the head changes position with respect to the environment, effectively anchoring auditory space to the position of the head.

In sum, spatial encoding in the different sensory systems operates by very different mechanisms. In vision, the pattern of activity on the retina already carries spatial information on the arrangement of visual events in the environment. As we anticipated in Chapter 1, this retinotopic organization is kept in many brain structures along the visual pathway. In touch, some of the spatial layout of the stimuli touching the body is captured by the ordered layout of touch receptors on the skin. This somatotopic organization is also maintained in the somatosensory pathway all the way to the cerebral cortex. Finally, for the cases of olfaction and hearing, there is no spatial information in the topography of receptors on the sensory epithelia (the olfactory epithelium and the cochleae, respectively). Space for these sensory mechanisms is somewhat of a reconstruction. In the case of hearing, for instance, it is built from auditory cues that the brain extracts from the spatial position of the sounds with respect to the head and ears.

One important aspect to remember is that this different way of capturing spatial information has consequences in terms of spatial resolution for the different sensory systems. Although the ability of the brain to infer auditory space based on auditory cues is truly amazing, the resulting spatial map is considerably less accurate than the one that can be obtained through vision or touch. Under optimal hearing conditions, humans can discriminate the position of a sound with a precision of a couple of degrees (Perrott & Saberi, 1990; 1 degree is approximately the size of your thumb nail, when your arm is fully extended in front of you). By contrast, the spatial acuity for the visual modality can

be as accurate as 0.01 degrees (Wandell, 1995) and the spatial acuity for the tactile modality is also in the order of fractions of degrees (Lederman & Klatzky, 2009). In brief, as
originally remarked by the psychologist William James more than a century ago, space is
'discernible in each and every sensation, though more developed in some than in other'
(James, 1890, p.135–6).

7.3 Merging multisensory spaces: the multiple coordinates problem

Dealing with the different spatial precisions of the multiple sensory systems is only part of
the problem. When attempting to merge multisensory information across modalities, the
brain has to solve a much harder task—the various sensory signals are all initially mapped
in different *spatial coordinates*.

To understand this problem, consider the simple situation of a chair in a room, as seen
from the perspective of three different observers (Figure 7.2a). Because each observer is
looking at the scene from his own point of view, if you were to ask them about the position
of the chair they would give you different responses. Observer A would say that the chair
lies approximately 30 degrees to his right, observer B would report the chair to be straight
ahead of him, and observer C would remark that the chair is approximately 30 degrees
on his left. Each observer is correct, because each observer is using a different system of
spatial coordinates, *centred* on their viewpoints.

Now suppose your aim is to draw the position of the chair with respect to a map of the
room, based on the answers from the observers. To achieve this goal, you would have
to know exactly where each observer stands in the room, and then use this information
to interpret and combine their different responses. In doing so, you would be making a
coordinate transformation, bringing the position of the chair as seen from the various
observers into a new system of coordinates, the room. If this coordinate transformation
is successful, you would end up knowing the position of the chair in a system of coordinates that is independent of the view-point of the different observers. Next, imagine
you have the different aim of guiding person C to the chair. In this different scenario,
knowing the exact position of each observer in the room is quite irrelevant, and the only
important information is where the chair is placed in the single spatial coordinate system
of observer C.

Now substitute the different observers with different sensory mechanisms and you will
be able to appreciate the complex spatial task that our brain continuously solves when
we use our senses to reconstruct the spatial layout of the environment. In Figure 7.2b, we
present the situation in which a mobile phone is ringing and vibrating in the left hand of
an observer, while the person's head is oriented to the left and his eyes are gazing directly
at the phone. The hand, the head, and the eyes are like the different observers described in
the previous example. The vibration originating from the mobile phone is stimulating the
palm of the left hand directly. For the head, the orientation of which defines the position
of ears with respect to the sound, the sound source is located on the right. For the eyes,

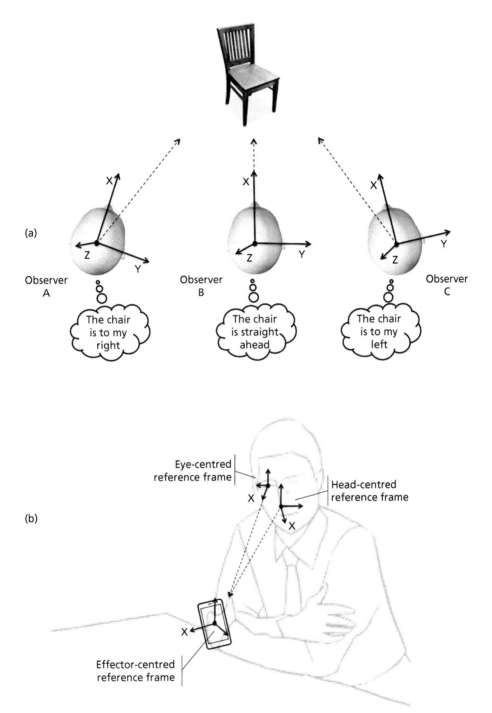

Figure 7.2 The coordinate transformation problem. (a) From the viewer-centred perspective of each observer the chair is in different locations with respect to the body. (b) From the perspective of each sensory channel the ringing and vibrating mobile phone has different coordinates.

the mobile phone is placed exactly along the line of gaze, in the portion of maximal retinal acuity (the fovea). In other words, like the different observers the different sensory systems represent the location of the phone in different coordinates: hand-centred (touch), head-centred (hearing), and eye-centred (vision).

How does the brain deal with this complexity? Two main accounts have been proposed and are currently under scrutiny in cognitive science. The first account suggests that in order to deal with the multiple coordinates of the incoming inputs the brain must convert the different types of spatial information into a *common reference frame* (Cohen & Andersen 2002). Such common representation could prove particularly useful for representing the spatial location of multisensory events in the environment. Plus, it may facilitate movement coordination across the different effectors (e.g. the eyes, the hand, the foot). However, building of a common reference frame would surely take time and would likely impose a continuous load on the cognitive system. The alternative perspective is that *multiple reference frames coexist,* and they concurrently influence behaviour depending on the current task (Buchholz, Jensen, & Medendorp, 2011). This view does not deny the importance of coordinate transformations, which remain always crucial when combining information across different reference frames. However, it proposes that the brain holds parallel representations of space, weights their appropriateness for the on-going scopes, and integrates them only when necessary. In this second account no common reference frame is necessarily built. One main advantage of this alternative perspective resides in its flexibility: the brain would use different estimates of the position of events in space, depending on the behavioural scopes and the past sensory-motor contingencies (i.e. previous co-occurrences of sensory and motor events; Heed, Buchholz, Engel, & Röder, 2015).

We now know that one key brain structure involved in handling the multiple coordinates for the different sensory systems is the posterior parietal cortex. Studies in non-human primates and other animals have shown that neurons in this brain region respond to different sensory channels and can represent space in different references frames (Andersen, Snyder, Bradley, & Xing, 1997). In addition, damage to this region in humans affects the ability to combine sensory and motor information. For instance, in the neuropsychological syndrome termed 'optic ataxia', brain-damaged patients are unable to plan and execute accurate movements to visual targets with their arms, despite the integrity of their visual and motor systems. The common interpretation of this disorder is that the lesion in the parietal lobe hampers the correct coordinate transformation required to bring the hand towards a target defined in eye-centred coordinates. Whether the parietal lobe holds a common reference frame or instead coexisting parallel reference frames, however, is a matter of debate. In favour of the common reference account, neurophysiological studies that showed that neurons in the parietal cortex can encode stimulus location regardless of the planned action (e.g. eye movement or hand-reach) or the stimulus channel (e.g. vision or hearing). These neurons have been documented in a fissure of the parietal cortex termed the intra-parietal sulcus (Cohen & Andersen 2002). At the same time, however, many neurons in the parietal cortex show responses that are suggestive of 'intermediate' reference frames, which may reveal a flexible and changeable spatial coding in these cortical neurons (Heed, Buchholz, Engel, & Röder, 2015).

Whatever the solution the brain finds when dealing with the problem of multiple spatial coordinates of multisensory events, it should now be clear that the introspective sensation of a unified and seamless space around us is—at best—only one of the possible spatial representation available. In the remaining sections of the present chapter, we develop the notions of multiple spatial coordinates starting from the case of space occupied by our own body, that is, of *personal* space.

7.4 **Personal space**

Personal space represents a paradigmatic example of the challenge posed by coordinate transformations in space processing. Whenever an event stimulates your skin (which is the physical boundary of your personal space), two frames of reference are potentially at play. The first frame of reference is *skin-based* and represents the position of the source of the tactile signal relative to your body surface; for instance, you know that something bit you on the dorsum of the right hand. The second frame of reference is *environment-based* and represents the position of the source relative to your surroundings; for instance, you learn that there was an insect in a certain position in the room. Thus, depending on which spatial reference frame is used, you learn either something about the state of the body (my skin was touched) or something about the state of the environment (there is something out there that touched me). In this respect, all somatosensory events occurring in personal space convey two pieces of information at once. The challenge of coordinate transformation refers to the need of managing the two frames of reference according to task demands. Coordinate transformations in personal space, for instance, can be difficult because the body is almost always in motion.

We continuously change posture and move in the environment; when a leg is moved forward to make a step or an arm is stretched to the side to grab an object, the relationship between personal space and external space changes. This can create conflicts between spatial coordinates in different reference frames. For instance, if the right hand crosses the midline to grab something on the left side, a tactile signal on the index finger of that hand would be coded 'on the right' with respect to skin coordinates, but 'on the left' with respect to a reference frame centred on the trunk. (Note that such a conflict does not emerge when the same tactile stimulus is delivered to the right hand resting on the right side of the body, i.e. in the typical anatomical posture.) As we shall see, this simple manipulation based on crossing the hands has proved especially useful for investigating changes in the spatial coding of touch, when examined in comparison with conditions with the hands uncrossed. The experimental elegance of this crossed vs uncrossed comparison lies on the fact that a tactile stimulus delivered at a specified location on the hand (e.g. the index finger) stimulates exactly the same patch of skin *regardless* of hand posture. Hence, any change in its processing must reflect the outcome of integration processes occurring centrally in the brain, after the position of the tactile stimulus has been combined with sensory (proprioceptive, visual), motor signal, or with memory information, to specify the different posture of the hands in space.

Early studies on the effects of crossing the hands have revealed that dealing with this conflict of coordinates can be difficult. For instance, imagine a situation whereby the right and left hands are touched in rapid succession, and participants are asked to decide which of the two hands was stimulated first. This type of judgement is known as the temporal order judgement task (TOJ; to learn more about this task see Chapter 8 on multisensory temporal processing), and in this case it requires to correctly code the location of the tactile signal. Seminal studies adopting this approach have shown that participants can resolve which hand was touched first even when the interval between tactile stimuli is as short as 30–70 ms. However, precise temporal order judgments occur only when the hands are in their typical body side (i.e. the left hand on the left, the right hand on the right). By contrast, if the hands are crossed, judging the order of the tactile signals becomes considerably harder. The interval between touches has to be 120–300 ms for participants to be able to solve which hand was touched first (Yamamoto & Kitazawa, 2001; Shore, Spry, & Spence, 2002). This cost of crossing the hands can be attributed to the fact that participants need to resolve which frame of reference (skin-based or trunk-based) is appropriate, before they can make their response.

Interestingly, vision plays a key role in modulating which representation is available for coding the location of touch, even when the visual input is entirely irrelevant for the task. Individuals who are blind from birth, and hence had no visual experience when developing personal space representations, show no cost of crossing the hands when performing a TOJ task (Röder, Rösler, & Spence, 2004). Instead, individuals who were sighted at birth and then lost sight in adulthood (i.e. late blind), show a comparable cost to that of typically sighted adults. This suggests that the cognitive mechanism responsible for updating the spatial coordinates of touch across reference frames is based on links established early in life between tactile and visual space. In early blind adults, for whom no such link develops, touch is processed by default in the skin-based reference frame, regardless of where the body is in space. Instead, in late blind adults, the long experience with the visual world calibrates spatial coding of touch is such that environment-based representation, which is largely based on visual inputs, is automatically activated. Remarkably, this interplay of different reference frames persists even when even vision is no longer available.

That vision is key in building representations of external space for touch does not imply that it is the only source of spatial information that can influence this process. Congenitally blind people would also be able to hit a mosquito landing on their body, and we can re-orient quite well towards objects that touched us on the back—a region of space that we never see. Maps of external space can also be built in the absence of vision, most likely using reference frames that we use when planning motor actions towards objects in space (Heed & Röder, 2011). One fine example of the importance of motor maps comes from a study based again on the TOJ paradigm (Hermosillo, Ritterband-Rosenbaum, & van Donkelaar, 2011). In each trial of this experiment, participants moved their hands from uncrossed to crossed postures, or vice versa. Tactile stimuli for the TOJ task were delivered to the two hands, just before the crossing/uncrossing action occurred. The rationale for delivering the tactile signals precisely at that time is that the brain computes a plan for the imminent action just before movement begins (motor planning). The motor plan contains, in particular, the end-point of the movement in space. What Hermosillo and colleagues found was that judging the correct temporal sequence of tactile stimuli delivered just before the hands changed from uncrossed to crossed posture was particularly difficult. By contrast, performance was better when tactile stimuli were delivered in the crossed to uncrossed condition. Thus, it seems that spatial coordinates for motor planning influenced the localization of the tactile signals.

Thus, updating spatial information across body postures is not as easy as it may seem. To convince yourself of the reality of this conclusion, you may want to try the Japanese illusion and the other phenomena that we describe in Practical 7.1. When experimenting with the Japanese illusion, for instance, you will notice that your ability to identify which finger was touched improves if you are allowed enough time to respond. Thus, one may argue that the brain needs time to change from one reference frame to another, and that under time pressure the process of conversion is not complete. Alternatively, it could be suggested that the brain has to juggle multiple concurrent spatial maps, and this creates confusion and leads to errors unless enough time is allowed. In these two questions, you should recognize the echo of the debate that we anticipated earlier, i.e. the possibility that the brain deals with multiple coordinates by slowly progressing towards a common reference frame vs the possibility that concurrent parallel references frames are always available and need relative weighting and coordination. In either case, it is clear that dealing with multiple spatial coordinates across sensory systems requires time.

Practical 7.1 Fooling perception with body postures

Two simple illusions can reveal how unusual body postures can fool perception and motor control. The first illusion is the so-called Japanese illusion (Burnet, 1904; Van Riper, 1935), which can be easily reproduced with the help of another person; it is illustrated in the top panel of Figure 7.3. To try the illusion extend your arms in front of you, crossing the right hand over the left one (Fig. 7.3). Rotate your wrists until the thumbs of both hands point downwards, then intertwine the fingers of the hands (Fig. 7.3b). Now, bring the joined hands towards your chest (Fig. 7.3) and keep rotating the hands until they are right in front of your face (Figure 7.3). Now ask the friend to point to one of your fingers, without touching it, and try to lift the indicated finger immediately. The complexity of this task should be apparent, as typically evidenced by a sense of frustration related to difficulty of moving exactly the finger we intended to move. The reason for this difficulty has precisely to do with the fact that the multiple crossing of the hands and fingers imposed by the Japanese illusion procedure result in a very unfamiliar posture.

Another interesting phenomenon, often used to reveal the difficulty of the cognitive system to take into account atypical postures, is the so-called 'Aristotle's illusion'. You can try it straight away after reading the following instructions. First, chose one hand and cross the middle finger over the index, as shown in lower panel of Figure 7.3. (You should also try crossing the middle and ring finger, as the illusory effects are typically stronger). Next, choose a small spherical object, such as a marble, or the small rubber at the back of your pencil, or even the tip of your nose. Close your eyes and gently rub the spherical object with the fingertips of the crossed fingers, making small circular movements. After a short while you should

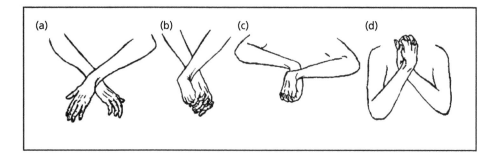

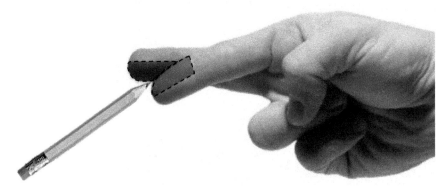

Figure 7.3 Illusions caused by unusual postures. (upper row) The sequence of hands and finger crossing that prepares the Japanese illusion; (bottom row) Aristotle's illusion, shown here with the crossing of the index and middle finger. The two shaded areas on the fingertips identify skin regions that are typically separate and have become adjacent only due to the atypical posture.

start experiencing the bizarre sensation that the touched object splits into two distinct ones. Now try a related experience. Uncross your middle and index finger, bring them in contact with one another, take one pencil and touch the skin between the two fingertips with the pencil tip without looking at your hand. In this condition, two different finger are touched and yet you should clearly perceive a single object. Now, cross again your middle and index finger, and repeat the experience. As before, the pencil will touch two distinct fingertips, but now you should experience the unusual sensation that the tip of the pencil has doubled.

The origin of these illusory sensations is easy to explain. It has to do with the difficulty of our brain of taking into account the highly unusual crossed-finger posture when processing tactile sensations (Benedetti, 1986; 1988). When the tip of the pencil touches the crossed fingertips, it stimulates regions of your skin that are typically on opposite sides of the two fingers (see grey-shaded areas on the fingertips). Thus, unless the brain effectively takes into account the postural change of the fingers (here conveyed only through proprioception because you are not supposed to look at your hands during these illusions), the somatosensory experience is more compatible with two distinct objects in the environment, rather than a single one. By contrast, when the pencil touches the uncrossed fingers, the stimulated skin regions are typically adjacent in external space coordinates. Hence, the brain resolves the perceptual experience as most likely related to a single object.

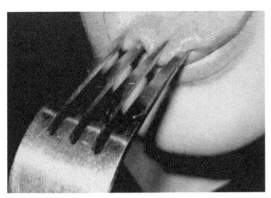

Figure 7.4 The illusion of the deformed fork.
Reproduced from Marc Egeth, Two New Illusions of the Tongue, *Perception*, 37 (8), pp. 1305-1307, doi: 10.1068/p6016 Copyright © 2008, SAGE Publications. Reprinted by Permission of SAGE Publications, Ltd.

Now try a final illusion (Egeth, 2008), most appropriate for entertainment during dinner and based on similar principles. Take a metal fork and invite a friend to stick out his tongue for this experience. Gently adjust the tip of your friend's tongue above and below the central prongs of the fork, as shown in Figure 7.4. Very likely he will report that the fork changed shape, with the central prongs deformed in the direction of the movements experienced on the tongue. Once again, atypical posture of a body part can lead our perception astray, affecting the perception of unseen objects.

Azañón and Soto-Faraco (2008) hypothesized that skin-based coordinates would be available first, whereas environment-based coordinates would emerge over time. To test this hypothesis, they introduced four different temporal gaps between the cue and target (30, 60, 180, and 360 ms). The results confirmed that for shorter cue-target intervals, a touch at the hand facilitated processing of visual targets that appeared on the anatomical side of the stimulated body part. For instance, if the right hand (resting in the left hemispace) was touched, visual discrimination was favoured for the LEDs placed in the right hemispace—i.e. the anatomical hemispace where the stimulated hand typically is (Figure 7.5). By contrast, when long temporal gaps were used (180 ms or more), tactile cues facilitated visual targets in the portion of space occupied by the hand. Thus, the stimulation on the right hand now favoured visual discrimination for the LEDs in the left hemispace. This important result has now been replicated and extended by several other studies (e.g. Overvliet, Azañón, & Soto-Faraco, 2011; Rigato et al., 2013; Soto-Faraco & Azañón, 2013) and the emerging pattern indicates that change of reference frame from skin-based coordinates to external-space coordinates likely starts within the first 100 ms and it is completed by 190 ms post-stimulus (Heed & Azañón, 2014). While this process is surely fast, occurring in the range of hundreds of milliseconds, it is clearly not instantaneous, and documents the effort that our brain puts into a seemingly trivial task as crossing the hands into unusual postures.

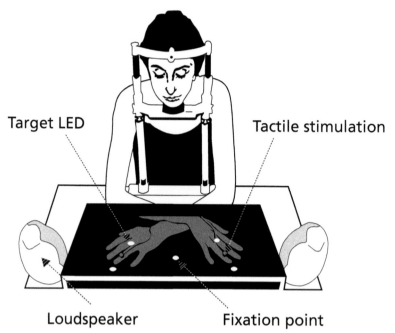

Target LED

Tactile stimulation

Loudspeaker

Fixation point

Figure 7.5 The set-up used by Azañón and Soto-Faraco (2008). White discs indicate the position of the LEDs (visual targets) for the up-down discrimination (a single LED illuminated in any given trial). The stimulators attached to the ring fingers indicate where tactile stimulation was delivered (a single hand was touched in any given trial). Loudspeakers served to mask the noise made by the tactile stimulators, so that their location could not be identified through hearing.

Reprinted from *Current Biology*, 18 (14), Elena Azañón and Salvador Soto-Faraco, Changing Reference Frames during the Encoding of Tactile Events, pp. 1044-49, doi: 10.1016/j.cub.2008.06.045, Copyright © 2008 Elsevier Ltd., with permission from Elsevier.

7.5 **Peripersonal space**

The distinction between personal space and extra-personal space is intuitive, as an iden-tifiable boundary exists between them (the skin). However, multisensory research has revealed that even the space beyond the boundary of our body is not continuous. Two examples will make clear two important distinctions within extra-personal space. First, not all the space around us can be reached and manipulated directly. Researchers have shown that people have a very precise idea of objects within reaching distance as op-posed to those which are not (Carello et al., 1989). This region of extra-personal space has been termed *reaching space*. As we shall see, reaching space can be updated when we handle a tool that extends reachability beyond the length of our limbs. Second, the space in the immediate vicinity of our body seems to possess a special status. Sharp objects or crawling insects trigger very different emotional and behavioural reactions when they are near our body, say less than 30 cm, compared to when they are farther away from it. This area of extra-personal space, so proximal to our own body that anticipates a potential tactile percept, has been termed *peripersonal*—literally the space near the person, from the combination of the Ancient Greek word for 'about, around' (*peri*) and the word 'personal'. An object in peripersonal space is also within reaching space; whereas an object within reaching distance is not necessarily near the body. Here will focus on peripersonal space, and expand the concept of reaching space in Tutorial 7.1.

The notion that the space immediately near the body has a different status with respect to the rest of extra-personal space is not new. It first appeared in the scientific literature in the 1950s when scientists studying animal behaviour started observing animals inside cages. The Swiss zoologist Heini Hediger (1908–1992) observed that when an animal approached another, there seemed to exist an invisible boundary around the approached animal (also described like an imaginary bubble by von Uexküll (1957). Trespassing beyond this boundary triggered avoidance or defence actions in the approached animal. Hediger (1955) termed this region the *flight zone*. Furthermore, the notion that the space immediately near the body has a special status has also been developed in the domains of social psychology, psychology of personality, and anthropology, giving rise to a discipline called *proxemics* (Hall, 1966; Sommer, 1959). The basic intuition of this discipline is that different cultures and individuals develop an untold consensus as to which interpersonal distance is appropriate in different circumstances. Somewhat similar to the case of caged animals, violating that untold space around each other's body triggers emotional and behavioural reactions.

Starting from the 1980s, however, neurophysiologists, psychologists, and cognitive neuroscientists offered an entirely new perspective on this space proximal to the body. Recordings directly from single neurons in the posterior parietal cortex of the macaque monkey, Finnish neurophysiologists Juhani Hyvärinen and Antti Poraren observed cells that were selectively activated by stimulation on the skin. This somatosensory response of the neuron was largely expected. To their surprise, however, a subgroup of these neurons also responded *before* the tactile stimulation begun. They were active also when a visual stimulus approached the region of skin that triggered the tactile response of the neuron. They soon realized that this was not the trivial consequence of some unwanted tactile stimulation, such as air movements caused by the approaching object. Indeed, hiding the approaching stimulus from the animal's view (while leaving everything else constant) eliminated the anticipatory neuronal response. Even more interesting, they observed that the neuronal response was influenced by the distance between the visual stimulus and the region of skin that evoked the cell response when touched. Hence, there are multisensory neurons that respond both to touch signals on a region of skin, and to visual signals approaching the same body part (Hyvärinen & Poraren, 1974).

To avoid conceptual confusions with the notion of space proposed by proxemics, this space near the body coded at the level of single neurons was termed 'peripersonal' by Rizzolatti and colleagues (Rizzolatti, Scandolara, Matelli, & Gentilucci, 1981). To fully appreciate the distinctive properties of these cells, it is useful to consider the example depicted in Figure 7.6, taken from a classic study conducted in the macaque monkey by the neurophysiologists Michael Graziano and Charlie Gross (Graziano & Gross, 1993). In their study, neuronal recording was conducted from a structure deep in the brain

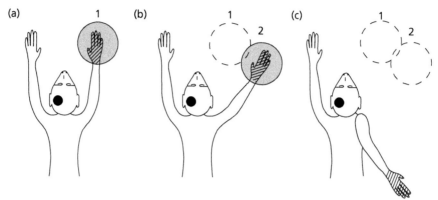

Figure 7.6 Peripersonal space in the monkey. Schematic representation of regions of visual and somatosensory space that affect the response of a putative visuo-tactile neuron. The grey circles indicate the 'visual receptive field' of the neuron; the grating on the hand indicates the 'tactile receptive field'. Note that the position of the visual receptive field moves from region 1 to region 2 as the hand changes position (compare A and B). When the hand is behind the back (C), visual stimulation within regions 1 or 2 no longer activates the neuron. The black circle indicates that single cell recording of neuronal response occurred in the left brain-hemisphere of the monkey, hence the visual and tactile receptive fields on the right side of the animal.

Reproduced from *Experimental Brain Research*, 97 (1), Michael S. A. Graziano and Charles G. Gross, A bimodal map of space: somatosensory receptive fields in the macaque putamen with corresponding visual receptive fields, pp.96–109, doi: 10.1007/BF00228820, Copyright © 1993, Springer-Verlag. With permission of Springer.

called putamen. In Figure 7.6, the skin region that activates the cell when stimulated by touch is indicated by the grating on the right hand of the animal—this is the *tactile* receptive field. In contrast, the grey circle schematically indicates the region of visual space that can evoke a response in the same neuronal cell—the *visual* receptive field. In panel A, the circle is located in the region identified by number 1, around the animal's hand. Importantly, the region of visual space that triggers the cell response changes when the hand is moved to a different location (as in panel B, in which visually evoked responses now occur for stimuli presented in the region identified by number 2). Thus, the visual receptive field of these neurons change with body posture, as if it were anchored to the position of the tactile receptive field on the hand. Neurophysiologists describe this visual receptive field as 'hand-centred'. Finally, if the hand is moved away from view (panel C), none of the regions of space that previously triggered the responses of the neuron when visually stimulated are effective.

Neurons with similar responses have now been documented in several brain regions (parietal cortex: Graziano & Gross, 1994; MacKay & Crammond, 1987; Duhamel, Colby, & Goldberg, 1991; premotor cortex: Rizzolatti, Scandolara, Matelli, & Gentilucci, 1981; putamen; Graziano & Gross, 1995). What is important to note here is that these brain regions are part of a network for planning and executing object-oriented actions in the environment. This is already indicative that encoding of peripersonal space in bi-modal neurons could be related to action planning, because it would allow anticipatory interactions between the body and the visual space immediately around it. To fully appreciate the importance of this multisensory coding for nearby objects it is useful to recall what we said in section 7.2 about coordinate transformations for multisensory processing and motor control. All visual objects are initially coded in terms of spatial coordinates of the retina. However, retinal coordinates are often of little use if one needs to act quickly. If you have to decide whether an object will hit your body, knowing that it is to the left or to the right with respect to fixation is not relevant. Mapping the approaching stimulus relative to the nearest body part is much more useful. The same is true if you want to intercept it. This 'gelatinous medium surrounding the body, that deforms in a topology-preserving fashion whenever the head rotates or the limbs move' (Graziano & Gross, 1993, p. 107) could thus serve the role of interface between our body and the immediately surrounding environment.

Building on the neurophysiological evidence discussed above, the Italian neuroscientists Giuseppe di Pellegrino, Alessandro Farné, and Elisabetta Làdavas were among the first to expand the notion of peripersonal space to humans. They reasoned that if visual stimuli near the body are coded within a visuo-tactile circuit, this should also be evident in behaviour. To explore this question they took a neuropsychological approach, studying patients with brain damage. In their very first study, they tested a 75-year-old man, Mr G.S., who suffered a lesion in the right-hemisphere caused by a stroke. When the experimenter briefly touched one of the two hands, G.S. had no difficulty in detecting the touches. (Note that both the patient's hands and the tactile stimulation were occluded by screens, see Figure 7.7a.) By contrast, when the two hands were touched simultaneously, G.S. perceived touches on the right hand (processed by the intact brain hemisphere) but extinguished touches on the left hand (processed by the damaged brain hemisphere; Figure 7.7a). So far, nothing new: this behaviour is typical of the neuropsychological condition termed 'tactile extinction', and was first reported by the German neurologist Hermann Oppenheim in 1885 (cited in Benton, 1956). Most interestingly, however, di Pellegrino and colleagues observed that extinction persists also when the screen covering the right hand was removed, and the experimenter twitched his finger *near* the right hand of the patient without touching it (Figure 7.7b). This is therefore visuo-tactile extinction, and it demonstrates a multisensory interaction that is compatible with multisensory coding of peripersonal space, for the visual stimulus near the right hand extinguished touch on the left hand in a very similar fashion to the condition in which two touches were presented. To explore this result further, di Pellegrino and colleagues asked the patient to move his right arm behind the back—a condition somewhat similar to the one tested by Graziano and Gross (1993) depicted in Figure 7.6c. When they repeated the visuo-tactile stimulation with this changed posture, G.S. was perfectly capable of detecting touches on the left hand, despite the visible movements of the experimenter's finger on his left side remaining identical to the previous visuo-tactile stimulation condition. Finally, no visuo-tactile extinction emerged when the patient's left hand was on the table but visual stimulation occurred at eye-level, more than 30 cm away from the G.S.'s left hand (di Pellegrino, Làdavas, & Farnè, 1997). These pioneering results supported the hypothesis

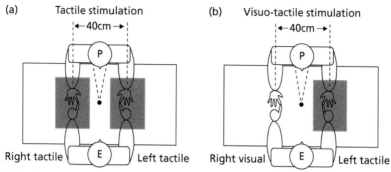

Figure 7.7 Peripersonal space in a brain-damaged patient. (A) Set-up for tactile extinction: the patient (P) rest his hands under opaque screens (grey rectangles), thus neither the hands nor the tactile stimulations delivered by the experimenter (E) are visible. When touched on both hands at the same time, patients typically report right touches (processed by the intact left brain-hemisphere) but fail to report left touches. (B) Set-up for the visuo-tactile extinction: the patient can now see his right hand and the finger of the experimenter approaching the hand. Although the right hand is never touched, this visual stimulation near the right hand can extinguish the touch delivered at the left hand.

Reproduced from Alessandro Farnè and Francesco Pavani, Left tactile extinction following visual stimulation of a rubber hand, *Brain*, 123 (11), pp. 2350–2360, Figures 1 a and b, doi: 10.1093/brain/123.11.2350 Copyright © 2000, Oxford University Press.

that visuo-tactile coding of experimenter's finger movements was only possible if the stimulation occurred near the hand, in G.S.'s peripersonal space.

This seminal study has been replicated in groups of neurological patients with tactile extinction (Làdavas, di Pellegrino, Farnè, & Zeloni, 1998; Làdavas, Farnè, Zeloni, & di Pellegrino, 2000; Farnè, Demattè, & Làdavas, 2003) and has been extended to other body parts such as the face (Làdavas, Zeloni, & Farnè 1998). Furthermore, the interest in peripersonal space in animals and humans motivated researches to seek behavioural signatures of peripersonal space also in neurologically healthy people. One such paradigm is based on the interference between tactile targets on the body and visual distractors (Spence, Pavani, & Driver, 2004); another one is based on the interaction between approaching (or receding) sounds and tactile targets (Serino, Bassolino, Farné, & Làdavas, 2007). For instance, in the classic version of the visuo-tactile interference paradigm (also known as the cross-modal congruency task, CCE), participants discriminate the position of single touches delivered to the thumb or index finger of either hand, while trying to ignore irrelevant visual stimuli that are either spatially congruent or incongruent with respect to the tactile target. Typically, a cost emerges when tactile targets are presented in combination with spatially incongruent distractors, revealing a multisensory interaction between visual stimuli near the hand, and tactile stimuli on the hand. The key aspect of this paradigm for the study of peripersonal space is that the amount of visuo-tactile interference depends on the perceived distance between the tactile target and the visual distractor. Spatial modulation of visuo-tactile interference is illustrated in Figure 7.8; the interference produced by visual distractors is larger when participants hold their hand

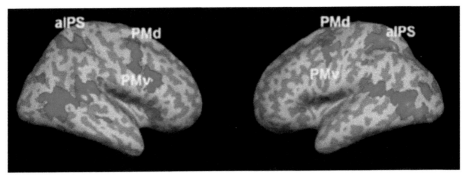

Figure 7.8 Peripersonal space in healthy humans. The interference between touches on the hand (black triangles) and distracting visual events (grey circles) is larger when the hand is near the visual distractors (A) compared to when the hand is farther away from them (B; adapted from Spence et al., 2010). This simple behavioural paradigm is useful for studying peripersonal space in humans. Visual stimuli approaching the hand are processed within similar brain networks in the human and monkey brain. An example of this network in humans as revealed through fMRI is shown in (C) and includes the anterior intraparietal sulcus (aIPS), the dorsal and ventral premotor regions (PMd and PMv, respectively) and the putamen (not shown in the figure).

Adapted from Claudio Brozzoli, Giovanni Gentile, Valeria I. Petkova and H. Henrik Ehrsson, fMRI Adaptation Reveals a Cortical Mechanism for the Coding of Space Near the Hand, *The Journal of Neuroscience: The official journal of the Society for Neuroscience*, 31 (24), pp. 9023-9031, Figure 2, doi: 10.1523/JNEUROSCI.1172-11.2011 © 2011, The Society for Neuroscience.

next to them (Figure 7.8a), compared to when they move their hand 30 cm away from them (Figure 7.8b).

Once again, this manipulation of posture is reminiscent of the one adopted in animals (Figure 7.6) and in patient G.S. (Figure 7.7), and points to the existence of a mechanisms in the brain that can code differently between visual stimuli near the body and visual stimuli away from the body. In recent years, this simple posture manipulation has proved effective to reveal neural correlates of peripersonal space in humans (e.g. Brozzoli, Gentile, Petkova, & Ehrsson, 2011; Brozzoli, Gentile, & Ehrsson, 2012; Makin, Holmes, & Zohary, 2007; Sereno & Huang, 2006; for a recent review see Brozzoli, Ehrsson, & Farnè, 2014). In one study, people were asked to lie inside the scanner for fMRI, watching a small sphere approaching repeatedly the surface of a small table placed on their hips. Critically, in one condition their rested their hand on the table, clearly visible in front of them, and the sphere approached it several times without touching it. In another condition, participants were asked to retract their hand and place it on their chest. Using a special approach to functional imaging termed *fMRI adaptation* it was possible to reveal the brain network that was active when the visual stimulation occurred near the hand (i.e. in peripersonal space). The network is shown in the Figure 7.8c and includes the premotor cortex (vPM: ventral pre-motor; dPM: dorsal pre-motor) and the parietal cortex (aIPS: anterior intra-parietal sulcus) in both brain hemispheres, as well as in the putamen (for a meta-analysis see Grivaz, Blanke, & Serino, 2017). Although drawing parallels between brain areas between humans and monkeys is always difficult, these regions correspond remarkably well to those regions of the monkey brain in which visuo-tactile bimodal neurons have first been described. Furthermore, there is now evidence that applying transcranial magnetic stimulation (TMS) to some of these regions (specifically, the vPM, or the posterior parietal cortex in which aIPS lies) can make behavioural effects linked to peripersonal space disappear (Serino, Canzoneri, & Avenanti, 2011). Recall that TMS is a stimulation technique used in cognitive neuroscience to create a temporary electrical interference in cortical regions, and can serve to test the causal role of the stimulated regions in a cognitive process. Intriguingly, Brozzoli and colleagues (Brozzoli, Gentile, Bergouuignan, & Ehrsson, 2013) have also documented that PMv is involved in encoding space near one's own hand and near another person's hand, suggesting that peripersonal space of others can be processed to some extent within the same neural circuitry that allow us deciding whether an object is near us or not.

It should be apparent by now that the space immediately near the body is much more than a just scientific or social convention: it is coded differently in the brain with respect to personal and extra-personal space, and it influences the way we perceive touch. Since the early studies of the 1990s, research on peripersonal space processing has flourished in three main directions. The first concerned the plastic nature of peripersonal space. We now know that peripersonal space can be reshaped by the use of tools, by the intention to act, by the nature of the approaching objects, and by the proximity of others. We discuss peripersonal space plasticity in Tutorial 7.1, presenting the prime example of peripersonal space expansion with tools. The second concerned the link between peripersonal space and the motor system. Note that this line of research emphasizes once again the notion that understanding multisensory interactions implies understanding their role in action. Several lines of investigation on this research topic are confirming the key role of peripersonal space as anticipatory interface for preparing actions as objects approach the body, and for preparing perception as the body intentionally approaches objects. Third, researchers have started to investigate peripersonal space in relation to more complex aspects of human cognition, such as the processing of social relationships or conceptual knowledge. In the final part of this section, we will briefly outline this fast evolving field (for reviews on the new perspectives related to the notion of peripersonal space see Brozzoli, Ehrsson, & Farné, 2014; or Blake, Slater, & Serino, 2015).

Tutorial 7.1 Expanding personal and peripersonal space with tools

In the 1970s the German artist Rebecca Horn started performing art experiments based on the idea that objects can extend body boundaries. In a famous performance, called 'Unicorn' (1970–1972), she asked a friend to wear a dress that included a long, white, conical structure on the top of her head. The performer was filmed early in the morning walking naked in a corn field, wearing only this horn-like body extension on her head. Following up on this idea, she then developed a 'Pencil mask' (1972): a mask that contained protruding pencils, 10 cm long, which she wore on her face to draw on a wall while making rhythmical movements of her head and body. In yet another performance, shown in Figure 7.9, she attached 1.7 metre long extensions to her fingers and touched the walls of a room while standing at its centre—a performance entitled *Touching the walls with both hands simultaneously*, 1974.

In the context of the present chapter, the extensions that allowed Horn to act beyond the natural reaching limit of her body raise two intriguing questions. The first question is whether it is possible to turn far (or extra-personal) space into near (or peripersonal) space—through tools. Did the impression of scratching both walls at once evoked by Horn correspond, for her perceptual system, to real perceptual expansions of reaching peripersonal space? The second question is whether using tools alters our internal representation of the body, producing metrical distortions of the body parts that manoeuvred the extensions, and producing re-calibrations that need to be taken into account by the motor system. This second question is also closely related to concepts we have discussed in Chapter 2. In particular, whether tools can become 'incorporated'—i.e. start to be perceived perceptually, cognitively, and affectively as parts of our own body.

The notion that tools or other body extensions can expand the perceived reaching and peripersonal space relates to everyday experiences like carrying a back-pack, holding an umbrella, or even driving a car. Indeed, novelist, philosophers, and scientists have described this experience in various narratives and anecdotes

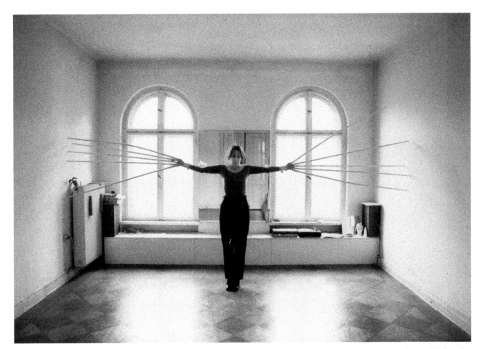

Figure 7.9 Extensions of the body as art. Performance artist Rebecca Horn experimenting with body extensions in *Touching the walls with both hands simultaneously*, from *Berlin Exercises* film, 1974.
© Rebecca Horn/DACS, London 2017. Photo: Helmut Wietz.

(Holmes, 2012). For instance, the neurologists Henry Head and Gordon Holmes (1911) remarked that 'a woman's power of localization may extend to the feather in her hat' (p. 188). Likewise, Gibson (1966) observed that simply using scissors to cut a sheet of paper could reveal how tactile sensations can extend to the blades, as if they were part of our own body (a suggestive image that reminds of a movie character for whom scissors were literally incorporated as bodily extensions—i.e. Edward Scissorhands, from the 1990 Tim Burton movie). Despite long-standing interest for tools as bodily extensions, the topic became the object of scientific scrutiny only in the late 1990s, with seminal work conducted at the Tokyo Medical and Dental University (Iriki, Tanaka, & Iwamura, 1996). In their study, Iriki and colleagues explored how the use of a rake to collect food pellets in extra-personal space changed the response of visuo-tactile neurons coding peripersonal space. They recorded from cells in the parietal cortex of macaque monkeys, which is one of the key cortical nodes of the peripersonal space network (see main text). At the beginning of the experiment, multisensory neurons responded selectively to tactile stimuli to the right hand of the monkey and to visual stimuli delivered in the space close to the hand. However, after two weeks of training with the rake, researchers observed that the region of space that evoked responses from multisensory neurons extended to the entire length of the tool. This suggests that coding of peripersonal space at the level of single multisensory neurons was plastic enough to expand beyond the physical boundaries of the body.

Shortly after this pioneering study in monkeys, several Italian researchers working in parallel expanded this investigation to humans (Berti & Frassinetti, 2000; Farnè & Làdavas, 2000; Maravita, Spence, Kennett, & Driver, 2002). For instance, Alessandro Farné and colleagues exploited visuo-tactile extinction (i.e. the phenomenon by which right-brain damaged patients fail to perceive a touch on the left hand if paired with a visual stimulus near the right hand; see Figure 7.5) to replicate the manipulation conducted by Iriki, Tanaka, & Iwamura (1996) in humans. They found that before tool use visuo-tactile extinction was primarily elicited by visual stimuli near the right hand. However, after a short period of active use of a rake to retrieve disks placed far from the body, visuo-tactile extinction was produced also when visual stimuli were presented near the tip of the tool (Farnè & Làdavas, 2000; Farnè, Bonifazi, & Làdavas, 2005; Farnè, Iriki, & Làdavas, 2005). After these early studies in neurological patients, several research groups have examined the mechanisms subtending peripersonal space expansion with tools in healthy humans, adopting a variety of experimental approaches and multisensory combinations (for a recent review see Martel, Cardinali, Roy, & Farnè, 2016). For instance, Angelo Maravita and colleagues (Rossetti, Romano, Bolognini, & Maravita, 2015) have examined skin conductance response (SCR) to a needle approaching and touching the hand, or approaching and touching a hand-held tool. Before tool-use, the autonomic response to the potentially painful stimuli measured through SCR increased selectively as the needle moved closer to the hand, peaking obviously for the stimulation that eventually touch the hand. Interestingly, however, this anticipation of pain changed after tool-use, expanding to locations that were previously ineffective in eliciting an SCR responses, as if they were of minimal risk for the body. Thus, tool-use can extend the affective/defensive boundaries of the body, in agreement with the view that peripersonal space is an interface of great relevance for anticipating interactions with the environment.

Although tool-induced plasticity is now well established, several questions are still extensively debated. For instance, it is unclear to what extent active tool use is necessary for triggering this expansion, in particular whether the systematic pairing of distal (visual) and proximal (tactile) sensations are sufficient to trigger peripersonal space plasticity. One paradigmatic example of a link between distal and proximal sensations in the absence of a physical tool is the use a computer mouse. When we operate a computer mouse we see visual events happening on the screen in extra-personal space, while we move and touch the mouse in peripersonal space. This creates a systematic linking of visual, tactile, and motor events, and yet there is no physical tool making a bridge between peripersonal and extra-personal space (Bassolino, Serino, Ubaldi, & Làdavas, 2010). Another open issue is to what extent the intuitive metaphor of peripersonal space expanding to include the tool corresponds to the psychological reality of the phenomenon. The alternative possibility is that tools bind personal and extrapersonal space, creating an intangible bridge between near and far.

However, there is increasing consensus that long-lasting tool use can induce stable modifications of peripersonal space. Andrea Serino and colleagues tested this hypothesis in a group of blind individuals who were regular users of a blind-cane and a group of sighted controls with no such experience (Serino, Bassolino, Farnè, & Làdavas, 2007). To probe peripersonal space extensions, they measured the interactions between touches to the hand and auditory stimuli delivered at the tip of the blind-cane. While 10 minutes of repeated use of the cane were necessary to create tactile-auditory interactions in the blindfold sighted controls who never used the cane, the same interactions were observed in blind participants immediately at baseline, as soon as they held the cane. This is compatible with the idea that repeated experience with the tool can result in stable modifications of peripersonal space. In other words, that our cognitive system maintains distinct representations of our body with and without the tool, and accesses them quickly as a function of behavioural needs.

More recently, research on tool use started to focus on a new question: whether body extensions can alter the internal representation of our own body. This is a different question because instead of focusing on the plasticity of the space near the body, it touches upon the notion of personal space and the concepts of body representations, which we also discussed in Chapter 2. The first study to address this issue was conducted by Lucilla Cardinali and colleagues (Cardinali et al., 2009), who measured arm representation before and after a 10 minutes of practice with a mechanical grabber. A mechanical grabber is the tool that street cleaners use to collect rubbish from the street while standing. Cardinali and colleagues recorded free-arm movement kinematics, measuring velocity and acceleration of the hand when participants reached and grasped an object located 35 cm from the body. These kinematic parameters changed after tool use, precisely in the same direction in which they would normally change if one were to compare the kinematics of people with naturally short arms with that of people with naturally long arms. Thus, participants acted as if tool-use increased their unconscious arm length! This interpretation was confirmed by an additional experiment in which Cardinali and colleagues measured arm lengthening directly, asking participants to quickly point to three anatomical landmarks on their right arm (elbow, wrist, and middle finger tip), using their left index finger. The results confirmed that overall arm length (i.e. the distance between the elbow and the tip of the middle finger) was indeed expanded after tool use.

The relationship between tool use and perceived body size has now evolved in several investigations that documented, for instance, that even imagined tool-use can result in perceived changes of arm length (Baccarini et al., 2014) or that only tools that introduce a significant 'gain' in reachability can transform the body representation. For instance, Sposito and colleagues (Sposito, Bolognini, Vallar, & Maravita, 2012) found that use of a 60-cm long tool can alter the perceived midpoint of the arm handling the tool, whereas no such change in arm length emerges after use of a short 20-cm long tool. Recently, a particularly important observation emerged from a study on right brain-damaged patients who cannot move their left arm (i.e. are hemiplegic) but experience the delusional embodiment of another person's arm as if it were their own (a condition known as somatoparaphrenia). Francesca Garbarini and colleagues (Garbarini et al., 2015) asked patients to estimate the midpoint of their left arm (as in Sposito, Bolognini, Vallar, & Maravita, 2012) before and after observation of the *experimenter* left arm handling and using a tool. Remarkably, patients who experience the delusion of using the tool with their own paralysed arm misjudged their forearm mid-point more distally, just like in the neurologically healthy participants handling long tools in Sposito et al.'s study. This evidence suggests that self-attribution (i.e. ownership) of the body part handling the tool is an important pre-requisite for inducing changes in body representation.

This concept has far-reaching clinical implications, as it can easily transfer to the applied domains of limb prostheses and distance-operated tools in telemedicine. Multisensory research is indeed quickly starting to develop also in this direction (e.g. Romano et al., 2015; D'Alonzo, Clemente, & Cipriani, 2015), addressing key questions such as the role of functional use (i.e. making the prosthesis an active and controllable tool) or the role of multisensory coupling in promoting the perceived incorporation of the prosthesis, and as a consequence its acceptance by the user.

The relationship between peripersonal space and action was already present in the early ethological observations that we mentioned at the beginning of the section (recall the notion of 'flight zone', i.e. a zone around the animal that triggers escape behaviour when trespassed). However, it has been specifically examined in relation to peripersonal space mostly in the last decade, initially in monkeys and more recently in humans. Graziano and colleagues observed that electrical micro-stimulation of the regions that contained neurons coding peripersonal space in the monkey brain triggered complex configurations of head, trunk, and limb movements (Graziano, Taylor, & Moore, 2002; Graziano & Cooke, 2006). These movements appeared as defensive or avoidance actions: the hand moved to the head, as if the animal wanted to protect the face; or it was retracted behind the back, as if the animal wanted to protect it from an anticipated contact. Recall, however, that no object was present in the environment and these reactions were triggered only by electrical stimulation of cortical neurons. Similar links between trespassing of peripersonal space and preparation of avoidance actions have been documented in humans. For instance, Makin and colleagues (Makin et al., 2009) asked participants to perform a simple button-press with the index finger of the right hand, while observing a three-dimensional ball suddenly falling above their hand or away from the hand. The ball never reached the hand and its movement was always irrelevant for the task. Nonetheless, its appearance reduced the excitability of the participants' motor system within the first 70–80 ms, specifically for the conditions in which the ball's trajectory aimed towards the hand. Makin and colleagues interpreted this motor system modulation as reflecting the suppression of an avoidance response triggered by the flying ball, to prevent interference with the on-going behavioural goal (i.e. button press). Related findings using approaching auditory (rather than visual) stimuli have also been documented (Serino, Annella, & Avenanti, 2009; Finisguerra et al., 2015).

These results suggest that peripersonal space could serve the purpose of an anticipatory interface for fast preparation of defensive and avoidance actions when unexpected stimuli approach the body. The adaptive nature of such a mechanism is apparent. For instance, we can all recall moments in life in which we started fast defensive or avoidance movements well before we became aware of an approaching danger. Our motor behaviour, however, is not only crucial to prevent injuries; it is also crucial for intentional actions towards objects. We reach for the cup, we intercept the flying ball, we walk to the opening in the room because this is what we intend to do. Can peripersonal space coding play a role also in these contexts, anticipating for instance the future sensory consequences of our intentional actions?

In 2009, Brozzoli and colleagues (Brozzoli et al., 2009) devised an experiment to test this question specifically. They asked participants to perform two concurrent tasks: first, perform a reaching movement towards a small wooden cylinder, when prompted by a tone; second, decide as quickly as possible whether a touch delivered on the right hand was to the thumb or the index finger. The target cylinder incorporated one LED at each extremity, and the LEDs flashed in synchrony with the touch on the hand in different moments of the trial. The interference between the visual stimulus and the tactile target (cross-modal congruency effect), is an indicator of the interaction between vision and touch in peripersonal space: interference being highest when visual stimuli are coded within peripersonal space. Crucially, however, the cylinder with LEDs was located 50 cm away from the hand—thus, in reaching space, but outside peripersonal space. The results of this study are shown in Figure 7.10. When visuo-tactile stimuli were delivered before participants were instructed to perform the action, the cost of the interfering visual stimuli was about 30 ms (see 'Before the action' panel). By contrast, when visuo-tactile stimuli were delivered at movement onset, the interference doubled to approximately 60 ms. Note that in the latter case, the hand barely changed position (see

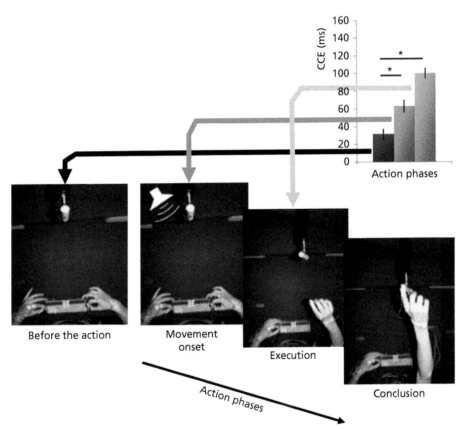

Figure 7.10 The paradigm adopted by Brozzoli et al. (2009). The interference of visual distractors (embedded in the to-be-grasped cylinder) on tactile distractors at the reaching hand (i.e. the crossmodal congruency effect, CCE) was minimal when stimuli were delivered before the action, increased at movement onset (despite the hand barely moving) and was maximal during execution.

Reproduced from the Claudio Brozzoli, Francesco Pavani, Christian Urquizar, Lucilla Cardinali, and Alessandro Farnè, Grasping actions remap peripersonal space, *NeuroReport*, 20 (10), pp 913-917, doi: 10.1097/WNR.0b013e32832c0b9b Copyright © 2009, Lippincott Williams.

Figure 7.10, 'Movement onset' panel), thus the physical separation between tactile targets and visual distractors remained almost unchanged with respect to the 'Before the action' condition. This increase in interference is compatible with the idea that participants expanded their peripersonal space to incorporate the target object at the moment they begin the action. Crucially, this modulation of interference did not emerge when the action was performed with the left hand, but tactile stimuli were delivered to the right hand. In sum, these results suggested that, in addition to playing a role in avoidance/defensive behaviour, peripersonal space could serve to anticipate the perceptual (somatosensory) consequences of our intentional actions.

While research on peripersonal space is evocative of proxemic space boundaries as studied by social psychologists in the 1960s, these two topics remained entirely separate for at least one decade. In recent years, however, researchers have attempted to measure peripersonal space in the context of social interactions. One of the first studies in this direction was conducted by Teneggi and colleagues (Teneggi, Canzoneri, di Pellegrino, & Serino 2013). They used touches on the participant's face and sounds approaching to (or receding from) the body. This paradigm is useful to estimate peripersonal space boundaries, because sounds perceived as occurring within peripersonal space are known to facilitate detection of touches in comparison to sounds perceived as beyond it. Critically, Teneggi and colleagues measured peripersonal space extension while participants faced either another person or a mannequin, standing approximately 1 metre away. The results showed that peripersonal space was smaller when facing another person, compared to facing the mannequin. In addition, if an economic game between the participant and the other person was introduced in the study, peripersonal space seemed to expand towards the other person—but only when the two were cooperating in the game, not in a non-cooperative condition. Although this study suggests that social variables can modulate peripersonal space, research on this topic is still in its infancy. Importantly, it remains unclear to what extent peripersonal space and social inter-personal space should be considered as a single spatial representation, or instead as distinct constructs: peripersonal space being a more sensory-motor representation, and inter-personal space being a more conceptual and cultural spatial boundary. One study that suggests that peripersonal and interpersonal spaces are functionally distinct has recently been conducted by Patanè and colleagues (Patanè, Iachini, Farnè, & Frassinetti, 2016). Taking advantage of the well-documented peripersonal space expansion with tools (see Tutorial 7.1), they measured peripersonal and interpersonal space before and after participants used a long rake to reach and retrieve tokens on a table. To measure peripersonal space, participant decided whether stimuli presented at different distances from the body were within arm distance or not. To measure interpersonal space, participants walked towards the other person (or saw the other person approaching them) and had to stop as soon as the proximity with the confederate became uncomfortable. The results showed that tool-use modulated peripersonal space, but not interpersonal space, suggesting these two spatial representations may be dissociable.

7.6 **Extra-personal space**

The previous sections discussed the multisensory and motor nature of the space occupied by the body (personal space) and of the space immediately adjacent to the body (peripersonal space). In Tutorial 7.1 we also discussed how peripersonal and reaching space can change when participants use tools. We will now turn to the region of space beyond the region around our body, which is generally identified as *extra-personal*. Everyday experience suggests that two sensory modalities crucially contribute to extra-personal space perception: vision and hearing. Vision conveys information about the position of surrounding objects with respect to our viewpoint, but also allows a reconstruction of the relative layout of objects in the environment. As shown in the schematic image of the ambient optical array presented in Figure 7.1, vision is limited by the frontal position of our eyes and, in any given moment, leaves a wide portion of space unexplored (e.g. the space above our head or the space behind our back). By contrast, hearing permits monitoring of the entire space around us, it can alert us to the many of changes occurring in the environment and can play an important role in fast reorienting of the eyes and the head towards sudden events. However, extra-personal space perception is not only built on these distal senses. As we shall see in this section, bodily sensations (e.g. proprioception and vestibular sensations) also play a role, primarily because—once again—our multisensory perception of space is almost inextricably intertwined with action planning and execution. Hence, information from proximal senses that help movement planning becomes part of the loop of our active perception of extra-personal space.

When reasoning about vision and hearing in extra-personal space, it is apparent that, most of the times, we pin down the sounds we hear to the locations we see. This is particularly evident when auditory and visual events are temporally correlated—your phone ringing and flashing at the same time. However, note that this can also happens when no audio-visual temporal correlation exists—your phone rings without flashing. Or consider the case of the sound coming from your radio when listening to the morning news. You pin the voice you hear to a location on the kitchen shelf, where the radio stands, despite there being no on-going visual changes that suggest this audio-visual pairing. By keeping perceptions of auditory and visual locations aligned our cognitive system achieves a more coherent and simplified representation of extra-personal space. For instance, a voice and a face in the environment become one multisensory event by effect of this spatial binding, reducing the complexity of the multisensory scene.

A classic example of audio-visual interaction in space perception is the experience we all have at the cinema. As we watch the film, all visual stimulations come from the screen in front of us, whereas sounds are typically produced by lateral loudspeakers. Yet, we do not experience a spatial discrepancy between the visible lip-movements of the actress and the sound of her voice: both seem to originate from exactly the same location on the screen, and instead of perceiving two separate events we perceive a single, meaningful compound. This phenomenon is one the many instances of the so-called 'visual capture of sound position' and reveals that our brain seamlessly integrates audio-visual inputs when perceiving external space. Precisely the same integrative mechanisms are also at play in the ventriloquist trick, in which the performer can effectively convey the impression that the puppet on his hand can speak. As we mentioned in Chapter 1, although the term ventriloquist hints at the possibility that the artist speaks with his stomach ('*venter*' and '*loqui*' are the Latin words for 'stomach' and 'to speak', respectively) the trick actually reflects a very different skill. The ventriloquist learns to utter words without apparent lip-movements, while controlling the lip-movements of the puppet in perfect synchrony with his concealed speech sounds. When this trick is played well, we attribute the concealed speech sounds to the most probable and temporally synchronous source, i.e. the visually salient lip movements of the puppet. Close your eyes and the illusion will vanish, revealing at once where the voice actually comes from. Ventriloquists are less common nowadays, but you can try the effect of closing your eyes next time you go to a cinema.

What is important to appreciate here is that the illusion is not just a belief that we consciously apply to our perceptual experience. Said otherwise, we don't hear the voice as coming from the puppet because we learned that speech usually originates from lip-movements. Many years of research has shown that visual captures of sounds, such as the ventriloquist illusion, are truly perceptual phenomena. They originate from the tendency of our brain to combine concurrent visual and auditory inputs, and they are rooted into multisensory integration mechanisms in our brain. One of the early experimental studies of the ventriloquist phenomenon, conducted by Paul Bertelson—the Belgian psychologist who has been one of the founding father of multisensory research—illustrates this point well (Radeau & Bertelson, 1974). Participants were enrolled in a study of sound localization and were asked to point with their index finger to the location of sounds delivered one after the other from unseen sources in front of them. After sound localization accuracy was measured, participants were asked to wear goggles fitted with prismatic lenses that shifted the visual field by 15 degrees (see Chapter 3). While wearing the prismatic goggles participants were instructed to pay attention to a series of paired auditory and visual stimuli. Although audio-visual stimulations were always delivered from identical spatial locations, the prismatic shift exposed participants to a systematic discrepancy between the two stimuli. Note that such a small discrepancy is barely noticeable, and participants were largely unaware of the experimental manipulation. After 120 trials (approximately 5 minutes), the prismatic goggles were removed and participants were asked to repeat again the sound localization task conducted at the beginning of the study. Although the task was again unisensory (i.e. it involved only sounds and no visual stimulation was delivered), sound localization was now biased in the direction of the visual shift previously produced by the prismatic goggles. This is an audio-visual capture after-effect, and it reveals the strong tendency of our brain to combine visual and auditory spatial information. This mechanism is so strong that even a small discrepancy, lasting no longer than 5 minutes, can quickly produce a recalibration of the less reliable auditory cues to match the more precise spatial information, even when participants were unaware of the discrepancy between lights and sounds.

The study of visual capture of sound has long history in experimental psychology (Thomas, 1941; Jackson, 1953; Howard & Templeton, 1966; Bertelson & Radeau, 1981) and was originally framed as an example of sensory dominance resulting from the higher spatial reliability of vision in comparison to hearing (Warren, Welch, & McCarthy, 1981). As we have already mention in previous chapters of this book (e.g. see Chapter 4 on multisensory objects), this concept has been largely revisited in favour of models of multisensory integration based on Bayesian models. A study conducted in 2004 by David Alais and David Burr was the first to reveal that this logic applies also to the ventriloquist illusion, showing that this multisensory phenomenon is the consequence of optimal in-tegration mechanisms, rather than a rigid dominance of vision over hearing. They pre-sented participants with pairs of visual, auditory, or audio-visual stimuli, and asked them to indicate which of the two (the first, or the second) was more on the left. Sound stimuli were clicks presented stereophonically by two speakers on the side of the screen, which could be delivered in different spatial locations with high precision. Visual stimuli were instead low-contrast blobs, which could be blurred to different degrees and hence made more or less difficult to localize. In audio-visual trials, clicks and blobs were combined to produce two successive multisensory events. Crucially, in multisensory trials a spatial conflict was introduced for one of the two events: clicks were displaced leftward and blobs were displaced rightwards. By estimating localization accuracy as a function of the degree of blurring of the blobs, Alais and Burr made three key observations. First, they repli-cated the classic visual capture of sound for the less blurred blobs, which were the most easy to localize. Second, they showed that the reverse phenomenon (i.e. auditory capture of vision) could be produced when the blobs were severely blurred, and hence become very hard to localize. Third, they managed to make neither sense dominate, by making the spatial precision of blobs comparable to that of the clicks. Thus, this important study revealed that perception was not mandatorily dominated by vision, but instead it fol-lowed relatively simple rules of optimal combination between the available multisensory stimulations. In sum, visual dominance in the ventriloquist phenomenon emerges as the outcome of the relative reliability of visual and auditory information in any given mo-ment. Typically vision offers the most reliable spatial signals, but when this changes even the adult cognitive system is flexible enough to adjust which sensory system must be followed.

It is important to emphasize here that, early on, researchers had the intuition that such a powerful and fast integrative mechanism should be hardwired in the brain. This mo-tivated a series of pioneering studies into the neural mechanisms underlying the tight link between visual and auditory space in animals. These studies targeted a very im-portant subcortical structure of the mammalian brain (the superior colliculus), as well as structures of the cerebral cortex (the posterior parietal cortex). The *superior colliculus* (SC) has the shape of two bumps in the brainstem of mammals, in the midbrain. Note that the homologue to the SC in the brain of birds and reptiles is a structure named *optic tectum* (OT). Despite being relatively small, the SC and the OT are of great rele-vance for multisensory space perception, because several sensory modalities converge there to contribute to overt orienting behaviour (e.g. turning eyes and head to a novel stimulus in the environment). The key features of the SC are concisely summarized in Tutorial 7.2, together with the principles that govern multisensory integration at the single neuron level.

Tutorial 7.2 Multisensory integration by single neurons: lessons from the superior colliculus

Investigations on the superior colliculus (SC) started in the late 1960s (Horn & Hill, 1966) and are still central to the field of multisensory perception (Stein, Stanford, & Rowland, 2014). There are at least two reasons why the SC is so important for the study of multisensory space perception. The first has to do with the fact that the SC receives and integrates signals from multiple sensory channels. Anatomically, the SC is organized in seven overlapping layers—pretty much like a layer cake. In the first three superficial layers, neurons respond only to visual signals. However, in the intermediate and deep layers, neurons receive signals from multiple sensory channels: vision, hearing, or somatosensation. Although some of these neurons are selective to only one sensory input (e.g. are vision-only neurons), many exhibit multisensory responses. Neurons responsive to all possible combinations of sensory inputs have now been described in the SC (Perrault & Rowland, 2012), with some cells showing bi-sensory responsiveness (e.g. visual-auditory, auditory-somatosensory, visual-somatosensory) and others characterized by tri-sensory responsiveness (visual-auditory-somatosensory). The properties of the multisensory neurons in the SC have been extensively examined by Barry Stein, Alex Meredith, and their collaborators and were first summarized in *The Merging of the Senses*, one of the most influential books in the field of multisensory perception and cognitive neuroscience (Stein & Meredith, 1993; Stein, Meredith, & Wallace, 1993; for recent updates on these findings see Stein & Stanford, 2008; or Stein, Stanford, & Rowland, 2014).

The second reason why the SC proved an ideal model for the study of multisensory space perception has to do with the fact that it contains *spatio-topically organized neurons*. This means that there is a clear and predictable correspondence between the position of stimulations in extra-personal space and the two-dimensional arrangement of the neurons within each layer of the SC. For instance, neurons at the most anterior portions of the SC respond to stimuli appearing in the space in front of you, whereas neurons at the most posterior portions of the SC respond to stimuli appearing towards your side (the left side if recording from the right SC; the right side if recording from the left SC). Neurophysiologists have also noted that spatial maps in different layers of the SC are aligned with one another. They measured neuronal responses across different layers using electrodes that penetrate vertically in the SC—just like a knife poking vertically into the layer cake. They found that neurons within the same vertical column responded to similar regions of external space (Stein, Meredith, & Wallace, 1993). This revealed that within the SC the brain codes for multiple maps of space, based on different sensory signals, keeping an ordered arrangement between them.

Finding space maps in the brain is not that uncommon for the visual and somatosensory signals. Recall that the retina itself has some sort of visual space map, and this ordered representation is maintained throughout the pathway that leads to the cerebral cortex. Likewise, the spatial organization of the receptors on the skin is evident in several brain structures, and we already described this somatosensory space map in other parts of this book. However, the auditory system is not inherently spatial and, indeed, neurons of the auditory cortex are not arranged according to some coding of auditory space (Brewer & Barton, 2012). Still, the SC contains maps for all of these sensory channels—including a map for auditory space—and keeps them in approximate spatial register with one another. The reason for this distinctive peculiarity of the SC is best understood if one considers that this brain structure is also involved in automatic orienting movements towards stimuli in the environment. Stimulation of the neurons in the SC deep layers triggers eye and head movements (Jay & Sparks, 1987) and, in some animals, even reorienting of the ears (Stein & Clamann, 1981). The overall picture that emerges from these studies on the SC is very striking: this small structure in the depth of the brain is fully equipped for serving as a multisensory integration hub, guiding orienting behaviour towards novel events in space, regardless of their sensory nature. Recall that the location of stimuli in the different sensory modalities are all initially encoded in different reference frames: visual stimuli are mapped in retinal coordinates, somatosensory stimuli are mapped with respect to the body and auditory stimuli are mapped with respect to head position. Thus, a structure that codes all these sensory signals in a shared reference frame is essential for orienting movements towards the events in the world.

By definition, multisensory neurons respond to more than one sensory signal. What is less intuitive is that many multisensory neurons do not simply 'sum' the responses they would produce for single sensory events. Instead, several of these neurons react to multisensory stimuli either by producing *supra-additive responses* (i.e. stronger outputs than the ones predicted by the summation of their unisensory responses) or *sub-additive responses* (i.e. weaker outputs than the one predicted by the summation of their unisensory responses). In this sense, multisensory neurons behave as non-linear integrators. An example of a supra-additive response at the single neuron level is shown in Figure 7.11. In this example, the multisensory responses of the neuron is 1207 percent of the unimodal responses.

The study of multisensory neurons in the SC have revealed some of the general principles that govern these non-linear responses. The first general principle has to do with the spatial arrangement of the concurrent multisensory events and is therefore known as *the spatial rule*. Like most sensory neurons, multisensory cells in the SC respond when the stimuli are delivered to a specific area of sensory space (i.e. the neuron's receptive field) and are silent otherwise. Figure 7.12 shows the visual and auditory receptive fields of an example multisensory neuron, within the polar representation of the entire visual field of the animal (e.g. a cat). Note that the visual receptive field (the dark grey area) and the auditory receptive field (the light grey area) overlap; they are in spatial register with one another. The letters V and A indicate the position of the stimulation with respect the visual and auditory receptive field. In panel (a) both stimuli fall within the region of overlapping receptive fields, a condition that is obtained when both stimuli are

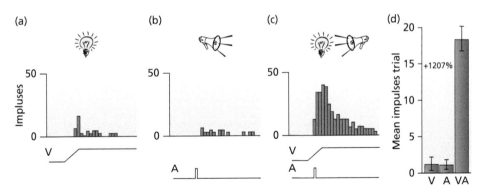

Figure 7.11 Supra-additive response in a single neuron of the superior colliculus. Bar-plots (a–c) show the cumulative responses of a single neuron when (a) the visual stimulus is switched-on, (b) the auditory stimulus is delivered, and (c) visual and auditory stimulation are delivered at the same time. Lines below each of the plots illustrate the onset of visual and auditory stimulation. The mean impulses recorded across trials is also summarized in (d). Clearly the VA stimulation produces a response which is more than the sum of the V and A responses alone.

Adapted with permission from Macmillan Publishers Ltd: *Nature Reviews Neuroscience*, 9 (4), Barry E. Stein and Terrence R. Stanford, Multisensory integration: current issues from the perspective of the single neuron, pp. 255-266, doi:10.1038/nrn2331. Copyright © 2008, Nature Publishing Group.

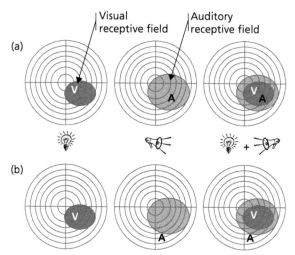

Figure 7.12 Visual and auditory receptive fields of an example multisensory neuron. Examples of (a) audio-visual stimulation falling within the multisensory receptive field of the neuron; (b) visual stimulation falling within the receptive field of the neuron and auditory stimulation falling outside the receptive field of the neuron.

delivered from exactly the same location in external space or from locations very close in space. By contrast, in panel (b) one stimulus falls within the receptive field of the neuron whereas the other falls just outside (in the example the auditory stimulus is just outside the visual and auditory receptive fields). What emerged from the study of SC neurons is that multisensory events that fall within the receptive field can trigger supra-additive responses (multisensory enhancement); by contrast, multisensory events that stimulate different receptive fields produce no response enhancement or even determine sub-additive responses (multisensory depression).

Just as spatial discrepancies between multisensory events can change the integrative response of SC neurons, the relative onset between multisensory stimuli also matters. This is known as *the temporal rule*. Neurons respond with multisensory enhancement when stimuli in different sensory modalities are delivered at the same time or approximately at the same time. By contrast, they show no enhancement or even depression, when the temporal interval between the stimuli becomes 'too long'. For SC cells 'too long' often means a couple of hundreds of milliseconds, although this temporal interval can be influenced by various factors, as we shall see in the section of this book dedicated to time perception (see Chapter 8). For now, it should suffice to say that studies on the SC neurons have revealed the existence of *temporal windows of integration*. On the one hand, these windows appear flexible enough to allow multisensory integration despite differences in speed of the energy reaching the sensory organs (light and sound travel at very different speed) and regardless of differences in time of transmission of the neural signals from sensory organs to multisensory neurons (pathways from the retina to the SC and from the cochlea to the SC are very different). On the other hand, temporal windows for integration are conservative enough to avoid merging together those sensory signals that were not concurrent.

The spatial and temporal rules make perfect adaptive sense when considering that one of the greatest challenges for our brain is to create unitary perceptual experiences. The brain must be able to bind together sensory stimulations that originate from the same event (e.g. the person speaking in front of us, for whom we see lip-movement and we hear speech sounds). At the same time, it must be capable of keeping multisensory information that do not belong together clearly distinct (e.g. the person in front of us and the voice coming from the radio). Under most circumstances, multisensory signals that originate from a single event have a common spatial source. In addition, they co-occur in time, frequently with related stimulation onsets and offsets across modalities (speech sound utterances are closely matched to single mouth movements). Within this adaptive perspective, also the third key principle for multisensory integration that emerged from the study of SC neurons is extremely interesting. This is known as *the inverse effectiveness rule* and captures the observation that intense unisensory signals will produce smaller integrative responses in the neuron, whereas weak signals will produce the strongest integrative outputs. What this means is that multisensory integrative responses are inversely related to the intensity of the unimodal sensory signals. In other words, multisensory enhancement would particularly benefit those sensory events that are barely noticeable when presented in isolation.

Multisensory neurons are ubiquitous, existing across many neural structures and across different species (Stein & Meredith, 1993). Yet, not all multisensory neurons are the same. Some are highly integrative and produce supra-additive responses given the appropriate stimulation conditions, just like we described in the above paragraphs. Others respond to multisensory stimuli without supra-additive responses, regardless of the stimulation conditions (Perrault, Vaughan, Stein, & Wallace, 2005). To what extent the principles observed for the SC can be extended to other brain areas remains unclear. A meta-analysis of the studies conducted in cats, for instance, indicates that the proportion and the functional properties of multisensory neurons differ between SC and cortical areas (Meredith, Allman, Keniston, & Clemo, 2012). In the SC approximately 63 percent of neurons are multisensory and, among these, 55 percent show super-additive responses with strong multisensory enhancements compared to the unisensory condition (88 percent increase, on average). By contrast, in other areas in the cat's cortex (anterior ectosylvian, rostral suprasylvian, and posterolateral lateral suprasylvian) a lower percentage of multisensory neurons was described (between 25 and 30 percent), with less supra-additive neurons (17 percent) and smaller multisensory enhancements (17 percent increase, on average). This could indicate that the mechanisms of multisensory process may differ between neural structures like the SC, which evolved to allow fast orientation towards novel events, and other brain areas involved in more complex behavioural responses. For instance, studies in the prefrontal cortex of primates—a cortical area that surely mediates more complex behavioural responses compared to the SC—Romanski and colleagues (Sugihara, Diltz, Averbeck, & Romanski, 2006; Romanski, 2007) noted that multisensory integration at the single neuron level was more common for semantically related audio-visual stimuli (such as face-vocalization pairs) than semantically unrelated ones (generic visual-auditory compounds).

This suggests that the potentials and the constraints for multisensory integration could differ across brain areas. One interpretation of this finding in terms of keeping a balance between two opposing needs, as a function of task-demands: merging sensory signals, and keeping them distinct (on this, see also Chapter 4 of this book). It should be always kept in mind that our brain must be equally capable of processing multisensory inputs in an integrative way, or to focus on the unisensory information primarily if the behavioural goal at hand requires it. In which way this interplay occurs and to what extent the rules for multisensory integration at the single neuron level operate for more complex cognitive abilities, such as speech perception or semantic processing, remain an issue for future research.

The other brain structure that has been in the focus of attention of scientists exploring the neural correlates of multisensory space perception is the *posterior parietal cortex* (PPC). This brain region has traditionally been described as 'associative', and it has long been known to play a key role in sensorimotor integration. The PPC receives multisensory and motor signals from several brain areas (Mountcastle et al., 1975; Hyvarinen, 1982; Andersen, Snyder, Bradley, & Xing, 1997). In addition, when damaged as a consequence of stroke, haemorrhage, or surgery it compromises the individual's abilities to represent space (Critchley 1953). The neurophysiology studies conducted on the PPC illustrate well the notion that the information available at the sensory epithelium (e.g. the retina or the skin) is not sufficient for reconstructing the position of the distal stimulus in the environment, a notion discussed throughout this chapter. In the 1990s, several research groups across the world showed that neural responses in PPC are often the results of integration of inputs from the receptor's surface and the proprioceptive and motor information that specify the position of the receptor in space (Cohen & Andersen, 2002). For instance, studying a portion of PPC known as lateral intra-parietal area (LIP), the North American scientist Richard Andersen and his colleagues showed that the response of several neurons was not just the result of the position of the visual stimulus in the environment. The neuronal response was also modulated in amplitude (i.e. it became stronger or weaker) as a function of the position of the eye in the orbit (Brotchie, Andersen, Snyder, & Goodman 1995). In other words, these neurons did not simply code the position of the visual stimulus in terms of retinal coordinates, but also integrated proprioceptive signals about the position of the eye in the orbit, or even the position of the head on the trunk. Recall that such information combination is essential to manage the coordinate transformation problem, as we discussed in section 7.3. For a recent review of the contribution of PPC to multisensory coding of space in monkeys and humans, see Bremmer (2011).

In the context of the audio-visual interactions described, it is worth noting that a retinal coding, modulated as a function of eye or head position, has also been documented at the single neuron level for *auditory* stimuli (Stricanne, Andersen, & Mazzoni, 1996). As we anticipated at the beginning of this chapter, the initial processing of the horizontal (azimuthal) position of sounds depends on the position of the head, not the eyes. A sound source straight ahead of you will generate a stimulation that reaches both ears at the same time and with comparable intensity. But if you turn your head 90 degrees to the left, the same auditory stimulation will now reach your right ear before the left ear, and will be louder at the ear facing the sound source. Thus, changing the position of the head on the trunk inevitably modifies the auditory cues that serve for localization of sounds in space. By contrast, none of the auditory cues are altered if your head is fixed and only your eyes move. So, why do auditory-responsive neurons also respond to the position of the eye in the orbit? The answer to this apparent conundrum is again to be found in the need to keep multisensory spaces aligned for the purpose of action. The hypothesis put forward by Cohen and Andersen (2002) is that the PPC generates a multisensory representation of space for action that adopts a common reference frame centred on the eye, irrespective of whether the stimulation is visual or auditory. Interestingly, while this could be the 'default' coding created in the PPC, the computational powers of this brain region also allow for several other reference frames to be created, as a function of which action is required at any given moment (a hand action, a whole body movement; for a computational description of this hypothesis, see Pouget, Deneve, & Duhamel, 2004).

Evidence that changes in eye position can alter the perceived location of sounds also comes from behavioural tasks in humans. Here is one study that tested specifically this hypothesis (Pavani, Husain, & Driver, 2008). Participants sat in front of five loudspeakers,

concealed from view behind a curtain, and listened in each trial a pair of sounds separated by 2.5 seconds. For each pair, participants decided whether the two sounds originated from same or different spatial locations. Crucially, while participants' heads were
fixed by a chin-rest throughout the experiment (thus preventing any change in the initial
coding of sounds at the ears), their eyes were either fixed to one side of the speaker array
(on the left or on the right) or moved from one lateral fixation to the other (e.g. from left
to right) during the long interval between the two sounds (see Figure 7.13). Once again,
note that changes in eye-position could not affect the initial input to the ears, as the relative position between the ears and the sounds always remained unchanged.

Nonetheless, the results showed that participants found it harder to make the same/
different judgement when intervening eye-movements were introduced between the
sounds, compared to when the eyes were held static. It could be argued that paying attention to the sounds while moving the eyes is a double task, and hence the difficulties
in this condition originate from increased mental effort. However, this was not the case,

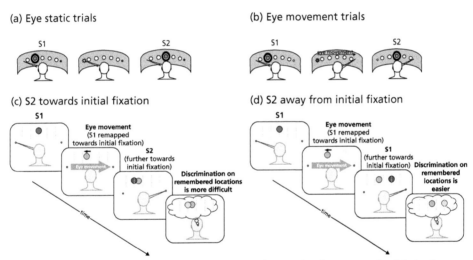

Figure 7.13 The experiment by Pavani et al. (2008). (a) Example of an eye-static trial: the first
sound (S1) is delivered 10 degrees to the left of the body midline), the second sound (S2) is
delivered along the body midline, the eyes fixate an LED to the left of the speaker array during
the entire trial. (b) Example of an eye-movement trial: S1 and S2 are delivered as in (a) but
an intervening eye-movement moves the eyes from left to right during the interval between
the two sounds. (c) Interpretation of the cost observed when S2 moves further towards initial
fixation with respect to S1: by effect of the intervening eye-movement the retinal position of S1
changes radically, remapping the memorized position of S1 further towards initial fixation; as
a consequence it becomes harder to tell the difference in spatial position if S2 is also delivered
towards initial fixation. (d) Interpretation of the better performance observed when S2 moves
away from initial fixation.

Reproduced from *Experimental Brain Research*, 189 (4), Francesco Pavani, Masud Husain, and Jon Driver, Eye-
movements intervening between two successive sounds disrupt comparisons of auditory location, pp. 435–449,
doi: 10.1007/s00221-008-1440-7, © Springer-Verlag, 2008. With permission of Springer.

because the disrupting effect of the eye movement only emerged for a specific condition. Figure 7.13 illustrate this for a condition in which the first sound (S1) is presented centrally, and the eyes move from left to right. Performance dropped when the second sound (S2) was delivered *towards* initial fixation (Figure 7.13c), but remained very good when S2 was delivered *away* from initial fixation (Figure 7.13d). This is compatible with a re-mapping of the memorized position of the first sound, which completely changed its retinal position by effect of the intervening eye-movement: S1 was to the right of fixation before the eye-movement, and 'jumped' to a position very much to the left of fixation after the eye-movement. This interaction between eye-movement, visual coordinates, and sound localization has been replicated in recent works (e.g. Krüger et al., 2016), and its neural correlates have been explored also at the level of the superior colliculus (for learning more about these interactions see the book by Jennifer Groh *Making Space: How the Brain Knows Where Things Are*, published in 2014).

7.7 **Conclusions**

Although space appears as unitary and continuous, it actually exists in our brain as a multitude of maps that differ as a function of initial sensory encoding and reference frames. In this chapter we have examined the evidence for this counterintuitive notion, with examples from experimental psychology and cognitive neuroscience, and we have described both the multiple spatial representations available to sensory systems, and the neural and functional mechanisms that integrate these distinct spatial maps. By focusing on three special multisensory representation—personal space, peripersonal space, and extra-personal space—we have shown that even when attempting to solve the position of a unisensory stimulus, multisensory and motor processes are always at play. Typically they help enhancing spatial precision of our perception, but they can also fool our unisensory estimate of object locations introducing systematic biases. This multisensory and motor perspective on space processing can be extremely useful for devising novel approaches to spatial learning or re-learning throughout life, for instance, as a basis for rehabilitation strategies for those individuals in which spatial processing is lost by effect of peripheral deficits (e.g. partial hearing or visual loss) or central damage (e.g. brain lesions).

Chapter 8
Time

8.1 The puzzle of time perception

Few domains of perception science are as puzzling as time. For instance, what are we actually perceiving when we 'perceive time'? Are we measuring a property of the physical environment, or experiencing a purely mental construct? In philosophical circles, this issue has been debated for centuries. Aristotle, for instance, asked whether time could exist 'if there were no soul' to experience time as it unfolds (*Physics*, Book IV, 218 b.C.), and Augustine concluded that 'it is in my mind ... that I measure time. I must not allow my mind to insist that time is something objective' (*Confessions,* XI.27). In *The Critique of Pure Reason* (1787), Kant argued that 'time is not an empirical conception'—in analogy with space, he argued that time is not something that we perceive, but rather an a-priori precondition for all experience. Whether you assume that time is objective or subjective, it is clear that time as measured by a clock does not necessarily match time as experienced in consciousness. For instance, the interval between 9 AM and 10 AM is the same every day, but it will likely 'feel' different during working days or during the weekend. This is sometimes called the Hans Castorp paradox, after the name of the protagonist of one the past century's literary masterpieces (see Box 8.1). If you think about it, these philosophical and literary preoccupations are not unfounded. Within the traditional notion of the five senses, different sensory mechanisms are devoted to recording information carried by specific energetic media: electromagnetic energy for vision, mechanical energy for touch and hearing, and chemical energy for olfaction and taste. We have already seen how problematic these taxonomic attempts can become when subjected to careful scrutiny (see Box 1.1 in Chapter 1). When time enters the stage, these problems become even more obvious, for there clearly is no specific physical energy that could be considered the medium carrying information about time, and hence no sensory receptors to perform the transduction of this medium. This has led contemporary theorists to argue that time must necessarily be a mental construction (Pöppel, 1997), and that rather than attempting to study 'time' perception, we should study time-related properties of events (Vicario, 2005).

With this recommendation as starting point, here we will examine five properties of events that are relevant to time perception, to reveal how they depend in fundamental ways on multisensory interactions. As a first step, we will examine *simultaneity* and *succession* between events. As we shall see, the ability to determine whether sensory signals in different channels have reached us at the same time plays a key role in triggering the perception of unity, i.e. the subjective feeling that the signals may originate from the same

Box 8.1 The Hans Castorp paradox

Thomas Mann's *The Magic Mountain* (1924) is considered a cornerstone of twentieth century German literature. Hans Castorp, a young man from Hamburg who is about to start his professional career, goes on a trip to visit his tubercular cousin at a sanatorium in Davos in the Swiss Alps. The planned brief visit turns into a seven-year long stay after Castorp is himself diagnosed with tuberculosis. The novel ends with the beginning of World War I, and with Castorp volunteering for the German army to face a probable death in the battlefield. Most of the book is devoted to describing Castorp's encounters and experiences in the unique environment of the sanatorium over this long period. The uneventful sanatorium life slows time down. However, Castorp's experience of time eventually results in a paradox. In his memory, the lengthy period becomes short, as if time had run faster rather than slower. The structure of the book's chapters reflects this asymmetry, with the first five chapters detailing evens that occur in the initial year, and the last two summarizing the remaining six and the closing of the plot. In this, Mann's novel may be considered both a meditation on psychological time (in its report of Castorp's experience of durations), and a quasi-experiment on temporal cognition (in its attempt to map time to chapter structure).

external object. Hence, the ability to perceive simultaneity may be of great importance in setting multisensory interaction priors (i.e. a priori assumptions on whether two or more sensory signals should be combined or not, see Chapter 4). On the other side of the temporal coin, how we perceive succession contributes to segregate events into distinct spatiotemporal units, and to order them into temporal chains. This in turn is central to our impression of causality: event A occurred just before event B, hence A may have caused B. The third property of events that we will discuss is their *temporal coherence*. As we shall see, when perceiving succession and simultaneity we are not particularly precise and often inaccurate. This fact has been amply documented, and it begs the question of how temporally coherent events could possibly emerge in consciousness. We will selectively review multisensory mechanisms that promote this fundamental feature of temporal perception despite imprecisions and inaccuracies in how we time-stamp events. The fourth property that we will address is *duration*. Duration is considered a key building block of the awareness of the unfolding of time (Pöppel, 1997), and studying it has rather naturally lead scholars to entertain the hypothesis of a 'mental clock.' What operations should be performed within a functional mechanism for tracking the passing of time? How would these be implemented in the brain? From the standpoint of multisensory processes, an important question here is whether we indeed use a single centralized clock, 'ticking' in the same way irrespective of the different sensory inputs, or rather we coordinate separate clocks for each sensory channel. Finally, we will consider how basic temporal features of events could combine, within and across sensory channels, to give rise to the perception of *rhythm*. Rhythm is central to several cognitive abilities, including sensorimotor coordination, the ability to predict the occurrence of future sensory events, and—last but not least—music. As we shall see, multisensory interactions have interesting implications for rhythm perception, and for the debated issue of multisensory Gestalten (which we have already discussed in Chapter 4).

In addition, two more conceptual points are in order to set the stage for the chapter. The first is the distinction between the ability to quantify time intervals and the ability to pin events to a moment in time. Gallister (2011) has called these two abilities the *interval sense* and the *phase sense*. The interval sense implies functional and neural mechanisms to keep track of durations that can then be compared. By contrast, the phase sense implies the existence of cognitive mechanisms that can time-stamp events in the continuous flow of experience. The distinction is important to understand how empirical questions about event features in time are operationalized in experiments. The second point is that time can entail very different scales: milliseconds (sometimes referred to as 'sub-seconds'), seconds, minutes, hours, days, years. Ideally, a psychology of time should address all of these, but in this chapter we will focus only on time in the sub-second and seconds range.

8.2 Simultaneity and succession

Imagine the following situation: you are sitting at a table, with an old book in front of you, and you decide to close it. In the precise moment when the two book's halves close against each other, a set of sensory signals becomes available and results in a constellation of percepts. You hear the sound of the soft collision between the two halves of the book when you close it. You see the visual consequences of this action in terms of changing shapes, motion, and of your own visible motor behaviour. You feel the impact as a vibration on your hands. Your smell the typical odour of old paper emanating from the pages. Multimodal perceptual experiences like this are common—perhaps you even remember experiencing something very similar when you last read an old book. So common, in fact, that we typically don't realize that they entail a set of complicated problems when considered from the standpoint of multisensory perception.

To appreciate the problem, consider the chain of events that needs to take place for our brain to receive all the available information about you closing the book. First of all, stimulus information from the environment is carried by some form of energy, which receptors transduce into neural impulses. The transduction process is very fast (approximately 1 ms) for auditory stimuli, and still quite fast for visual stimuli (about 30 to 40 ms) and somatosensory stimuli (between 15 and 30 ms, depending on which body part has been stimulated (Bergenheim, Johansson, Granlund, & Pedersen, 1996; von Békésy, 1963). For olfactory stimuli, in contrast, transduction is considerably slower as it may take up to 100 to 150 ms (Hummel, Knecht, & Kobal, 1996). This means that sensory signals within different channels will not become neural impulses at the same time, even if they originate from the same physical event. To complicate matters further, consider also that different media (i.e. physical energy) carry information through space at different velocities. Odour molecules typically diffuse slowly in the air, sound waves propagate in the air at approximately 330 metres per second, light travels at 300 *million* metres per second, and mechanical events on the skin do not need to travel at all, they exert their action directly on the skin's surface.

Once we combine the effects of the different transduction times and of the different propagation speeds, simultaneity becomes a complicated concept indeed. An event may generate physically simultaneous visual and auditory signals. Typically, however, these signals will not reach the brain at the same time. For an audio-visual stimulus *near* the body, although light will travel faster, sound will still reach the ears relatively quickly and, because transduction is faster in auditory receptors in comparison to photoreceptors, signals will reach the auditory cortex *before* they reach the visual cortex. However, exactly the same event occurring *far* from the body would result in opposite processing advantages. Because visual signals travel at the speed of light, over a longer distance they will reach the photoreceptors quickly and before the auditory signals reach the ears. Therefore, photoreceptors will begin transduction considerably earlier than auditory receptors, and this will result in brain responses occurring earlier in visual than auditory cortices. One could try to calculate the exact distance at which differences in transduction and energy propagation time are in perfect balance, such that the multisensory signals reach the primary sensory cortices at exactly the same time. This distance has been termed the *horizon of simultaneity* and has been estimated for vision and hearing to occur approximately at 12 metres from the observer (Pöppel, 1997). However, the horizon of simultaneity obviously does not predict perceived simultaneity—most conversations occur at much shorter distances that 12 metres, and yet we do not perceive the person talking to us as being out of sync.

Given these premises, one might doubt that simultaneity and succession can be perceived at all. No doubt, we perceive that some events occur at the same time and that others do not, but several experimental psychologists of the past have indeed argued that these percepts are, at best, rough guesses that can be dramatically inaccurate. For instance, the French psychologist Henri Piéron maintained that a rigorous impression of simultaneity can be experienced only for stimuli presented within the same sensory channel, whereas this is not possible for stimuli delivered to different channels (Piéron, 1952). A similar idea was also expressed by Paul Fraisse (1964), a student of Henry Piéron and Albert Michotte. Following in his mentors' footsteps, Fraisse went on to become the founding father of the psychology of time. Half a century of carefully planned psychometric research has shown that our ability to tell whether two multisensory events are simultaneous or sequential is influenced by many variables, such that perceived simultaneity and succession do not always correspond to physical simultaneity and succession (for review, see Keetels & Vroomen, 2012).

To illustrate the dissociation between perceived and physical time, let us consider a study conducted by van Eijk and colleagues (van Eijk, Kohlrausch, Juola, & van de Par 2008). In each trial of this experiment, participants were exposed to visual and auditory stimuli separated by different delays, and were asked to perform three different types of task. In some blocks, the instruction was to judge which perceptual modality was presented first, vision or hearing. This task is known as a *temporal order judgement* or TOJ (see also Chapter 7 for a description of this method in the unisensory context of tactile processing). In other blocks, participants were asked instead to judge whether the two stimuli were presented at the same time, making a forced choice between 'synchronous' and 'asynchronous.' This is a *simultaneity judgement* task and it is often abbreviated SJ2, because only two responses are allowed in each trial. Finally, in some other blocks participants made simultaneity judgement with three possible responses: 'synchronous', 'auditory first', or 'visual first.' This is abbreviated as SJ3, because three responses are allowed in each trial. The employed stimuli were also changed across experimental sessions: in one session, the stimuli were a visual flash and an auditory click; in another session, they were a computer simulation of a ball falling vertically and bouncing on a flat plane, paired with the sound of its impact. Thus, van Eijk and colleagues examined simultaneity and succession when task demands changed, and when stimulation changed. If estimates of simultaneity and succession depended only on the physical stimulation, neither task demands nor stimulation type should have played a role. However, this turned out clearly not to be the case.

The results of the van Eijk experiment are illustrated in Figure 8.1, separately for the flash-click stimulus and for the bouncing ball stimulus. Plotted in each graph is the performance of participants in the TOJ and in the SJ2 task, as a function of the delay between

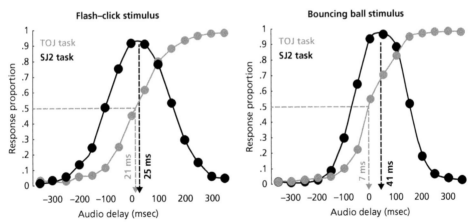

Figure 8.1 The results of the study by Van Eijk and colleagues (2008). The black bell-shaped curves show performance in the SJ2 task (simultaneity judgement, with only two responses 'simultaneous' vs 'not-simultaneous'); response proportion refers here to the proportion of 'synchronous' responses. The grey S-shaped curve show performance in the temporal order judgement (TOJ) task (i.e. which event came first); response proportion refers here to 'visual first' responses. Note that the estimate of the point of simultaneity (the peak of the bell curve for the SJ2 task, the point corresponding to 0.5 response proportion in the TOJ task) do not match in the two tasks. Moreover, note that changing the nature of the stimuli (flash-click or bouncing ball) modulates this discrepancy.

the visual and the auditory stimulus (for the sake of clarity we have omitted the results of the SJ3 task). Consider the black bell-shaped curves first, which show the proportion of 'synchronous' responses in the SJ2 task. The proportion is very low when visual and auditory stimuli are separated by more than 250 ms (i.e. participants never think that the two stimuli were simultaneous at this temporal separation). In contrast, the proportion becomes high when the stimuli are delivered more or less at the same time (i.e. participants very often believe that the two stimuli were simultaneous). By projecting the peak of the curve onto the x-axis (see black dashed arrow in Figure 8.1), we can locate one estimate of the delay that best yields perceived simultaneity. We note that participants perceive the two events as synchronous when in fact the visual stimuli lead the auditory ones by a small interval. However, this error depends on the nature of the delivered stimuli: it is larger for the bouncing ball (41 ms; right plot in Figure 8.1) in comparison to the flash-click stimuli (25 ms; left plot in Figure 8.1).

Consider now the grey S-shaped curve, which shows the proportion of 'visual first' responses in the TOJ task. The proportion is near 0 when the auditory stimulus leads by 200 ms or more (i.e. participants never think that the visual stimulus led the auditory one). In contrast, it rises to near 1 when the visual stimulus leads by 200 ms or more (i.e. participants most often think that the visual stimulus led the auditory one). In this S-shaped curve the perceived simultaneity can be estimated by reading the value on the x-axis that corresponds to a proportion equal to 0.5, that is, when participants are equally likely to say that visual precedes auditory, or that it lags it. This can therefore be taken as another estimate of the delay yielding perceived simultaneity (see grey dashed arrow in Figure 8.1) Note that again the nature of stimulus affects the temporal judgement (subjective simultaneity for the bouncing ball is 7 ms; but for the flash-click it is 21 ms). Furthermore, it is evident that changing the task (TOJ vs SJ2) alters the perceived simultaneity between the two events: the measures obtained with two methods diverge.

The results of van Eijk and collaborators reveal that perceived simultaneity does not necessarily correspond to physical synchronicity. This finding has been replicated using audio-visual stimuli in many other studies, and these studies have confirmed that perceived simultaneity usually occurs when the visual stimulus anticipates the sound by a small interval (e.g. Dixon & Spitz, 1980; Slutsky & Recanzone, 2001; Zampini, Shore, & Spence, 2003; Vatakis & Spence, 2006). Why this is the case has not been definitely established. One possibility is that this effect reflects an adaptation of multisensory mechanisms to a regularity of the natural environment. Think of the last time you saw lightning and heard thunder. The events producing the visual and the auditory signals were of course synchronous, but as light travels much faster than sound, we usually see lighting first. In general, physically synchronous signals will tend to result in visual experiences leading auditory experiences, especially if the signals originate at some distance from the body. Multisensory perception may somehow 'take into account' this regularity by displacing perceived simultaneity to situations when vision is in fact leading hearing (King & Palmer, 1985). Alternatively, the visual-lead bias could reflect a physiological constraint, namely, that transduction times are faster for auditory compared to visual signals. As we have seen earlier, if signals originate near the body, the differences in transduction times will cause auditory signal to reach cortex first. Perhaps the visual-lead bias reflects an imperfect compensation of this second regularity. But note that the two regularities are not mutually exclusive. Perhaps both have been incorporated, and the observed biases are the outcome of an imperfect internal calibration.

Most importantly, the van Eijk study shows that contingent variables—which task is performed, which stimuli are presented—can modulate the perceived simultaneity of events (and therefore, presumably, that visual-auditory calibration is flexible). The difference between the TOJ and SJ2 tasks observed by van Eijk and colleagues could reflect different expectations that were triggered by the two tasks. In TOJ, participants presumably focused on the delay between the two signals, which may have led them to expect that they would not be synchronous. By contrast, in SJ2 they presumably focused on the impression of unity that the two signals conveyed, leading to the opposite expectation. Likewise, discrepancies in performance between the flash-click and the bouncing ball stimuli could be due to different expectations elicited by the two multisensory events. The flash-click stimuli were arbitrarily paired stimuli, and synchronicity could not be anticipated. By contrast, the bouncing ball stimuli were more 'naturalistic' and allowed participants to anticipate the presentation of the sound by looking at the ball approaching the horizontal line of bounce. Thus, expectancy induced by the task or by the stimuli could have contributed to the changes in perceived simultaneity. In Tutorial 8.1 we discuss another possible variable that could have affected the simultaneity/succession judgment, namely the way attention was allocated to the involved sensory channels.

Tutorial 8.1 Prior entry

Interest in *prior entry* predates studies of experimental psychology (Boring, 1950). Its origin is traditionally ascribed to a fight between astronomers at the Royal Greenwich observatory in the UK. Around the turn of the nineteenth century, astronomers attempting to measure stellar transits (i.e. the exact time when a star passed a meridian) adopted the so-called 'eye-and-ear' method. The method consisted in observing the star through a telescope with the meridian indicated by a vertical wire, while at the same time listening to the ticking of a clock. By remembering the position of the star at the beat just before and just after the crossing of the vertical reference, astronomers were capable of estimating the exact moment in which the stellar transit occurred (Mollon & Perkins, 1996). The precision of this measurement was assumed to be in the order of 100 ms. In the winter of 1796, however, the Astronomer Royal at that time, Nevil Maskelyne, discovered that measures taken by his assistant, David Kinnebrook, differed from his own by as much as 800 ms. The discovery lead to a quarrel, and Kinnebrook was eventually dismissed from his role. Admittedly, Kinnebrook also refused to marry a lady who was Maskelyne's protégée (Mollon & Perkins, 1996), but this aspect of the story remained in the archives, whereas the dispute over stellar transit times became a topic of scientific investigation.

Why did the two astronomers gave such different measurements although they were using the same method? The most accredited interpretation originates from the work of another astronomer, Bessel (1822), who shortly after the Maskelyne–Kinnebrook affair noticed that many other astronomers diverged in their estimates of stellar transit when using the 'eye-and-ear' method. Instead of attributing these mistakes to negligence, he speculated that different individuals allocate attention to different perceptual modalities when performing multisensory tasks. Moreover, Bessel hypothesized that a stimulus in the attended modality (visual or auditory) enjoys a temporal advantage in processing and therefore obtains priority in accessing to awareness. In other words, the difference between any two astronomers could reflected the tendency of one to pay attention to the stars observed, and the other to pay attention to the clock's ticks. Resulting differences in temporal judgements may thus been caused by different strategies in allocating attention. The intuition that attended objects or events may reach awareness faster that unattended ones proved correct, so much that Edward Titchner (1908), one of the pioneers of experimental psychology, listed it among the seven laws of attention and termed it the *prior entry* phenomenon (for review see Spence & Parise, 2010).

Almost a century later, interest in prior entry and its multisensory implications are still a matter of investigation. For instance, Spence, Shore, and Kline (2001) presented participants with visual-visual, tactile-tactile, or visuo-tactile stimulus pairs, each in one hemifield (e.g. vision on the left, tactile on the right). In some blocks, the proportion of visual and tactile stimuli was unbalanced (e.g. 50 percent of V-V stimuli; 50 percent of V-T stimuli, but no T-T stimuli), and participants were instructed to attend to the most probable modality. In other blocks the proportion of visual and tactile stimuli was balanced (e.g. 25 percent of V-V stimuli; 25 percent of T-T stimuli; and 50 percent of V-T stimuli) and participants were instructed to attend to both modalities at once. Participants were asked to judge the temporal order of each pair of stimuli, reporting whether the first stimulus appeared on the left or on the right. The results of one of the experiments conducted by Spence, Shore, & Klein (2001) are shown in Figure 8.2, and illustrate well the consequences of attention on perceived timing. Overall, the plot shows that the visual and tactile signals were perceived as occurring at the same time when vision had a temporal advantage with respect to touch. This effect is typically interpreted as the consequence of faster neural processing of the tactile signals compared to the visual ones, such that the visual signals need to be delivered some interval before the tactile for simultaneity to emerge. When instructing participants to divide their attention between the

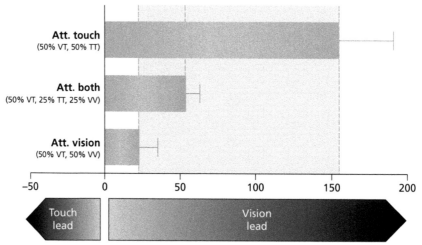

Figure 8.2 The results of Spence, Shore, and Klein (2001; Experiment 2). When attention is allocated to both modalities, vision lead by about 50 ms. However, this effect is halved when attention is allocated to vision, and rises to over 150 ms when attention is allocated to touch. Note that the *x*-axis in the plot shows the PSS, i.e. the relative timing between visual and tactile events at which participants were unable to estimate which side came first—hence, the two stimuli were perceived as occurring at the same time (see main text for explanation of the PSS).

two modalities, this interval was approximately 50 ms. Directing attention selectively to vision or select-ively to touch, however, changed this interval depending on the attended modality. Attending to vision decreased the vision-lead effect to less than 25 ms, whereas attending to touch alone expanded the effect to over 150 ms.

The observation that orienting attention to a specific modality changes perceived multisensory timing has now been extended to other combinations of sensory modalities. For instance, Massimiliano Zampini and co-workers have documented the same phenomenon between vision and hearing (Zampini, Shore, & Spence, 2005), and even between vision and nociception (Zampini, Sanabria, Phillips, & Spence, 2007). Furthermore, we now know that prior entry effects can also emerge when attentional resources are dir-ected to a specific spatial location, rather than a specific modality, before the appearance of relevant target stimuli. One elegant multisensory demonstration of this phenomenon was provided by Shinsuke Shimojo using the 'line-motion effect' (Shimojo, Miyauchi, & Hikosaka, 1997). When a flash of light (i.e. a spatial attention cue) is delivered shortly before the appearance of a line, the line is typically perceived to expand from the cued side towards the other, even when it was in fact presented all at once. This effect again reflects the prior-entry phenomenon: because of the spatial cueing one extremity of the line access aware-ness before the other, and the resulting percept is the apparent unfolding of the line in time. Interestingly, Shimojo and colleagues observed that exactly the same line-motion effect could be induced also when a beep was presented from left or right space (auditory cue), or when an electro-tactile stimulation was applied to the right or left hand (somatosensory cue) resting on either side of the screen on which the line was delivered. In sum, individual preferences to attend one modality over the other, instructions to monitor one specific sensory modality or spatial cues can result in prior entry effect that alter our sense of time over multisensory stimuli.

Although prior entry is well established, several issues remain unanswered. For instance, one open question concerns its neural implementation. Intuitively, one would expect that prior entry effects should emerge as changes in the speed of neural processing in the brain. This position was proposed in the mid of the twentieth century by the Gestalt psychologist Wolfgang Köhler who claimed that 'experienced order in time is always structurally identical with a functional order in the sequence of correlated brain processes' (Köhler, 1947, p. 62). Evidence in support of this claim were provided a decade ago using event-related potentials (ERPs). Vibell and colleagues (Vibell, 2007) measured ERPs while participants performed a visuo-tactile TOJ task, in blocks in which attention was direct attention either to vision or to touch (similar to the study by Spence, Shore, & Klein, 2001; see Figure 8.2). The authors noticed that the voltage peaks of two of the visual evoked potentials (the first positive peak, P1; and the first negative peak, N1) were anticipated when participants paid attention to vision (P1, 147 ms; N1, 198 ms) compared to when they paid attention to touch (P1, 151 ms; N1, 201 ms). This result is indeed compatible with the notion that attention speeds up perceptual processing in the attended modality. However, it should also be noted that the effects were in the order of few milliseconds (on average 3 to 4 ms) whereas the effects measured in behaviour are almost two orders of magnitude larger (see Figure 8.2 in which the difference between attending to vision and attending to touch modulated the PSS by approximately 150 ms). This huge discrepancy between neural and behavioural data should—at the very least—invite extreme caution when considering the effect measured by Vibell and colleagues as the neural homologue of prior entry. In fact, it suggests once again that the temporal perception of events cannot be reduced to just neural trans-mission times as we have argued throughout this chapter.

Having established that perceived simultaneity and succession are influenced by many psychological variables, let us now return to the plots shown in Figure 8.1. If you consider the bell-shaped curves that plot the simultaneity judgements, it is clear that participants show a degree of uncertainty as to whether stimuli are synchronous or not. On average, they start to provide 'simultaneous' responses when the stimuli are still separated by tens of milliseconds. For instance, when the separation is 150 ms and flash-beep stimuli were used (left plot), participants judged these to be simultaneous in about 20–30 percent of responses. This is not just an averaging artefact, as it emerges also when analysing participants individually (not shown). Thus, participants experience a degree of uncertainty when trying to establish whether the two events happened at the same time or in succession. This uncertainty is interesting, because it can be used within a statistical model to estimate the *differential threshold* (DT), which in this case would be the temporal offset needed by participants to be able to reliably classify successive signals as such (reliably usually meaning 'at least 80% of the times').

The DT is a measure of sensory precision (the smaller the threshold, the more precise you are in classifying), and this represents a valuable piece of information, both for researchers studying time perception across modalities, and for professionals operating in several practical contexts. For instance, it has been studied by engineers interested in broadcasting (e.g. Finger & Davis, 2001; Fedina & Glasman, 2006) because it captures the degree of de-synchronization that observers can tolerate when hearing voices and viewing lips (in a poorly dubbed movie, in a slow-connection videoconference). Specifically, if the delay between auditory and visual stimulation is below the DT, it will remain unnoticed. In contrast, if it exceeds the DT, it will lead to frustrating mismatches that could become an obstacle to speech understanding. As for perceived simultaneity, the DT also varies with task demands and stimulus features. We will consider two of examples of such modulations: the influence of the spatial separation between the sources, and the influence of to the nature of the stimulation.

That differential thresholds change as a function of the spatial separation between the sources of sensory signals has been often reported, suggesting an intriguing link between time and space. For instance, Paul Bertelson and Gisa Aschersleben (2003) showed that DTs for beeps and flashes are lower for sources at distinct spatial locations, in comparison to presentations where they are both at a common central location. Likewise, Keetels and Vroomen (2005) manipulated the spatial separation between sources of audio-visual signals and observed that participants were better at discriminating temporal order when these were farther apart than when they were close. (see also Zampini, Shore, & Spencel, 2003). Two different explanations have been put forward to account for these interactions between space and time (Spence & Squire, 2003). The first has to do with a sort *assumption of unity* induced by spatial proximity. Elements that are near each other tend to form a perceptual unit (the Gestalt law of proximity, see Chapter 4), and sensory signals that are coded as originating from the same location are more likely to be treated as originating from the same event (Chapter 7). It would therefore be plausible to expect that signals that are unified would be harder to discriminate on all perceptual dimensions, including their position in time. A different explanation is instead linked to the notion of *information redundancy*. The idea here is that placing of correct time-stamps could be aided by the possibility of pinning events to different locations in space. For instance, observers attending a visual event delivered in the right hemifield, followed by an auditory event delivered in the left hemifield, can encode that the visual stimulus as 'first' and 'to the right,' and the auditory event as 'second' and 'to the left.' In comparison with a condition in which both events occur at the same spatial location, this redundancy of temporal and spatial markers could help establishing a criterion for decision.

Whatever your preferred explanation, that space changes our sensitivity to auditory offsets has important practical implications. It means, for instance, that in contexts where it is important to convey an impression of temporal unity (think video-conferencing), one should keep the sources of multisensory signals as close as possible (i.e. the speaker and the screen). Vice versa, in contexts where it is important to emphasize succession one should keep the sources as spatially distinct as possible. This may happen, for instance, in a multimodal interface for human–computer interaction. Suppose you touch a button to cause a global change of the environment (say, go to the next input window), and that a sound is provided to signal that the request has been carried out, whereas another sound is presented as an error signal if your request cannot be executed. It will be useful within such a context that the success sound be perceived as successive to your action (and therefore as applied to the global environment), whereas failure be perceived as intrinsic to your action. These simple multisensory rules are often violated in multimodal interfaces, with confusing and sometimes maddening effects on user behaviour, as many of us know well from using cash machines.

The complexity of the stimulus situation is another factor that changes how precisely we can perceive simultaneity. This was first shown in a classic study (Dixon & Spitz, 1980) that compared different audio-visual events. Specifically, some of these stimulus events consisted in the face of a person reading a text, whereas others in a hammer hitting a peg. All videos started in synchrony and were brought increasingly out of synch (with either the auditory or the visual stream leading in time). Participants responded as soon as they detected an asynchrony. This study revealed an unexpected effect of the type of event. In the audio-visual speech videos, asynchrony was perceived when the voice was delayed by 258 ms or more with respect to the images, or when it preceded the video by 131 ms. By contrast, when the video showed the hammer hitting the peg, the asynchrony was perceived when the sound preceded the images by 75 ms or followed them by 187 ms. This means that observers failed to notice temporal discrepancies over an interval that spanned more than one-third of a second when judging audio-visual speech, but were considerably more precise when judging the audio-visual hammering action.

It is now generally accepted that DTs are higher for stimuli of greater complexity, in comparison to simpler ones (Jones & Jarick 2006; Stekelenburg & Vroomen 2007; Vatakis & Spence 2006; Vatakis, Ghanzanfar, & Spence 2008). For instance, Vatakis and Spence (2006) compared temporal order judgements of different types multisensory stimuli: audio-visual speech, audio-visual music, or audio-visual actions. Examples of these would be a video of a person visible from the waist upward, uttering the sentence 'Keep up the good work'; of a person playing music on a guitar, or of a person visible from the waist up hitting a soda can with a wooden stick. Using these materials, Vatakis and Spence found that DTs were larger for speech in comparison to actions (160 vs 120 ms, respectively), as had already been reported by Dixon and Spitz (1980). In addition, they found that the DTs were even larger for the music stimuli (about 250 ms). In general, the magnitude of the DTs for all these complex stimuli was considerably larger than those observed with noise bursts and light flashes (about 65 ms; Zampini, Shore, & Spence, 2003), with audiovisual syllables (105 ms; Stekelenburg & Vroomen, 2007), or hand claps (64 ms; Stekelenburg & Vroomen, 2007).

In sum, perceiving simultaneity and succession in multisensory conditions turns out to be quite complicated. We sometimes judge as simultaneous events that are, in fact, asynchronous; and vice versa. While well established, this conclusion is, however, at odds with how we experience spatiotemporal events in different perceptual modalities. We experience multisensory events as temporally coherent, unified sources of percepts, and these unified perceptions serve us well in our bodily interactions with these events. Scientists investigating multisensory time perception typically resolve this issue invoking the notion of *window of temporal integration,* i.e. a degree of temporal tolerance that is applied to multisensory events and allows for their integration even when they are not perfectly synchronous.

In a nutshell, the idea of a window of temporal implies that multisensory interactions can take place even when different sensory signals are not physically synchronous. Instead, multiple signals interact if their timing is within a certain temporal window. Examples of this notion have been reported within different domains, both linguistic and non-linguistic. You may recall from Tutorial 1.1 (Chapter 1) that an interesting example of audiovisual interactions in speech perception is the McGurk effect (see Box 8.2). Soto-Faraco and Alsius (2007) have shown that participants can experience the McGurk effect even with audio-visual parings that they perceive as asynchronous. On each trial of this study, participants were presented with a brief videoclip showing the close-up of a mouth uttering a phoneme. By varying the delay between the video and the audio traces, the experimenters produced different physical asynchronies. Immediately after each presentation, participants performed two tasks: a temporal order judgment ('was the voice first or second?') and a phoneme discrimination ('ba, da, or else?'). This resulted in two concurrent measures of audio-visual timing: one related to the perception of simultaneity, and another related to the optimal McGurk effect. Although one would expect that events perceived as asynchronous would be less prone to integration, and therefore to a less salient McGurk effect, the results of Soto-Faraco and Alsius (2007) disconfirmed this prediction. Participants instead reported a strong McGurk effect even in many conditions that were perceived as asynchronous as inferred from the TOJs.

Empirical support for a window of temporal integration is also found from studies using non-linguistic materials. For instance, Shimojo et al. (2001) used the so-called 'stream-bounce' task (Sekuler, Sekuler, & Lau, 1997), which you may recall from our discussion in Chapter 4. In the stream-bounce effect, two discs are moved on the computer screen, each moving downward along one of the screen diagonals. When the discs meet at the centre of the screen, a sound is played. The resulting perception of movement changes depending on whether the tone is integrated with the visual stimuli or not. If it is integrated,

Box 8.2 The McGurk effect and the multisensory nature of spoken language

We communicate using our body, our voice, and by abstract visual symbols in writing. The mental functions subtending these abilities constitute fundamental cognitive interfaces for presenting our social self, sharing internal states, and generally interact socially with other humans. Although our behaviour at large is a form of communication—we approach, avoid, smile, frown, laugh, whine—human language is undoubtedly the main vector of our interpersonal communication with other humans. For most people, this is a rich multisensory experience that emerges from the continuous integration of auditory, visual, somatosensory, and motor signals. The topic of interpersonal communication and human language is terribly vast, and this box can offer only a glimpse. Among the research areas that we have not the opportunity to develop in this book, language is surely one that could easily become a book on its own. There is, however, at least one multisensory effect in language perception that cannot be left out of this book, if anything because it is one of the most cited perceptual illusion of the psychological literature, and an icon of multisensory research: the McGurk effect.

More than 30 years ago, Harry McGurk and John McDonald (1976) described an impressive demonstration that the perception of spoken language is more than just processing the auditory input at the ears. The effect is known as *the McGurk effect* (sometimes also called 'ba-ga-da' effect). In the typical version of this effect the voice of a person uttering the /ba/ syllable is recorded. Next, the same person is filmed while producing the /ga/ syllable. When considered in isolation, the auditory and the visual syllables are largely unambiguous, i.e. listeners systematically report hearing /ba/ in the audio trace, and seeing /ga/ in the video trace. However, when the audio and video are delivered together, like in a dubbed movie, an unexpected perceptual effect emerges. In most cases, people report hearing the /da/ syllable, which did not exist in the sensory stimulation. In brief, what you see modifies what you hear (see Figure 8.3; if you wish to try this illusion, you can find many well-prepared examples on the internet; just type 'McGurk effect demo' in your search engine).

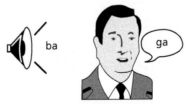

Figure 8.3 The McGurk effect. The audio of a person saying /ba/ is paired with the video of an actor saying /ga/. This audio-visual stimulus frequently produce the illusory impression that the uttered syllable is in fact /da/.

Box 8.2 Continued

The McGurk effect shows that spoken language is more than just an auditory experience, and it is a fine example of how multisensory integration creates novel percepts that did not exist in the environment. Since the original demonstration of the effect, a large set of studies have examined its robustness and have explored its perceptual boundaries. For instance, we now know that the McGurk effect persists even when the heard voice belongs to a male, and the seen face belongs to a female person or vice versa; Green et al., 1991). The effect emerges also when participants repeat the audio-visual syllables, instead of identifying them (Gentilucci & Cattaneo, 2005). In addition, it can be obtained with combinations of audio-tactile inputs, touching the video of the actor uttering /ga/ while hearing /ba/ through closed headphones (Fowler & Delke, 1991; see also Gick & Derrick 2009 for further example of audio-tactile interactions in speech perception). These results, together with many others that we do not discuss here for brevity, indicate that perceiving spoken language is a rich multisensory experience. It can involve hearing, sight, and somatosensation; it emerges in a largely automatic fashion, across different types of tasks; and—most importantly—it changes our recognition and categorization of the information obtained through the separate sensory channels. One important aspect to remark is that the McGurk effect has been documented in all the languages in which it has been investigated (Massaro et al., 1993), and it seems to emerge only when the auditory stimuli are processed specifically as spoken language. If the normal sounds of language are transformed into sinusoidal tones that mimic speech (the so-called *sine-wave speech*; see examples at http://www.scholarpedia.org/article/Sine-wave_speech), the McGurk effect tends to disappear when the listener does not recognize the sounds as syllables, and emerges again if the participants are taught to recognize the syllable hidden in the modified sound (Tuomainen et al., 2005). These results indicate that the McGurk effect likely entails perception of spoken language, and not just generically sound. It is as if our brain had a multisensory mechanism specifically dedicated to the processing of spoken language.

The McGurk effect is paradigmatic in showing the contribution of multisensory perception in many instances of human communication. Consider, for instance, the effort we make when try to understand someone speaking a foreign language. If you can hear the speaker but you cannot see her lips, typically it is harder to understand what is being said. You may have experienced this difficulty last time you used a foreign language over the phone, and perhaps you noticed how listening in this situation proved more difficult compared to face-to-face situations. Or, in case you wear glasses, you may recall the experience of hearing better with glasses on than without them. Research has documented the advantage of seeing the face and lips of the speaker starting from the 1950s. Sumby and Pollack (1954) showed that listening in noise—a minimally challenging situation for typically hearing people, but a frustratingly difficult experience for most hearing-impaired individuals—considerably

Box 8.2 **Continued**

improves when combined auditory and visual input is available, compared to an auditory only situation. For instance, in their hardest scenario Sumby and Pollack made participants listen to a series of 256 bisyllabic words, embedded in noise (signal-to-noise ratio -30 dB in favour of noise). They observed that the percent of words correctly identified was between 0 and 5 percent when listeners faced away from the speaker (auditory only condition), but performance increased to about 40 percent when participants watched the speaker's facial movements as he spoke (see Figure 8.4).

A familiar context for experiencing the multisensory nature of spoken language is the cinema. We already referred to this situation when describing the ventriloquist illusion, but here we would like to emphasize another aspect of this common experience. In many countries, there is the habit of dubbing foreign movies into the local language, pairing the speaking face of the actor on the screen with words spoken in a different language. In Italy, for instance, agent 007 orders his cocktail shaken but not stirred by uttering 'Un Vodka-Martini —agitato non mescolato' with the

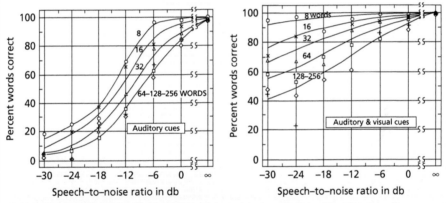

Figure 8.4 The advantage of seeing the speaker when hearing in noise. All curves show performance (percent words correctly reported) for the different conditions of the experiment (i.e. spoken streams of 8, 16, 32, 64, 128, or 256 words), as the speech-to-noise ratio decreases from -30 dB (speech less loud than noise) to 0 dB (speech and noise equally loud). The left panel shows performance when listeners faced away from the speaker (only auditory cues to speech comprehension were available). The right panel shows performance when listeners watched the speaker's facial movements as he spoke (auditory and visual cues available). When auditory cues alone are used performance is very poor at -30 dB and ameliorates progressively as the loudness of speech relative to noise increases. By contrast, when visual cues are also available performance is already above 40 percent correct in the -30 dB signal-to-noise ratio.

Adapted with permission from W. H. Sumby and Irwin Pollack, Visual Contribution to Speech Intelligibility in Noise, *The Journal of the Acoustical Society of America*, 26 (2), pp. pp.212–215, doi: 10.1121/1.1907309 Copyright © 1954, Acoustic Society of America.

Box 8.2 Continued

voice of Italian actor Pino Locchi. Seen in the perspective of this box, you may think that this should be a massive source of McGurk effects: the words uttered by the dubbing actor should be systematically altered by the mismatching visual utterances of the actor in the movie. Yet, this does not happen. One explanation for this is that the overall semantic context of the movie dialogues strongly constrains what can be heard. These is evidence that the McGurk effect does not emerge if meaningful words instead of syllables are used as stimuli (Easton & Basala, 1982), or at least it is much weaker (Delke, Fowler, & Funnel, 1992). Furthermore, the McGurk effect works well with different consonants, but is not equally stable when changing vowels in the stimuli (Green & Gederman, 1995). In addition, a very important factor is the perceived synchrony between the auditory and visual signals. Skilled dubbing actors can produce the impression of a remarkable correspondence between their own spoken utterances and the lip movements of the actors in the movie. This is also possible because dialogues are not simply translated for dubbing, they are carefully adapted attempting to match as closely as possible the length of sentences or even the length of single words, to obtain the maximal correspondence between spoken and seen messages. Nonetheless, it is a common experience for those who actually know both languages (i.e. the original language of the movie, and the language used for dubbing) to experience the frustration of perceiving the two languages at the same time. This could reflect the difficulty of integrating across vision and hearing when the two channels convey distinguishable spoken messages and, as a consequence, even small discrepancies appear as more salient. Indirect support to this interpretation comes from a study by Vatakis and Spence (2007), in which the authors showed that the temporal window for audio-visual integration with language stimuli is broader when the auditory and visual component are congruent (e.g. the /ba/ syllable is both seen and heard), compared to when they are incongruent (e.g. the /ba/ syllable is heard, while participant sees the video of a person pronouncing /da/). Hence, perceiving incongruences in the flow of audio-visual speech could limit multisensory integration for linguistic stimuli.

Over the years, several different accounts have been put forward to explain the McGurk effect. Here we will focus on two classic views. The first one builds on the so-called *motor theory of language perception* (Liberman et al., 1967). According to this theory, originally proposed by the North American psychologist Alvin Liberman, speech perception is not based on the correct identification of specific sounds, but instead reflects the listener's ability in identifying the articulatory gestures that subtend word production. The 'auditory object' we perceive are movements, rather than sounds; which we encode taking advantage of implicit knowledge of the motor patterns that we ourselves use when articulating sounds. The McGurk effect is coherent with the motor theory, because it shows that

Box 8.2 Continued

extra-auditory information related to the visible articulatory gesture can modify speech perception. This theory, however, does not explain why the articulatory gesture associated with /ga/ (perceived through the visual channel) should change the heard sound to /da/, rather than conveying precisely the articulation we observed (i.e. /ga/). This issue is less problematic when seen from the perspective of a different explanation of the McGurk effect: the *fuzzy logical model of perception* or FLMP.

This model has been developed by Dominic Massaro, a psychologist based at UCLA Santa Cruz (Massaro, 1987). According to FLMP, information originating within a single sensory channel or from multiple channels, contributes to various degrees to the definition of the resulting percept. The degree of support resulting from each source of information is quantified in the model with a number between 0 and 1. In some cases, a specific piece of information can be entirely unambiguous with respect to the percept (support = 1), but in most cases the various pieces of information contain ambiguities (support < 1). Let's now apply this logic to the McGurk effect (although note that the FLMP is general and could be applied, in principle, to any perceptual process). If we consider the three consonants involved in the classic McGurk effect (i.e. 'b', 'd', and 'g'), and taking into account some rules of phonetics for consonants (i.e. some consonants are vocalized but others are not; some consonants have a visible place of articulation whereas others are less visible), it is possible to predict which syllable will receive strong vs weak support from the auditory and visual signals. Suppose that strong support means 0.9, weak support means 0.1, and intermediate support equals to 0.5. The /ba/ syllable would receive strong support from the auditory signal, because it is vocalized, but weak support from the visual signal, because it is barely visible on the lips (i.e. 0.9 from hearing × 0.1 from vision = 0.09). On the contrary, the /ga/ syllable would receive weak support from the auditory signal, because it is barely vocalized, but strong support from the visual signal, because it is clearly visible on the lips (i.e. 0.1 from hearing × 0.9 from vision = 0.09). Both signals, however, provide intermediate support to the /da/ percept, which is both vocalized and visible (i.e. 0.5 from hearing × 0.5 from vision = 0.25). As a result, the /da/ percept will dominate, and the audio-visual combination will result in the perception of a consonant that was in neither of the signals. As some of you may have noticed the notion of 'support' in the FLMP model closely resembles the concept of likelihood in the Bayesian approach to multisensory integration (see Chapter 4, section 4.3). To assert that a sensory signal S strongly supports perceptual interpretation X, is equivalent to saying that the probability of S given the X distal state of affairs is high. As a matter of fact, Massaro and Friedman (1990) showed that the FLMP model is formally equivalent to a Bayesian model of multisensory integration.

the sound is perceived as evidence of contact between the two balls, and participants re-port the impression that the two balls 'bounced' one against the other. By contrast, if the sound is not integrated with the visual stimulation, the two balls appear to 'stream' one over the other, without any contact. Shimojo and collaborators varied the delay between the visual impact and the sound systematically. Although the bouncing interpretation (i.e. the signature of audio-visual integration) was maximal when the sound was delivered approximately 50 ms before the object coincided, integration was also observed even for sounds delivered 250 ms before collision and up to 150 ms after collision. This indicates once again a remarkable tolerance for physical asynchronies in multisensory integration, revealing that the brain can ignore detectable temporal discrepancies when this brings the world in synch.

8.3 How do we achieve temporal coherence?

The assumption that a window of temporal integration exists is intuitive and, as we have seen, supported by empirical data. However, it is almost a concept of common sense—if we can integrate despite the difficulty of perceiving synchrony, we must have a window of tolerance when it comes to multisensory processing. The key question thus becomes which cognitive mechanisms our brain implements to make this possible. Keetels and Vroomen (2012) list and discuss a number of mechanisms that may lead to perceived temporal coherence across modalities, and thus serve as a window of temporal integration. Here we will focus on a subset of those mechanisms (interested readers can refer to the original article for a more comprehensive description). Importantly, these mechanisms should not to be considered mutually exclusive, in fact it is very likely that future research will help clarify their interactions.

A first mechanism that could promote temporal unity is *temporal recalibration*. The idea here is that the brain can progressively adapt to discrepancies in the timing of multisensory signals, eventually recalibrating their relative mental time-stamps. For instance, Fujisaki and colleagues (Fujisaki, Shimojo, Kashino, & Nishida, 2004) continually exposed parti-cipants to asynchronous tone-flash stimuli during an adaptation period of approximately 3 minutes. The asynchrony between tones and flashes remained constant throughout this adaptation phase (either the sound or the visual stimulation led by 235 ms). After adaptation, participants were tested using the 'stream-bounce' paradigm described above (p. 224). This test phase revealed that the optimal audio-visual delay producing the bounce percept was shifted in the same direction as the temporal lag used during adapta-tion (see also Vroomen & Keetels, 2004). One important finding that emerged from this study is that the effects of temporal recalibration can generalize to different, unadapted stimuli. For instance, after adaptation to asynchronies between a tone and a flash, partici-pants showed a shift in the stream-bounce phenomenon. This generalization of temporal recalibration has been documented also in other conditions. For instance, some studies (Navarra et al., 2005; Vatakis, Ghazanfar, & Spence C, 2008) asked participants to search specific target words within continuous speech streams in which the lips and the voice of the speaker were either synchronous or asynchronous (with the audio presented 300 ms after the visual information). While engaged in this linguistic task, participants were also asked to perform a temporal order judgement (Navarra et al., 2005) or a simultaneity judgement (Vatakis, Ghazanfar, & Spence, 2008) on non-linguistic stimuli—flashes or burst of white noise—overlaid on the video streams. Exposure to the asynchronous linguistic stimuli degraded performance also on the non-linguistic task. Specifically, the ability to tell the relative time-stamps of flashes and noises decreased, resulting in larger DTs. This can be interpreted as the evidence that adaptation recalibrated the perceptual criteria for simultaneity of flashes and noises, despite the fact that adaptation was to asynchronous audio-visual speech. Note that this recalibration may consist in readjusting the limits of a window of temporal window of integration.

Examples of temporal recalibration have also been reported for other multisensory conditions, and even in relation to actions (see Box 8.3 for other examples of visuo-motor recalibration). However, much remains to be understood about the involved mechanisms. One question regards the scope of the recalibration process. Given repeated exposure to asynchronous sensory signals in two different channels, will recalibration be confined to those signals or it will generalize to other signals in other channels? Initial reports suggested that adaptation could generalize across channels (e.g. from audio-tactile to visuo-tactile), suggesting that temporal recalibration might occur at a sensory-aspecific stage (Hanson, Heron, & Whitaker, 2008). However, later studies reported more limited generalization effects (Di Luca, Machulla, & Ernst, 2009; Harrar & Harris 2008). For instance, Di Luca and colleagues (2009) exposed participants to asynchronous audio-visual stimulation and found that temporal recalibration occurred for the audio-visual pairs (as expected), and generalized to audio-tactile and visual-tactile pairs only depending on the way in which the multisensory stimuli were presented.

. There have also been suggestions that audio-visual pairings may be more prone to recalibration compared to audio-tactile and visuo-tactile pairings (Keetels & Vroomen, 2012). This may be expected because the relative timing of audio-visual stimuli is often altered by the effect of distance (we discussed this problem in section 8.2), whereas pairings involving tactile stimuli occur directly on skin and for this reason they may not require compensating for different latencies.

A second mechanism that could promote temporal coherence across modalities is *temporal ventriloquism*. As suggested by the term itself, this mechanism is assumed to be the temporal analogue of the spatial ventriloquist's effect that we described elsewhere in this book (see Chapter 7). In spatial ventriloquism, a visual signal 'captures' an auditory signal in space, such that we hear the sound as if it came from the location of the seen puppet's mouth. In temporal ventriloquism, an auditory signal captures a visual signal *in time,* such that we perceive the timing of a visual signal to be the same as the timing of an auditory signal. (Incidentally, this mechanism also contributes to the success of a ventriloquist performance, as it promotes the impression that the puppet's voice and lip movements are synchronous, even if the performer is not producing them at exactly the same time.) More generally, the hypothesis is that temporal asynchronies can be compensated by a

Box 8.3 Time recalibration and agency

Exposure to systematic delays between sensory channels can induce temporal recalibration. After adapting to the delays, participants start to perceive the two stimuli are closer in time than they are physically (Fujisaki et al., 2004; Vroomen & Keetels, 2004). One intriguing prediction of temporal recalibration is that events that were synchronous before adaptation should appear as asynchronous at post-adaptation. Said otherwise, there should be a temporal aftereffect of adaptation (see Chapter 3). Evidence for this phenomenon has been reported for motor-visual adaptation in a study by Cunningham and colleagues (2001). They asked participants to play a simple video game which consisted in piloting a simulated airplane, at different speeds between trials, in a screen full of obstacles. The participants controlled the plane by using a computer mouse. The experiment was divided in three phases: at pre-adaptation and post-adaptation, the plane moved almost instantaneously when the mouse moved; whereas during the adaptation phase there could be a delay. Precisely, for half of the participants there was a 200 ms delay between the mouse movements and the airplane movements on the screen (experimental group). For the remaining half, no delay was introduced and the mouse and airplane movement remained synchronous (control). As expected, participants in the experimental group initially found it difficult to take into account the delay when manoeuvring the plane. However, by the end of the adaptation phase they were capable of guiding the plane, suggesting that recalibration of the motor-visual signals had occurred. This recalibration was clearly evident in the post-adaptation phase, when the original synchrony was reinstated. Participants in the experimental group crashed the plane in obstacles much more often than the control group, as if they were now unable to cope with the actual synchrony of motor and visual events. Most interestingly, participants in experimental group spontaneously reported that mouse and plane movements seemed simultaneous towards the end of the training. By contrast, at post-adaptation the plane seemed to move before the mouse moved. Albeit anecdotal, this after-effect is most remarkable because it suggests that temporal recalibration can produce an apparent reverse of causality: events caused by my intentions that appear to occur before I even made the action. Although exposure to repeating temporal discrepancies can induce temporal recalibration that challenge the sense of agency, it is important to remember here that in most instances we actually bind in time our motor actions and their sensory consequences. We have discussed this phenomenon, termed *intentional binding*, in Chapter 3 presenting the clever experiment by Haggard, Clark, and Kalogeras (2002).

mechanism that shifts in time the time-stamp of a stimulus in one sensory channel (say vision) at (or towards) the time-stamp of a stimulus in a different sensory channel (say hearing). In contrast to temporal recalibration, temporal ventriloquism has been hypothesized to be a temporal shift that occurs immediately, in the absence of adaptation;

whereas temporal recalibration emerges as an after-effect, after a phase of adaptation to asynchronous stimuli.

One of the first demonstration of temporal ventriloquism was reported again by Shinsuke Shimojo and colleagues (Scheier, Nijhawan, & Shimojo, 1999) using a visual TOJ task. Participants in the experiment judged the temporal order of two lights presented above and below fixation. Although the lights were the only relevant stimuli in the task, entirely irrelevant sounds were also present. In one condition, the sounds were presented one before and the other after the two lights—using a AVVA temporal sequence. In another condition, the sounds were delivered between the two lights—using a VAAV temporal sequence. The prediction was that sounds delivered before and after the lights could 'capture' the time-stamp of the two visual events and introduce larger temporal separation between them. By contrast, the sounds delivered between the lights could have reduced the temporal separation between the visual targets. The results supported this prediction, showing that the task was easier in the VAAV condition (visual DT = 24 ms) compared to the AVVA condition (visual DT = 39 ms).

Since this first demonstration, temporal ventriloquism has been documented by several other researchers, using similar or different paradigms to the one adopted by Scheier and colleagues (e.g. see Freeman & Driver, 2008; Morein-Zamir, Soto-Faraco, & Kingstone, 2003; Vroomen & Keetels, 2006). These follow-up studies showed that temporal ventriloquism is largely unaffected by the relative location of the visual and auditory stimuli (Vroomen & Keetels, 2006), suggesting that temporal shifts may emerge independently of a principle of unity related to spatial correspondence. Furthermore, there is evidence that temporal ventriloquism does not emerge if auditory and visual stimuli are separated by more than 200 ms (Morein-Zamir, Soto-Faraco, & Kingstone, 2003). Finally, temporal ventriloquism has been documented also with multisensory pairings other than hearing and vision, suggesting that it could be a general mechanism in multisensory processing. For instance, Keetels and Vroomen (2008) examined whether touch could also alter the perceived time-stamp of visual events. They successfully obtained a tactile-visual temporal ventriloquism and replicated also the observation that the spatial co-location or spatial discordance of the stimuli did not alter the phenomenon.

It is also noteworthy that temporal ventriloquism has been used to reduce masking in the visual channel. Specifically, Vroomen and Keetels (2009) used it to modulate the four-dot masking phenomenon, in which identification of a brief visual stimulus (the target) is impaired when an annulus of four dots (the mask) is presented shortly afterwards (Enns & DiLollo, 1997). Because this visual masking phenomenon is sensitive to the temporal interval between the target and the mask, Vroomen and Keetels (2009) ingeniously added a task-irrelevant sound just before the target, and just after the mask. As in the AVVA condition used by Scheier and colleagues (Scheier, Nijhawan, & Shimojo 1999), the prediction was that the two visual events (the target and the mask) would have become more separate by effect of temporal ventriloquism. In agreement with this prediction, identification of the visual target was easier when the two sounds framed the target and the mask, compared to when only one sound was delivered before the target, or no sound at all was added. Although the behavioural effects in this paradigm were rather small, they suggest that the effects of temporal ventriloquism are not just a recalibration of the time-stamp of the sensory events. The effects can also influence the way in which sequential visual events interact with one another.

A third mechanisms for keeping temporal coherence across modalities is *temporal renormalization*. The existence of a temporal renormalization process has been hypothesized from observations on patient P.H., the first fully documented neurological case of acquired difficulty in perceiving the synchronicity of audio-visual streams (Freeman et al., 2013). Mr. P.H. started hearing people's voices *before* he could see their lips move when he was 67 years old. At first, he thought this was a problem with his TV set, or an effect of poor dubbing of the television programme. 'I told my daughter her living room TV was out of sync,' he reported to *New Scientist* magazine in 2013. 'Then I noticed that the kitchen telly was also dubbed badly. Suddenly I noticed that her voice was out of sync too. It wasn't the TV, it was me.' In addition to reporting difficulties with the temporal coherence of lip movements and voices, he also experienced his own voice happening before the felt movements of his mouth and jaw. Interestingly, understanding speech in noisy environment had also become harder for P.H., as one would expect given the key role of multisensory integration in speech perception (Sumby & Pollack, 1954). Neuropsychological examinations confirmed that P.H. had no specific functional impairment, no obvious neurological abnormality, and only a mild hearing loss. High resolution magnetic resonance imaging, however, revealed two small lesions in the brain stem: one in the left sub-thalamic nucleus, and the other in the pontine nuclei. Both lesions are compatible with the P.H.'s functional anomaly. The lesion in the pontine nuclei in particular could have impacted on the anatomical pathway that brings information from the ear to the inferior colliculus—a fundamental node of early auditory processing.

Elliot Freeman and colleagues studied P.H. in 2013, probing different aspects of audio-visual timing by several tasks. The main task replicated the paradigm described at the end of section 8.2 (Soto-Faraco & Alsius, 2007), which involves concurrently assessing both the perceived temporal order of audio-visual speech stimuli and the McGurk effect. On each trial of this task, P.H. saw a brief movie showing an actor's mouth uttering a phoneme, and was requested to give a timing judgement and a phoneme judgement. The results confirmed that P.H. experienced an audio-visual temporal mismatch: A visual lead of 210 ms was required before he could experience the voice and the lip movements as synchronous. Most interestingly, the audio-visual mismatches which brought the strongest McGurk phenomenon were *reversed* with respect to the one measured in the temporal order judgement task. For P.H. the optimal effect of vision on hearing the phoneme was achieved when hearing led vision by 240 ms. What this means is that P.H. experienced different alterations of audio-visual speech timing depending on whether the task entailed integration ('what' was said) or temporal order estimation ('when' each sensory signal occurred).

Why would a brain lesion produce opposite results in different measures? According to Freeman, what happened to P.H. is that his lesion introduced speech-specific slowing of hearing relative to vision. As a consequence of this, the brain re-adjusted the relative timing between events to counterbalance the slowed auditory processing. To illustrate this concept Freeman and colleagues used a multiple-clock analogy. Imagine that you are in a room filled with many clocks, each independently subject to inaccuracies, and you have to estimate the correct hour. How would you proceed? Probably, you would not trust any arbitrarily chosen clock; instead, you would create your estimate based on some 'central indicator'—i.e. the average time as computed from all the clocks. The good side of this method is that, assuming that the differences between the clocks are random, this average will approximate the true time as the number of clocks you consider increases. Now imagine that one clock is particularly slow (as the auditory speech perception mechanisms damaged in P.H.). This single clock will lower the average timing and will make all other clocks in the room appear fast. Yet, combining all the inaccuracies (small and large, over- and under-estimating) of the different clocks will allow you to maintain a near-veridical time estimate overall. Freeman and colleagues suggested that this is a key cognitive mechanism involved in keeping temporal coherence in multiple sensory events, and termed it *'temporal renormalization.'* Importantly, they also suggested that renormalization is not specific to just a single atypical individual (P.H.), but it exists in *everyone*. This prediction found initial support in the performance of healthy controls tested in the same paradigm as P.H. (Freeman et al., 2013) and is now under further scrutiny in follow up studies of the same group (Ipser et al., 2017).

8.4 **Duration**

Percepts last for certain amounts of time. *Duration* is a fundamental property of events, and it poses great challenges for cognitive neuroscience, both when investigated within single sensory channels or with a multisensory approach. As introduced at the beginning of this chapter and in Box 8.1, perceived and physical durations rarely match. Physical duration is always the same independent of context, but perceived duration can be altered by many contextual factors, such as attention, alertness, emotional arousal, and even the event's probability of occurrence (Zakay & Block, 1997). As we will now see, often these factors involve multisensory interactions.

To appreciate duration distortions within and between sensory channels, consider the following example from a study by Virginie van Wassenhove and colleagues (van Wassenhove, Buonomano, Shimojo, & Shams, 2008). Each trial of this experiment comprised five consecutive stimuli, delivered either to hearing or vision individually, or to both channels at the same time. Stimuli 1, 2, 3, and 5 in the stream were all 500 ms long, whereas the 4th stimulus (the target) varied in duration only, or in duration *and* feature. For vision, a feature change could be, for instance, an expansion of the target disc, while all other stimuli in the stream remained of constant size (Figure 8.5a). For hearing, a feature change could consist in an upward modulation of the target sound frequency, whereas all other sounds in the stream remained of constant frequency (Figure 8.5b). In multisensory conditions, participants were instructed at the beginning of the block as to which stream had to be attended to (Figure 8.5c), but, and this was a key feature of the

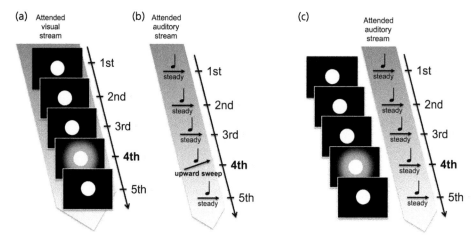

Figure 8.5 Some of the conditions used in the study by van Wassenhove et al. (2008). Each trial comprised five successive stimuli, and the target was always the fourth one. In critical trials, the target varied in duration and feature. For instance, in the visual unisensory condition (a) the target was a disc of expanding size, among discs of fixed size; or in the auditory unisensory condition (b) the sound was an upward frequency-modulated sweep, among steady tones. During audio-visual trials (c), participants were instructed to attend only one of the two streams (indicated here by the shaded grey ribbon). Note that all stimuli in the attended stream had the same features, whereas the feature change existed only in the non-attended stream.

study, duration and feature changes were only introduced in the *unattended* stream. In other words, all stimuli in the attended signal were 500 ms long, including the target. In the example shown in Figure 8.5c, the attended stream is auditory, and the unattended stream is visual. Note that only the visual stream contains a duration and feature change (the expanding disc). The task was straightforward. Throughout the experiment and irrespective of conditions (unisensory or multisensory), participants had to monitor the fourth stimulus and decided if it was 'shorter' or 'longer' in comparison to the other stimuli in the stream.

The first important observation of this study emerged from unisensory conditions: feature changes in these streams produced changes in perceived duration. For instance, the expanding disc appeared to last longer than an unchanging disk of the same duration. Vice versa, a disc of constant size, when embedded in a stream of expanding discs, appeared to last for a shorter time. However, these effects of time dilation and compression did not emerge following all feature changes. For instance, a visual target decreasing in size did not produce distortions of subjective time. The second key observation made by van Wassenhove and colleagues (van Wassenhove, Buonomano, Shimojo, & Shams,

2008) concerned the interactions between different channels in multisensory conditions. Specifically, the auditory duration of events was distorted (shortened or lengthened) by information in the unattended visual channel. However, the reverse not observed: perceived duration of visual events was only minimally affected by concurrent auditory stimulation. This suggests the existence of asymmetrical multisensory interactions when processing event duration.

Multisensory interactions in duration perception have been documented also by other research groups, both using different sensory channels and exploiting different experimental paradigms. For instance, a recent study by Yue and colleagues (Yue, Gao, Chen, & Wu, 2016) examined event duration for visual or auditory targets, when these were paired with task-irrelevant odours. The targets were continuous visual stimuli or continuous tones lasting 1 or 4 seconds. Participants were asked to reproduce the duration of each presented target, marking the beginning and the end of the interval with two key-presses. The task-irrelevant odours that accompanied the presentation of the targets were jasmine, lavender, garlic, or a no-odour baseline. As frequently observed in these tasks, shorter durations were overestimated, whereas longer durations were underestimated. This effect is known as Vierordt's law, from the early observations on time perception published in 1868 by the German physiologist Karl von Vierordt. Interestingly, however, some odours also affected perceived durations. For instance, participants produced longer intervals after the lavender odour, compared to when they were exposed to jasmine and garlic. The mechanisms underlying this effect remain elusive, as all three odours could have diverted attention from the visual/auditory targets, or could have exerted influences on emotional valence and arousal. Nonetheless, the results of Yue and colleagues show that even entirely irrelevant odours seem to alter perceived duration, at least in some cases.

Studies on perceived duration across the senses are very useful when trying to understand how our mind could attempt to estimate time quantities (i.e. durations). As anticipated in the first section of this chapter, there are neither receptors in our nervous system that can directly solve this task for our cognitive system, nor forms of energy in the environment whose quantity could translate into duration. In the attempt to solve this conundrum, psychologists have introduced the notion of *internal mental clocks*. Internal clock models typically assume the existence of a pacemaker, an accumulator, and a switch (Allan 1979; Gibbon, Church, & Meck 1984; Treisman 1963). The *pacemaker* generates discrete events at a fixed frequency; the *accumulator* counts how many of these events occur in a given time; the *switch* determines whether the accumulator is activated (i.e. whether we are tracking event duration or not). While it remains unclear how these functional models could be implemented in the brain, they proved useful to conceptualize some of the distortions observed in subjective duration. For instance, changes in perceived duration as a function of participant's arousal have been linked to changes in the rate of the pacemaker—if you are more aroused, your pacemaker runs faster. Similarly, changes in duration perception as a function of the attentional resources allocated to the target have been associated with changes in the efficiency of the switch mechanisms—if your attention is diverted from the relevant sensory event, you are less ready to start tracking the ticks of the pacemaker.

One key related point is whether the internal clock model is inherently multisensory. Is there a single centralized clock, operating regardless of the sensory channel encoding the target; or there are instead multiple internal clocks, each somewhat related to the involved sensory channel? Although the perspective of a single 'centralized' clock has been dominant for over three decades, the prevalent position nowadays is for 'distributed' timing models (Buhusi & Meck, 2005; Bueti, 2011). Distributed models assume that multiple mechanisms are implemented throughout the brain to process time and durations, some are specific for each sensory channel and others are shared and centralized. Evidence in support of sensory-specific clock mechanisms originated, for example, from the observation that duration is frequently overestimated for auditory compared to visual stimuli presented for exactly the same physical time. This effect is most pronounced for durations of 1 second or less (Goldstone & Lhamon, 1974; Wearden, Edwards, Fakhri, & Percival, 1998), and it is instead less evident for durations of several seconds (3–5 s; Block & Gruber, 2014). Using the internal clock perspective it could be hypothesized that the auditory clock has a faster pacemaker compared to the visual one (Wearden, Edwards, Fakhri, & Percival, 1998), or alternatively that the auditory clock has a slower operating switch compared to the visual clock. However, the results described above (van Wassenhove, Buonomano, Shimojo, & Shams, 2008; Yue, Gao, Chen, & Wu, 2016) also indicate that the information provided by the multiple sensory clocks must converge and interact at some stage. Otherwise it would be impossible to observe modulations of one sensory channel over a different one. Hence, the proposal of hybrid model in which parts of the internal clocks are sensory specific, whereas others are sensory independent.

Figure 8.6 provides a schematic representation of this notion presenting three possible descriptions of internal clock models: a completely sensory-specific model, a completely sensory-aspecific model, and an hybrid version (van Wassenhove et al., 2008). In the completely sensory-specific model (Figure 8.6a) the pacemaker, the switch, and the accumulator are all assumed to be specific to each sensory system. In this model, the only stages that are shared across sensory channels are attention modulations (assumed necessary to activate the switches for tracking auditory or visual durations) and the memory components (required to estimate duration of the experienced events with test duration held in memory). Here interactions across sensory systems are possible only at a very late memory stages. By contrast, in the completely sensory-aspecific model (Figure 8.6b) the pacemaker, the switch, the accumulator, and the memory components are all shared. Irrespective of which channel process the sensory event (in the example, vision or hearing), common processing stages are always activated and interactions in duration perception across the senses can emerge at any step of the process. Finally, the hybrid model presented in Figure 8.6c (adapted from Rousseau & Rousseau, 1996, and cited in van Wassenhove, Buonomano, Shimojo, & Shams, 2008; Supplementary Figure 1)

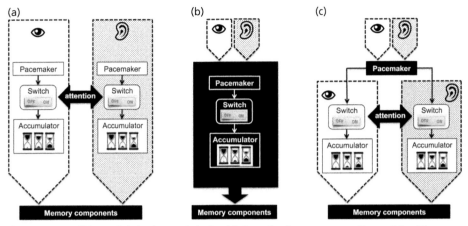

Figure 8.6 Possible models for internal clocks. (a) Completely sensory-specific model, with no shared stages between sensory systems. (b) Completely sensory-aspecific model, with all clock mechanisms shared across sensory channels. (c) Hybrid model, in which the pacemaker is assumed sensory-aspecific, whereas all other components are sensory-specific. In all diagrams, sensory-aspecific stages are marked with black background.

Adapted from Virginie van Wassenhove, Dean V. Buonomano, Shinsuke Shimojo, and Ladan Shams, Distortions of Subjective Time Perception Within and Across Senses, *PLOS One*, 3 (1), e1437, Supplementary Figure 1, doi: 10.1371/journal.pone.0001437 © 2008 van Wassenhove et al. This work is licensed under the Creative Commons Attribution License (CC BY 2.0). It is attributed to the authors Virginie van Wassenhove, Dean V. Buonomano, Shinsuke Shimojo, and Ladan Shams.

assumes that the pacemaker is sensory-aspecific, but the switch and the accumulator are sensory-specific. Again, attentional modulations and memory components are mechanisms shared across sensory channels.

Further evidence for interactions between sensory channels in duration perception emerged also from paradigms that attempted to train temporal abilities across sensory channels. Pioneer in these approaches was the North American researchers Michael Merzenich, whose contributions to the cognitive neurosciences of plasticity and learning span from neurophysiological studies in the macaque monkey to behavioural research in humans. His work has set the basis for several methods for training and rehabilitation, proving the great translational potentials of cognitive neuroscience research for issues of daily life. Merzenich himself founded two companies, Scientific Learning and the Posit Science Corporation, whose business mission is to provide services and products for 'brain training' and 'brain fitness'. In one of his early studies on time perception, participants were trained to discriminate the duration of brief temporal intervals (75 or 125 ms) defined by pair of vibrations delivered to one hand. Note that, unlike the studies described above, this paradigm measured duration judgement for 'empty' intervals (i.e. not the duration of a persisting event, but the empty temporal interval comprised between two successive events). Furthermore, this research focused on durations of milliseconds, rather than seconds as before. Merzenich and colleagues trained participants on 900 trials each day, for a period of 10–15 days. After training, participants improved their duration discrimination thresholds, and were able to generalize this learned ability to vibrations delivered to the untrained hand. This implies that the training was not confined to a specific set of tactile receptors, nor limited to a specific brain hemisphere. Most interestingly, participants were also able to generalize their learning to auditory stimuli (Nagarajan et al., 1998) when similar temporal intervals were tested, revealing some transfer of duration discrimination across sensory channels.

In the two decades after the pioneering observations of Merzenich and colleagues, researchers have debated about the actual possibility of extending this learning to other combinations of sensory channels, or if similar results can be obtained for longer durations (e.g. in the range of seconds). Initial attempts to transfer training from hearing to vision for durations in the sub-second range have been unsuccessful (e.g. Grondin & Ulrich, 2011; Lapid et al., 2009). However, at least two studies (Bratzke, Seifried & Ulrich, 2012; Bratzke, Schröter, & Ulrich, 2014) obtained transfer of temporal discrimination training from the auditory to the visual channel, but not vice versa. This reveals a potential asymmetry in temporal processing, which is consistent with the notion that the auditory system may serve a pivotal role in time perception (to learn more about this notion, read Tutorial 8.2 on the role of the auditory cortices for temporal processing). Bratzke and colleagues argued that these discrepant findings in the literature could reflect the existing uncertainty as the optimal conditions for implementing efficient training across sensory channels. For instance, in one study that failed to show training from hearing to vision (Grondin & Ulrich, 2011) participants were trained and tested in a single long session lasting over 3 hours, with limited breaks during the session. By contrast, the study that measured effective transfer of training between sensory channels (Bratzke et al., 2012) distributed the training sessions across several days. Interestingly, also the consolidation time allowed after training seems to play an important role for multisensory training. When participants were tested 5 minutes or 25 hours after the end of training, transfer of training to the visual modality was significantly larger after 1 day of consolidation (this differential effect of consolidation time did not emerge for unisensory training). Thus, multiple variables—including fatigue, duration of consolidation, or absence of appropriate feedback—could contribute to the presence or absence of training generalization. This calls for a systematic research programme dedicated to the potentials of training across modalities and invites caution when reading about the success (or failure) of brain training programmes—a concept that clearly applies beyond the specific domain of temporal processing.

Taken together, these results point to models of duration processing that are neither fully centralized (i.e. a single clock, irrespective of sensory channel) nor fully segregated temporal processing mechanisms (i.e. independent clocks, intrinsic to each sensory system). Instead, they suggest that that hybrid models in which parts of the processing are sensory specific and others are more centralized could best capture the complexity of time perception.

Tutorial 8.2 Does time perception rely on hearing?

One recurrent perspective in the time perception literature is that hearing plays a pivotal role in temporal computations, irrespective of which sensory event is being processed. In this theoretical account, temporal computations are neither entirely sensory-independent, linked to a centralized system that can be accessed through the different sensory systems, nor entirely sensory-specific, relying on segregated mechanisms embedded within each sensory channel. Instead, sensory-specific mechanisms related to hearing would serve sensory-independent purposes. For instance, it has been proposed that information from other sensory systems (e.g. vision) is converted into an auditory code whenever temporal computations are required (e.g. Guttman et al., 2005; Kanai et al., 2011). This perspective has traditionally been motivated though the higher temporal resolution of the auditory channel compared to the visual or somatosensory ones. In addition, throughout this chapter we have presented examples of the dominance of auditory over visual or tactile information when solving temporal tasks. In the last decade, new support to the hypothesis that hearing plays a key role in time perception is starting to emerge from neuroimaging and neurostimulation studies. Convergent results suggest that the auditory cortices play a causal role in temporal tasks performed on visual or somatosensory stimuli.

The observation that the auditory cortices are involved in temporal processing was initially serendipitous. In one of the first fMRI studies on the functional anatomy of time perception in humans (Coull et al., 2004), a number of brain areas were recruited when participants compared the duration of pairs of *visual* stimuli. Among these areas the authors reported also the right temporal cortex. Note that term 'temporal' here has nothing to do with 'time perception': it is just a neuroanatomical label, used to identifies the brain lobe located under the temporal bone of the skull. Coull and colleagues commented that 'the observed temporal cortex activation may reflect strategies related to auditory imagery' (p. 1508). Functional neuroimaging, however, does not allow us to establish causal relationships between brain activations and behaviour. Brain imaging studies can determine whether a region is *involved* in the task, but they cannot determine whether that brain region is *necessary* for the task. A different tool used in cognitive neuroscience research, transcranial magnetic stimulation (or TMS), has instead the potentials to determine such causal relationships. TMS is a brain stimulation technique that creates transient perturbation of neural activity and, when paired with behavioural measurement, can help determine whether the stimulated brain region is necessary for the task performed by the subject.

In a study conducted in 2011, Kanai and colleagues used TMS over two different cortical sites, the primary visual cortex or the right primary auditory cortices, while participants performed auditory estimation tasks on visual or auditory stimuli. In each trial, participants were asked to compare the duration of two consecutive stimuli lasting around 600 ms, and report which one was longer. The results showed a remarkable dissociation. When TMS was delivered over the primary visual cortex, duration estimates of visual stimuli was affected, whereas performance for auditory stimuli was unimpaired. By contrast, when TMS was delivered over the right auditory cortex, performance decreased both for auditory and visual stimuli. This result is surprising because it indicates that stimulation of a sensory-specific brain region (the auditory cortex) can produce sensory-independent behavioural effects. If considered within the context of mental clocks models described in section 8.3, this result suggests a novel hybrid model in which time processing mechanism embedded within the auditory system are recruited when processing visual stimuli (this model is not shown in Figure 8.5).

Another striking example of the role of the auditory cortex in temporal duration processing comes from a TMS study conducted by Nadia Bolognini and colleagues around the same years (Bolognini et al., 2010). Participants received tactile stimuli at the right or left index finger, and performed either a temporal discrimination task (detect and respond to longer duration stimuli, and ignore the short duration ones) or a spatial discrimination task (detect and respond to spatially long vibrations, and ignore the short ones). TMS was applied over the left auditory regions or over the primary somatosensory cortex, shortly after the stimulation (60 ms) or at longer intervals (120 or 180 ms). Using TMS at different time intervals from the stimulation is an efficient method for exploring *when* a specific brain regions is relevant for the performed task. As expected, when TMS was delivered over the primary somatosensory cortex shortly after stimulus presentation, performance decreased. This impairment emerged for both the spatial and temporal task, and simply reflects the involvement of the somatosensory cortex when processing tactile stimuli. More interestingly, performance modulations were also observed when TMS was applied at longer intervals (180 ms) over auditory areas. Notably, these modulations were specific for the temporal task, suggesting again a causal role of the auditory cortices when temporal computations are required.

Another interesting approach to examine if time perception relies on hearing is study the behavioural and neural correlates of this function in individuals who are profoundly deaf from birth. People born deaf have never had the opportunity to experience temporal durations or rhythm through the auditory system, or to converted multisensory stimuli into an auditory code when performing temporal computations, or to calibrate time perception for what they see or feel with respect to their auditory experience. If hearing and the auditory cortices are so critical for temporal processing, then deaf people should be impaired in temporal tasks. This hypothesis has been advocated by several researchers, and it is currently known as the 'auditory scaffolding hypothesis' (Conway et al., 2009). It argues that sound provides a supporting framework—a scaffolding—for time perception and for sequencing behaviour.

This prediction found consistent empirical support only in relation to duration perception (Bolognini et al., 2012; Kowalska & Szelag, 2006). For instance, Bolognini and colleagues (2012) tested congenitally deaf participants in the temporal and spatial tasks described in Bolognini et al. (2010). When assessed in these behavioural tasks, deaf participants performed as well as the hearing controls on spatial discriminations, but worse than controls on temporal discriminations. Most interestingly, the neural correlates of duration perception were explored also in this group using TMS. While TMS over primary somatosensory cortex produced similar results in deaf and hearing controls, the recruitment of the auditory cortex was very different between groups. Unlike hearing controls, TMS over the auditory cortices in deaf participants interfered with performance only when delivered shortly after the stimulation (60 ms). This is most remarkable, because it suggests that already 60 ms after stimulation, the somatosensory input was processed in the *auditory* cortex of congenitally deaf people. This result is compatible with notion of a plastic recruitment of the un-stimulated auditory cortices for processing tactile and visual stimuli (Merabeth & Pascual-Leone, 2010). However, it also suggests a potential mechanistic explanation for the deficit of deaf participants when performing the temporal task. Specifically, the plastic reorganization of the auditory cortex in deaf individuals may have subtracted resources for temporal processing, diverting an originally neural module for temporal duration processing towards somatosensory processing. In other words, maladaptive neural plasticity may have hindered the typical recruitment of auditory circuits for sensory-independent temporal computations.

Interestingly, other domains of temporal perception seem intact in deaf individuals compared to hearing controls, or in fact even improved. This dissociation is compatible with the notion, discussed in the various sections of this chapter, that time is a multifaceted phenomenon. The study by Iversen and colleagues (2015) on visual and auditory rhythm perception that we introduced in section 8.5, included also a group of early deaf participants. Synchronization of movements to the visually bouncing ball proved in the deaf group as good—or even better—than that of hearing controls. The ability of deaf participants in perceiving the rhythm of these moving visual stimuli, as the behaviour in additional tests involving static flashes, closely resembled that of hearing participants when processing auditory rhythm. Thus, at least for this aspect of time perception, the lack of auditory experience does not seem to detrimental for temporal computations. Because recent fMRI work (Bola et al., 2017) showed that perception of visual rhythm in early deaf people recruits regions of the auditory cortex that are typically engaged in auditory rhythm processing in hearing individuals, it would be tempting to relate this preserved/enhanced ability of deaf people to this preserved neural circuit. The interesting side of this possibility is that this auditory node of the network could not have matured under the influence of auditory inputs in deaf individuals. Hence, it could be a genetically determined node for processing rhythm in the auditory cortices.

8.5 **Multisensory rhythm**

The last aspect we consider in this chapter is the multisensory perception of rhythm. Perceiving rhythm through different sensory channels—hearing, vision, or somatosensation—is a fundamental ability in our life. Rhythm is relevant to many sensorimotor interactions with the environment, necessary for music perception and production, and central to many socially binding behaviours such as dancing or moving in synchrony. The ability to perceive rhythm is also closely linked to our ability to predict future events, as stimuli that repeat according to regular rhythmic structures can be anticipated. Charles Darwin (1871) hypothesized that rhythm perception takes place in all animals, and believed that perceiving rhythm might depend on some form of neural synchronization to the external environment. However, he was probably wrong on both aspects. First, exactly which non-human species perceive and synchronize to rhythm remains to be ascertained. We now know that species closer to us phylogenetically, such as the Rhesus monkeys, synchronize to rhythms with less accuracy than humans (Zarco et al., 2009). By contrast, more distant species such as the cockatoo birds show remarkable synchronization to music. Patel and colleagues (2009) have demonstrated that Snowball, an Eleonora cockatoo (*Cacatua galerita eleonora*), was able to dance in time with music in the absence of any previous training. If you are curious to see Snowball dancing, take a moment to appreciate the remarkable ability of this bird to synchronize to the rhythm of a song (simply search for 'cockatoo dancing Patel' on your browser). Second, rhythm perception does not seem to emerge simply because the central nervous system synchronizes to rhythmicity in the external stimulation—a phenomenon often referred to as 'entrainment.' As we shall see in this section, our phenomenal experience is not merely the result of the stimulation in the environment and higher-order organizational principles often emerge. In other words, as described in Chapter 3 with visual examples, rhythm can be considered a perceptual Gestalt (see Tutorial 4.2 in Chapter 4) that, interestingly, can emerge across elements in different perceptual modalities.

But let's start with the basics. Consider the fundamental building block of rhythm perception—the ability of participants to perceive multiple elements in a sequence. In a series of influential studies published at the beginning of the year 2000, Ladan Shams, Yukiyasu Kamitani, and Shinsuke Shimojo presented participants with sequences of visual stimuli, that were either delivered in isolation (unisensory condition) or paired with a variable number of 1 to 4 beeps (multisensory visual-auditory condition). The visual stimuli were flashing discs, and their number was varied from 1 to 4. The number of beeps was also varied from 1 to 4. Participants had to report the number of flashes they had seen. In the unisensory condition, they participants could do this quite accurately. However, in the visual-auditory conditions they were often tricked by the concurrent beeps. For instance, if they had been shown two flashes but heard three beeps, they often reported seeing three flashes. In general, when the number of beeps exceeded the number of flashes, participants perceived more flashes than had been actually presented—a phenomenon referred to as 'fissions,' because the discs seemed to multiply due to the effect of the sounds. By contrast, when there were less beeps than flashes, participants perceived less flashes—a phenomenon referred to as 'fusions', because multiple discs appeared to have collapsed due to the effect of sounds (Shams et al., 2000, 2002). Follow-up studies (McCormick & Mamassian, 2008; Mishra et al., 2013) confirmed the validity of this observation, showing, among other things, that these multisensory fissions and fusions are not merely changes in response criterion (i.e. a tendency of participants to report the number of heard beeps, instead of the number of seen flashes) but reflect genuine changes in the perception of the visual numerosity of the flashes. Furthermore, it has been shown that similar effects can be obtained when pairing visual stimuli with touches on the fingertip (Violentyev et al., 2005), and that the illusion is strongest in children aged 6–7 years and decreases progressively with age. This is consistent with the proposal that hearing is most important in young age than later in development (Nava & Pavani, 2013).

Along the same line of reasoning Recanzone (2003) examined the ability of participants to discriminate rates of presentation for visual or auditory streams presented in isolation (unisensory) or paired with congruent or incongruent multisensory signals. In the main experiment of this study, trials consisted of two sequences of four auditory stimulus tones and/or four flashes (see Figure 8.7). The first sequence was always presented at 4 Hz, whereas the second sequence was presented either at the same temporal rate (4 Hz) or at different rates (from 3.5 Hz to 4.5 Hz). Participants were instructed to compare the two sequences and decide if the second sequence was presented at a higher or lower temporal rate than the first one. Crucially, the task was performed on visual or auditory stimuli (target sequence), with or without distractors presented in the unattended sensory system (e.g. target visual, distractor auditory). In the multisensory conditions, the rates of the attended and unattended streams were either matching or mismatching. Figure 8.7 illustrates these experimental conditions for trials with a visual target sequence. The first important result that emerged from this study was that the ability to discriminate temporal rates was better for auditory compared to visual target streams. These findings reveal once again the higher precision of the auditory system when temporal computations are necessary. The second key finding was that auditory rates influenced the perception of visual rates, but the reverse did not apply. For instance, when the target visual sequence changed its rate on a trial-by-trial basis while the distractor auditory sequence was always delivered at 4 Hz (as in Figure 8.7d), participants were quite capable of perceiving the changing visual rates. Thus, the presence of auditory distractors impacted on the perception of visual rates, whereas visual distractors had no measurable effect on the perception of auditory rates.

Rhythm perception, of course, is much more than perceiving temporal rates. The complexity of rhythm perception is well captured by concepts originally developed in music theory, which describes rhythm in terms of hierarchically organized structures involving four distinct perceptual features (Radocy & Boyle, 2012). The first of these is the *beat*, which corresponds to the perception of a periodic pulse in the sound sequence. Musical beats are what we typically mark by foot tapping, head bobbing, or dance movements when listening to music (Patel & Inversen, 2014). Beats are the basic units of time in a

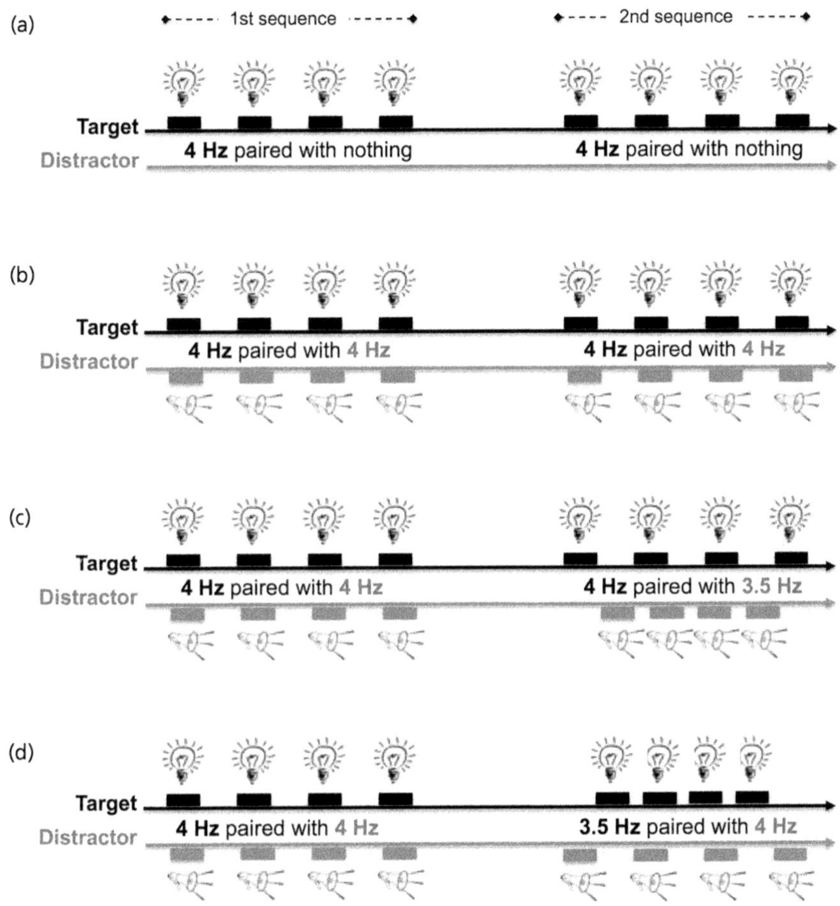

Figure 8.7 Schematic representation of the conditions used in Recanzone (2003). In these example trials the target stream was always visual, but in the actual experiment participants were presented across blocks with targets in the visual or auditory modality. Furthermore, stimuli of the first and second target sequence were presented with same or different rates. Example trial in (a) the unisensory condition; (b) the multisensory congruent condition; (c) the multisensory incongruent condition with rate changes introduced only in the distractor stream; (d) the multisensory condition with rate changes introduced only in the target stream.

Data from Gregg H. Recanzone, Auditory Influences on Visual Temporal Rate Perception, *Journal of Neurophysiology*, 89(2), pp. 1078–1093, DOI: 10.1152/jn.00706.2002, 2003.

rhythmic sequence, and can be explicitly marked in a music piece by a bass or drum line, or remain implicit. In this case, listeners are usually capable of inferring or extrapolating the beats from the global rhythmic structure (Kramer, 1988). The second feature is *tempo*, which is the speed at which beats repeat in time. In musical notation, tempo is usually indicated by metronome indications in beats per second, or by descriptive Italian terms, such as *andante* or *allegro*. The third element is *accent*, which is a special emphasis on certain beats of the sequence. In rhythmic musical structures, a beat can be accented by varying several different features, including intensity, duration, or pitch of a note. Finally, the combination of beat and accent results in the emergence of the *metre*, which is the cyclical grouping of beats into units. Metre is the fundamental high-order structure that listeners experience in rhythmic sequences.

In music, metre is typically stressed through accents on the beats, as in the case of isochronous patterns that can be made to appear 'march-like' if the accent is placed every two beats, or conversely they can become 'waltz-like' if the accent is placed every three beats. However, metre can also emerge in non-musical contexts and, importantly, even with no accents. Consider for instance, what happens when you listen to a mechanical clock, i.e. to an isochronous sequence of identical 'ticks.' Mechanical clocks are somewhat difficult to come by these days, but if you have ever had one in the room, you may you have noted that the ticks are not heard as if they were all the same. Instead, some ticks seem more salient (louder, longer or both) than others. As a result, one does not hear 'tick-tick-tick-tick- …,' but rather one hears 'tick-tock-tick-tock-….' This phenomenon, known as the 'tick-tock' effect, has been known and studied since the nineteenth century (Bolton, 1894). The tick-tock effect is important, because it shows two things: that metre is a fundamental feature of temporal unit formation, perceived even in non-musical sequences; and that metre can emerge as a consequence of subjective accenting applied on physically identical auditory sequences.

Despite the importance of metre in temporal unit formation, we now know that the perception of metre is not equally efficient in all sensory channels. For instance, given the same rhythmic sequence, hearing will typically more effective than vision in conveying a sense of beat. A nice demonstration of this general principle was provided by Patel and colleagues (2005). In their study, these researchers presented adults with isochronous or non-isochronous rhythmic patterns, delivered as sequences of tones or as sequence of flashes. The task was to tap in sync with the perceived beat. While participants were well capable of tapping to the beat when listening to the auditory sequences, they had great difficulties with visual sequences when the rhythm was non-isochronous or when the isochronous rhythm had a fast tempo. The authors concluded that motor synchronization to beat perception may 'have a special affinity with the auditory system' (p. 226). While this finding has been replicated by other research groups (McAuley & Henry, 2010; Grahn et al., 2011), there is now evidence that *moving* visual stimuli may be as effective as auditory stimuli in conveying a sense of beat. This has recently been documented by asking participants to tap in synchrony to an animated bouncing ball that moved up and down in silence, or to tap in synchrony with a sequence of sounds (Iversen et al., 2015). Surprisingly, when tapping to the visually bouncing ball participants performed as accurately as with the sequence of tones, suggesting that synchronization to visual rhythms is in fact possible, at least in the conditions of this study (which used only isochronous rhythms). However, even in these results there was an asymmetry between vision and hearing. The isochronous auditory rhythm resulted in a stable, binary metrical structure—as in the 'tick-tock' effect described above. By contrast, no such binary percept emerged when participants synchronized to the visually bouncing ball. This initial evidence suggests that moving visual stimuli can produce a sense of beat, but do not necessarily grant access to more complex high-level structures of rhythm perception.

Metre perception is also possible through somatosensation (Brochard et al., 2003; Huang et al., 2012). For instance, Huang and colleagues (2012) ran a series of experiments on the ability to discriminate rhythms in streams of auditory or vibro-tactile stimuli. These were built according to a march-like rhythm, with a critical tone (or vibration) every four beats, or according to a waltz-like rhythm, with a critical element every three beats. Between these fixed metrically important elements, the experimenters also added random tones (or vibrations) as well as rests (silences), to make the target streams more ambiguous and rhythm categorization more difficult. In the first experiment, participants experienced unisensory streams—auditory or tactile—in which the metrically important elements were either accented or unaccented. The accent consisted of an increase in volume of the metrically important elements. In these unisensory conditions, participants were able to perceive the metric patterns (march-like vs waltz-like) in unaccented streams with 82 percent accuracy when the stream was auditory and 75 percent accuracy when the stream was tactile. Furthermore, both unisensory abilities improved with accent cues. This shows that metre can be perceived through passive touch almost as well as through hearing. Interestingly, the authors also tested participants in multisensory conditions in which the sensory channels were made to convey either congruent or incongruent metric cues. In these conditions, the target stream was delivered through one sensory channel (e.g. hearing), while the other channel (touch) marked either the metrical notes of the same rhythm (congruent trials) or the metrical notes of a different rhythm (incongruent trials). With congruent metrical cues, metre recognition improved to 90 percent correct. By contrast, with incongruent metrical cues performance dropped to 10 percent if incongruent auditory cues were presented, but only to 60 percent if incongruent tactile cues were presented. Again, hearing proved the dominating sensory channel for the perception of rhythm.

A final very interesting condition tested by Huang and colleagues (2012) intermixed the auditory and tactile streams, with metrically important beats assigned to a single channel, or assigned to separate channels in equal proportions. In these conditions, neither unisensory stream was coherent enough to determine the metre—in other words, thus metre perception could only emerge if participants were able to unify the alternating auditory and tactile elements into a multisensory pattern. When all the metrically important beats were assigned to a single channel, participants were more than 70 percent accurate in recognising metre. Strikingly, however, performance remained above chance (60 percent accurate) even when half of the metrically important cues were assigned to one channel, and the remaining were assigned to the other channel. As noted by Spence (2015), the perception of metre in a sequence of intermixed auditory and tactile events is a form of multisensory unit formation (see Chapter 4) or, in Spence's terminology, *intersensory Gestalt*. Huang's results thus contrast with the long-held belief that rhythms cannot be perceived from multimodal elements (e.g. Fraisse, 1964). It would be interesting to test whether a similar result can also emerge if auditory or tactile stimuli were inter-mixed with visual events, or if multisensory rhythm is instead specific to hearing and touch alone.

Given the asymmetries we reported in perceiving rhythms between vision and hearing, it would be important to understand whether hearing could serve as a guide for training rhythm perception in the visual modality. This question is relevant from the theoretical point of view, as it could shed further light on the potentials of multisensory training for unisensory perception (see also Chapter 9 on this point) and because it could re-veal interactions between sensory systems when processing time. In 2015, Barakat and colleagues addressed precisely this question by testing the ability of adults in a visual rhythm discrimination task, before and after two sessions of visual, auditory, or audio-visual training. The basic task consisted in attending to pairs of rhythmic sequences, each built from the concatenation of three short (50 ms) and four long (200 ms) elements separated by 100 ms intervals, and deciding whether they were same or different. During training, participants practiced either with unisensory versions of the task, with just visual stimuli (blinking discs) or just auditory stimuli (beeps), or trained with a multisensory version using audio-visual stimuli (synchronous discs and beeps). The results showed that training of visual rhythm was indeed possible and, furthermore, it emerged as long-term perceptual learning effect, as the post-training measurements were completed 24–48 hours after the training exercise. However, they also revealed that this performance im-provement only emerged with the auditory or the audio-visual training. Practice with the flashing discs alone did not improve visual rhythm perception. This result is somewhat surprising, as it suggests that training on exactly the same stimuli used for testing can be ineffective, whereas training on a different sensory system could be successful. However, it is yet another example that hearing could play a key role in temporal computations (see Tutorial 8.2 for further discussion of this point).

As a final note on this topic, it is important to remark that multisensory interactions in rhythm perception have been documented also in relation to multisensory body-related signals (vestibular, proprioceptive, tactile), and very early during human development. In a classic study, Phillips-Silver and Trainor (2005), exposed a group of 7-months infants to rhythmic auditory sequences of 2 minutes. The sequences were rhythmical, but metrically ambiguous as they were built without accented beats. The crucial manipulation consisted in bouncing the infants either on every second beat or every third beat, thus accenting a duple or triple rhythm respectively. After the bouncing phase, the experimenters pre-sented infants with auditory rhythms that now contained accented beats, to mark duple or triple metres. The results showed that infants attended for longer periods to the metre that corresponded to the one they experienced in the bouncing phase, compared to the other one. This suggest that the multisensory experience of bouncing disambiguated the original auditory sequence towards one of the two metres. Critically, if infants were not bounced and remained on their mother's lap while they observed the experimenter dan-cing to one of the two metres, no preference for one of the rhythms emerged. Follow up experiments on adult participants suggest that this phenomenon may specifically rely on vestibular cues related to head movements. The preference for rhythms experienced through body movements emerged when the whole body was rocked using an adult-sized seesaw, or when the head was moved, but not when the movement involved the legs alone (Phillips-Silver & Trainor, 2008). The hypothesis of a key role of vestibular cues has further been strengthened in a study in which direct electrical stimulation of the vestibular nerve modulated perception of ambiguous auditory rhythmic sequences (Trainor et al., 2009).

Chapter 9

Attention and Learning

9.1 A multifaceted gateway to awareness

The concept of attention is intuitive but also elusive. We often explain the behaviour of others by referring to some notion of attention—'he failed the test because he was not paying attention,' 'she gave the speaker all her attention'—and we routinely use the term when we interact with others—'pay attention to what I say'. In this respect, as famously put by the psychologist William James, everyone seems to have an intuitive idea of what attention is (James, 1890, p.404). However, what we really mean by attention often eludes us, and further consideration reveals that our intuitive notion of attention could, in fact, correspond to many different cognitive mechanisms. Among those that have been studied extensively by psychologists and cognitive neuroscientists are the ability to focus on relevant information among concurrent distractors (*selective* attention), the ability to split processing resources between concurrent stimuli (*divided* attention), the ability to alternate resources between two different tasks or streams of information (*alternate* attention, or task-switching ability), the ability to focus on the same task for a prolonged period of time (*sustained* attention), and the general preparation to process and respond to the events in the environment (properly called *alertness* or *arousal*). Indeed, the multifaceted nature of attention has proved to be a real challenge for scientist trying to capture its cognitive and neural mechanisms.

As acknowledged in a recent authoritative book (Nobre & Kastner, 2014), developing a precise terminology and working towards an accepted taxonomy are important aims within current attention research (p. 1206). Terminological issues aside, however, it is clear that attention represents a gateway to awareness. To appreciate what this means, consider what happened just now, as you were reading the first lines of this chapter. Did you notice that sitting produced noticeable tactile sensations on your body, resulting from your weight on the chair? Did you realize that there were several sounds in the room? Perhaps the humming sounds of some electrical device or air-conditioning system, the distinctive taps of someone using a laptop or a smartphone, or the always present noises of city traffic? Most likely, you did not, although you would certainly agree that the stimuli that could have caused you to experience these sensations *were* there, and they were likely stimulating your sensory channels. Apparently, your attention was not directed towards them, and because of this they remained outside your awareness.

The notion that attention is a gateway to awareness has been put forward by many authors (Mack & Rock, 1998; Rensink, O'Regan, & Clark, 1997; Simons & Chabris, 1999), and several examples available on the world wide web prove this point eloquently. For instance, highly visible details of a scene can be changed from the first and the second view of a scene. When the two views are shown in alternation, most viewers do not notice these changes if there is an interruption in between. For instance, studies have inserted a blank field between the images, or added distractors in the form of 'mudsplashes' where the changes occur, or swapped the images while an eye movement is being executed. Using the latter manipulation, it has been reported that many viewers do not notice that two people in a photograph exchanged heads (Grimes, 1996). These dramatic failures to notice obvious changes in a scene have been termed *change blindness*. Change blindness has been shown to occur even if viewer are actively searching for a change, or if they are informed that distractors will be introduced for the purpose of making changes less noticeable (Rensink, O'Regan, & Clark, 1997; Simons & Rensink, 2005; see demos at http://nivea.psycho.univ-paris5.fr). Transport for London has exploited the surprising outcome of change blindness demonstrations to raise public awareness on how easily we can fail to see cyclists while driving (search for 'test your awareness: whodunit' on YouTube). Even more striking are examples of the related phenomenon termed *inattentional blindness*. Inattentional blindness occurs when highly noticeable events are not noticed by viewers engaged in some other demanding task (Mack & Rock, 1998; Simons & Chabris, 1999; Simons & Levin, 1998; see demos at http://www.simonslab.com). From the multisensory perspective of this book, we stress that examples of change blindness and inattentional blindness have also been documented for auditory (e.g. Vitevitch, 2003; Eramudugolla, et al., 2005; Pavani & Turatto, 2008) or tactile events (Gallace, Tan, & Spence, 2006, 2007) and even across sensory channels (Auvray, Gallace, Tan, & Spence, 2007; Gallace, Auvray, Tan, & Spence, 2006). Box 9.1 provides more details, including a striking multisensory example of inattentional blindness across vision and hearing.

In this chapter, we provide an introduction to the key issues in the study of multisensory attention. We will start by considering the possibility of allocating attention deliberately to stimuli from different sensory channels, and by comparing this with the possibility of grabbing an observer's attention across sensory channels. This broad distinction between *orienting attention* according to one's internal goals and *having one's attention oriented* by stimuli in the environment has proven very useful for the initial characterization of attentional mechanisms (Posner, 1980; Theeuwes, Atchley, & Kramer, 2000). The basic notion is that goal-driven (endogenous) attention orienting allows us to deliberately allocate processing resources towards events or locations that are relevant for behaviour. This is potentially a long-lasting process, and its duration depends on the person's ability to sustain the same goal and attentional set in time. Instead, stimulus-driven (exogenous) attention orienting involves the transient 'grabbing' of processing resources by unexpected and salient sensory events (Yantis & Jonides, 1984). This is a short-lived process that can take place automatically, and for this reason it can even counteract behavioural goals and expectations. Although we will broadly refer to this distinction, we will also discuss the interplay between these two mechanisms. Next, we will discuss what happens when we orient attention in contexts when space is not relevant (i.e. non-spatial multisensory attention). We will examine the interplay between attention and multisensory processing by

Box 9.1 The invisible gorilla, the chalkboard, and the inaudible gride

The 'invisible gorilla' is one of our favourite demonstrations of inattentional blindness. It was first published in a scientific journal at the end of the past century (Simons & Chabris, 1999), and rapidly became popular in magazines and internet media. In this demonstration, viewers are asked to participate in a (mock) attention test. Imagine a video of two teams exchanging passes of two basketballs. One team wears white shirts, the other wears black shirts. Your task is to keep a tally of the passes of the white team only, and to keep things more interesting, to provide separate counts for aerial (the ball flies in the air from the hands of the first to hands of the second player) and bouncing passes (the ball bounces on the floor before reaching the second player). At one point during the video, a furry, black gorilla walks in from one side, reaches the centre of the scene, turns towards the camera, beats its chest, and leaves from the other side. The gorilla (actually, a woman wearing a costume) is in the scene for several seconds and walks though the players, sometimes even occluding them. It is a bizarre, supremely noticeable event, and all viewers notice it—but only if they were not taking the attention test. A large majority of the viewers who *do* try to keep a tally of passes instead completely miss the gorilla. In class demonstrations, we have repeatedly observed that the percentage can be as high as 90 percent. In the published report, the figure varied somewhat according to several manipulations. For instance, it was around 60 percent in conditions comparable to those you can see on the internet, but skyrocketed to 92 percent if the teams and the gorilla were filmed separately and then shown as digitally edited semi-transparent video streams.

The invisible gorilla was originally an invisible woman carrying an umbrella. This refers to a manipulation in several selective looking studies performed by the group of Ulric Neisser, one of the key figures in experimental psychology of the past century (for a review of these studies, see Neisser, 1979). In most versions of these studies, observers viewed superimposed videotapes of ball games and performed some attentionally demanding task. After a few seconds, a woman carrying an umbrella was presented walking across the scene, in a third partly transparent video that was superimposed on the other two. And of course, very few participants noticed the woman. Neisser's studies were inspired by famous studies on auditory selective attention performed in the 1950s and 60s (Cherry, 1953), which first suggested that unattended auditory information will often fail to reach consciousness, and in turn inspired classic work on inattentional blindness in simple visual displays and on inattentional *deafness* in auditory events (Mack & Rock, 1998). The invisible gorilla was therefore not a radically new discovery. However, it was probably the first demonstration that inattentional blindness could occur in fully natural conditions: In the basic demonstration, there were no transparent superimposed video streams but a continuous, uninterrupted scene of a complex real-life event.

Box 9.1 **Continued**

It may be noted, however, that these studies investigated inattention to unisensory stimuli. In real life, of course, visual signals often occur in synchrony with related signals in other sensory channels. For instance, an event may generate a visual and an auditory signal at the same time. Would you be cured of your inattentional blindness by the concomitant stimulation of the auditory channel? Or, vice versa, of inattentional deafness when a visual stimulus is also presented? There is surprisingly little research on this question, but at least two papers suggest a first answer. In a clever study, Wayand, Levin, & Varakin (2005) created a video of a basketball-counting game very much like the original gorilla video, but added a soundtrack. Instead of a gorilla, they inserted a woman that walked to a chalkboard and scratched her nail on it. The 'gride' was clearly audible; even worse, it was, as such sounds are, very unpleasant to hear. Participants were requested to keep a tally of passes, and then they were asked to rate the pleasantness of five sounds, including the gride, and to identify them. The results indicated that about 60 percent of 108 participants in the experimental group did not see the woman entering the scene, and did not hear the gride. Interestingly, participants who missed the gride did not give it higher pleasantness ratings, nor were they more likely to identify it, in comparison to controls who saw the video without the woman scratching her nails on the chalkboard. This may indicate that the gride did not have an implicit effect on the participants who failed to notice it, as one would expect that such an effect would unconsciously prime internal representations of the sound, facilitating its later identification, and possibly perceived pleasantness.

Thus, it appears that, at least in these conditions, noxious auditory stimulation fails to enter consciousness, or to evoke a degree of implicit processing, not only if auditory attention is strongly engaged (as in attentional deafness studies), but also in a multisensory situation where visual attention is engaged by the pass-counting task. A possible caveat is, however, that in the Wayand study the soundtrack included bouncing sounds, shoe squeaks, and other game-related noises. It may be, therefore, that both visual and auditory attention were engaged by the pass-counting task. In an (unpublished) informal class demonstration, one of us (NB) tried a simpler manipulation. Viewers counted passes in the original silent gorilla video, but a sound was added when the mock-gorilla beat its chest (a thump-thump-thump digitally synthetized sound, in synch with the beating). In this condition, 14 viewers out of 15 did not notice the gorilla. This may be taken as indicating that inattentional blindness occurs even with multisensory stimulation signalling the unexpected event. More formal tests of this possibility, and discussions of their implications for multisensory attention, may well be worth future consideration.

discussing the evidence that indicates that under many circumstances attention promotes multisensory integration. Finally, we will discuss implications for multisensory learning and memory.

9.2 **Paying attention in a multisensory environment**

Charles Spence, a leading expert in the field of multisensory processes, reports the following anecdote about the origin of some of the most important and pioneering studies of multisensory attention. When he was a student at Oxford, Spence was looking for an undergraduate thesis project. He met a junior research fellow at Christchurch College, Jon Driver, who suggested a meeting in his flat in the centre of Oxford to talk things over. By chance, the audio on Driver's TV was malfunctioning at the time, and Driver had connected the TV to the hi-fi, such that auditory signals from the TV came from a different location in space than the visual signals on the screen. And again by chance, when Spence got there the TV was on—and the two started noticing things. Sometimes, this spatial separation between the visual and auditory sources was barely noticeable. In other occasions, however, it led to a perceivable disconnection between the two sensory streams. These unusual experiences attracted their scientific curiosity and led to an undergraduate project that aimed to reproduce the effect in the laboratory (Spence, 2014). This in turn led to a highly influential series of studies (Spence & Driver, 2004), which set the basis for many of the current studies of the cognitive and neural mechanisms of multisensory attention.

Several of the early experiments conducted by Spence and Driver closely mimicked the television setup in Driver's flat (Driver & Spence, 1994; Spence, Ranson, & Driver., 2000). Importantly, however, their scientific interest did not focus on the visual capture of the location of sounds, which occurred in some conditions (this is the ventriloquist effect, which we already discussed in several chapters of this book). They instead sought to understand to what extent people can pay attention to a stream of auditory inputs (e.g. spoken words) at one location in space, while focusing their visual attention to a different location. In one experiment, for instance, participants were instructed to listen to pre-recorded triplets of words (e.g. 'olive, notice, topic') and repeat them immediately after their presentation (Spence et al., 2000). Target word triplets were always delivered from a speaker directly behind participants. At the same time, a concurrent stream of distracting word triplets was presented in front of them, on the left or right side. This additional auditory stream was completely irrelevant for the task and yet it made listening and understanding more difficult. Note that this set-up reproduces a situation that we often experience in daily life, in which the voice of a speaker that is relevant to us is heard together with other overlapping voices—a condition often termed the 'cocktail party situation.'

The cocktail party situation has classically been exploited by experimental psychologists to investigate people's ability to select relevant information in the context of distracting inputs (Cherry, 1953; Broadbent, 1958). Crucially, in the Spence and Driver studies, two video monitors were also added to the set-up, in front of the participant. The active monitor and the loudspeaker delivering irrelevant word triplets were either in the same location (e.g. both on the right of the observer; see Figure 9.1a) or in different locations (e.g. the active monitor on the right, the loudspeaker delivering distracting triplets on the left; see Figure 9.1b). The multisensory prediction was that participants would find it harder to ignore the distracting *auditory* stream of word triplets when they attended to a *visual* stimulus placed at the same position in space (compared to the arrangement in which auditory and visual stream occurred in different locations). In some experimental blocks, the monitor showed the video of the person speaking the target words (speaking-lips condition), adding a visual stream which was actually relevant to the task at hand. In other blocks, the active monitor only showed a video of the same person

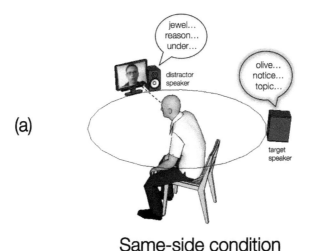

Same-side condition

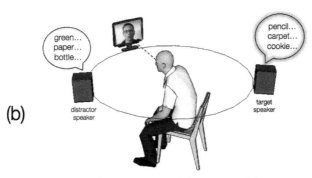

Different-side condition

Figure 9.1 The experimental set-up in Spence et al. (2000). (a) Video and audio on the same side relative to the participant. (b) Video and audio on different sides. For clarity only the active monitor is shown in the image. The participant's gaze is always directed to the active monitor.

making meaningless lip and jaw movements (chewing lips), thus contributing only task-irrelevant visual information.

Participants found it easier to repeat the relevant words when they concurrently observed the lip movements, compared to when they observed chewing lips. This is the well-known multisensory advantage of jointly hearing and seeing a spoken message (Sumby & Pollack, 1954; incidentally, this is also the reason why short-sighted people sometimes report an improvement in their hearing when they put on their glasses). More importantly, the experiment also showed that participants were indeed worse at repeating the target auditory message and ignoring the irrelevant auditory stream when they fixated the monitor *near* the distracting sounds. In other words, having the auditory distractors delivered from a location that was also visually attended made interference worse (Spence et al., 2000).

A series of follow-up experiments extended these original observations, using an even simpler set-up that allowed generalization of the result beyond language processing. In the new set-up, Spence and Driver used white noise bursts as auditory targets, and brief flashes of light as visual targets (Spence & Driver, 1996). In each trial of the experiment, sounds were delivered from one of four speakers, placed at upper or lower locations, to the left or right of the participant. Visual targets were delivered from LEDs placed in the centre of each loudspeaker (see Figure 9.2). Participants sat in front of this apparatus, with their eyes and head oriented towards a central LED, and indicated the elevation of every target (up vs down) as quickly and accurately as possible, regardless of side (left or right), and presentation modality (hearing or vision). Sometimes, participants were instructed to expect both auditory and visual targets on the same side of space. At other times, they were instructed to expect auditory targets on one side and visual targets on the opposite side. Presumably, when expecting auditory and visual targets on the same side of space participants allocated attention towards the same location in both modalities. By contrast, when expecting auditory and visual targets at different locations they had to split attention between the two hemispaces.

Spence and Driver aimed to contrast two different accounts of multisensory attention. The first was that separable mechanisms for orienting attention exist for different sensory channels. According to this idea, when visual targets are presented to the right, a mechanism for allocating attention in visually based space is engaged. At the same time, when auditory targets are presented to the left, there is an analogous mechanism for allocating attention in auditory-based space. Thus, participants should have no problem allocating visual attention to one side and auditory attention to the other. The alternative account was that there is a single mechanism for orienting attention that operates on inputs from all sensory channels. According to this second idea, it is the very same brain mechanism that orients attention to the right in visually based space and to the left in auditory space. Thus, when the task requires processing both, participants should not be able to split attention between vision and hearing. Rather, when a visual channel is cued for, say, the right side, this should cause attentional mechanism to similarly orient to the right within the auditory channel, and vice-versa. These two accounts are sometimes called the *modality-specific* and the *supra-modal* account of multisensory attention

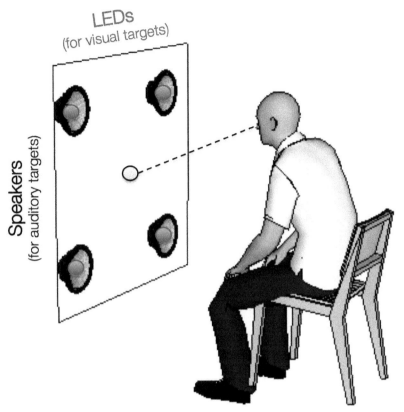

Figure 9.2 Schematic representation of the experimental set-up in the elevation-discrimination studies. Visual stimuli were delivered from one LED at a time (shown as red circles in the centre of each speaker). Auditory stimuli were delivered from one loudspeaker at a time.

(Duncan, Martens, & Ward, 1997; Farah et al. 1989). We prefer to avoid using these labels, for the reasons detailed in section 1.6 of the first chapter.

The experiments of Spence and Driver showed that voluntary attention was neither entirely linked across different sensory channels, nor completely specific for each sensory channel. People found it easier to respond to visual and auditory targets when they occurred in the same spatial location. However, they also managed to some extent to split their multisensory attention across opposite hemispaces (left and right). Importantly, the latter condition was harder to sustain and led to poorer performance. The suggestion they put forward was that attention resources across sensory modalities are 'separable-but-linked' (Spence & Driver, 1996). To better understand this notion, imagine two objects linked by a spring. One object represents your auditory attention, the other represents your visual attention. To some extent, you can force the two objects to different locations in space. However, as soon as your active effort of keeping them separate decreases, the spring will tend to bring them close to one another again. We emphasize that the links in orienting attention between sensory channels are not limited to the case of auditory and visual attention. For instance, similar results have been found when participants divide their attention between visual and tactile targets (Spence, Pavani, & Driver, 2000) or between auditory and tactile targets (Lloyd, Merat, McGlone, & Spence, 2003).

Understanding which of these contrasting accounts of multisensory attention is most accurate in explaining human performance has relevant implications for daily life. For instance, an account of attention orienting in which sensory channels operate in a linked manner implies that, while driving a car, it is hard to pay attention both to the visual stimuli in the road in front of us and to the spoken words of a conversation listened through a mobile phone head-set. By contrast, fully independent mechanism of attention orienting across sensory channels would suggest that dividing attention between the road and the heard conversation bears little or no cost for our performance on either task. The results of Spence and Driver's study suggest that splitting our multisensory attention while driving a car is indeed possible, but comes at a cost, both in terms of actual driving performance and in terms of fatigue. This kind of experiment has been conducted using driving simulators, and you can read more about them in Box 9.2. But note that many other real life situations tap on similar issues. Consider the typical situation of a teacher speaking to a class while projecting animated slides on the screen. It is surely possible to split attention between the spoken message and the slides, but this becomes more and more difficult when both the visual and auditory stream are demanding, when they are not related, or when they originate from different locations in the classroom.

9.3 Grabbing attention in multisensory conditions

Approximately at the same time when Spence and Driver started investigating how we split endogenous attention between locations and modalities (as described in the previous section), they, along with others, launched the study of exogenous multisensory attention. In the typical unimodal exogenous spatial-orienting paradigm, two successive stimuli are presented to the observer. The first is task-irrelevant, whereas the second is the target the participant is waiting for. In earlier pioneering studies, Posner and colleagues had found that targets delivered at the same location as the preceding irrelevant stimulus are processed more efficiently (e.g. faster and/or with greater accuracy), in comparison to targets delivered at different locations with respect to the irrelevant stimulus (Posner, 1980). This processing advantage is short-lived and can be measured only for inter-stimulus-intervals less than about 200 mss (Müller & Rabbit, 1989). The key multisensory question was whether an irrelevant stimulus presented in one sensory channel (say, auditory) could trigger exogenous orienting effects that could benefit a subsequent target in a different sensory channel (say, visual), delivered at the same location.

So, for instance, in a typical experiment adapting the Spence and Driver elevation-discrimination task, participants were asked to respond to the elevation (up vs. down) of visual targets delivered to the left or right of fixation (Spence & Driver, 1997). Each visual target was anticipated by an auditory stimulus, delivered either on the same side as the target or on the opposite side. Importantly, unlike the endogenous paradigms described

Box 9.2 Using a phone while driving

Many of us take, or make, phone calls while driving our car. According to traffic regulations in many countries, this is safe as long as the mobile phone is used in combination with a headset or some connection to the car's hi-fi. This rests on the assumption that the phones affect driving inasmuch as they limit your control of the steering wheel. You have to hold the phone with one of the hands, and therefore you have only one left to hold the wheel. (If you are not driving an automatic transmission vehicle, this will also interfere with shifting gears). This may be true, at least to some extent, but that this is the main source of safety issues related to mobile phones and driving is debatable. A study conducted in the USA by the National Highway Traffic Safety Administration (NHTSA) showed that even hands-free set-ups for in-car mobile phone use increase the risk of accidents by 38 percent (ABC News, July 21st, 2009). Thus, using your phone while driving may imply more than just limiting how you can use your hands at any given time. Presumably, phones do more than that: they might interfere with cognitive processes underlying driving, and a large part of these processes are likely to involve multisensory attention.

The topic discussed in this chapter can offer useful insights into this very relevant practical problem. For instance, listening to a mobile phone conversation while driving tends to draw visual attention away from the road ahead of us. Listening to a conversation is an auditory task, sometimes even a demanding one. Regardless of whether we hold the phone with our hand or use a headset, we will pay auditory attention to a region of space near our head. Similarly, if we use an in-car speakerphone, we will be paying attention to a sound that originates from somewhere in the car. In all cases, auditory attention will be engaged in a very different location with respect to the road ahead of us. As suggested in this chapter, studies of multisensory spatial attention reveal that resources across sensory systems are 'separate-but-linked.' In other words, whenever we allocate auditory resources to one portion of space (e.g. on the near right side of our body) it becomes increasingly difficult to keep the same amount of visual resources in a different region of space (e.g. the road far ahead to the left of gaze). Engaging in a phone conversation could thus limit our attention resources for the main task we should be doing—a non-negligible risk when we are responsible of the trajectory of an object weighing several tons that moves at high speed.

It has been shown experimentally that directing visual and auditory attention towards different parts of the car interior can prove difficult. For instance, in a now classic study, Spence and Read (2003) tested a group of participants using a car simulator that reproduced the demanding conditions of driving in city traffic. In addition to paying attention to the road and driving the car, participants were asked to listen and repeat words presented on speakers inside the simulator. In different conditions,

Box 9.2 Continued

words were spoken from a loudspeaker placed directly in front of them, or from a speaker placed to their left (the experiment was run in the UK so the car simulator was a right-hand drive). To make listening even more difficult, a third speaker placed behind the driver was used to deliver additional spoken words that were irrelevant to the repeating task. Results showed that performance in the repeat task was much better when words were spoken from the loudspeaker in front of the driver, compared when they were spoken from the side. In other words, it was easier to pay auditory attention to the most-similar location to the location where visual attention was also allocated. This result fits well with a multisensory account of mobile phone issues while driving.

But if auditory signals not coming from the location relevant to driving (the road ahead) can be dangerous, what about having a conversation with passengers in the car? Shouldn't this also be dangerous? We know of no accident statistics relevant to this matter, but a recent paper (Gaspar et al., 2014) suggests that conversations with passengers are, in fact, much less dangerous than mobile phone conversations. The reason? Multisensory shared experience, apparently. In the study, researchers set up four scenarios in a driving simulator: driver alone, driver conversing with a peer in the simulator, driver conversing with a remote peer through a hands-free phone, and driver conversing with a remote peer who could see the road and the driver's face on video. The mobile phone condition yielded the higher rate of simulated collisions; conversely, no conversation or having a conversation with a peer in the simulator yielded comparable collision rates. Most interestingly, chatting with the remote peer who could see what the driver saw, as well as the driver's face, also yielded low collision rates. Reportedly, sharing the experience of the driver (either by being there, or by video) passengers tended to modulate the conversation to the traffic conditions, to make more frequent references to traffic events, and to generally 'help' the driver by reducing distractions when appropriate. This conclusion fits nicely the informal observation that talking to passengers in the back seat *is* quite distracting. Sitting in the back, they get only a limited view of traffic, and are less able to modulate the conversation appropriately (and even less so if in the back of your cars are your kids).

Although multisensory constraints may be only part of the attentional difficulties related to mobile phone use while driving (for further discussions of this topic, see Kunar, Carter, Cohen, & Horowitz, 2008), they provide useful practical indications (for a review of the multisensory issues involved in driving, see Ho & Spence, 2017). If you have to make a phone call while you are driving, make sure that you use an in-car speakerphone and try to balance the speakers so that the voice seems to come from the space in front of you. Or, even better, pull over and make the call while you are not driving!

in the previous section, participants were instructed to pay attention to visual targets *only*. They were explicitly informed that auditory stimuli were completely irrelevant for the task and never conveyed useful information about the upcoming location of the target. In this paradigm, the auditory stimuli were presented with equal probability on either side of fixation. Thus, there are as many visual targets preceded by an auditory stimulus at the same location (often termed as 'valid' or 'congruent' trials) as there are with an auditory stimulus presented from the opposite location (termed 'invalid,' 'uncued' or 'incongruent' trials). The finding was that participants were faster and more accurate when processing visual stimuli that occurred on the same side as the preceding sound (see also McDonald et al., 2000; Koelewijn, Bronkhorst, & Theeuwes, 2009). Later studies extended this result by showing that auditory grabbing of visual attention has an impact also on the perceived timing of the stimulus (visual stimuli on the side of the sound are perceived earlier, compared to visual stimuli occurring at the same time but on the opposite side of the sound; McDonald et al., 2005) and its contrast (Stramer et al., 2009).

It is now well established that multisensory exogenous attention-orienting can occur for *all* combinations of successive visual, auditory, or tactile stimuli (Spence & McDonald, 2004; Spence, 2010). It is also clear that one key factor in determining whether these orienting effects will emerge is the perceived spatial correspondence between the successive stimuli. Despite orienting effects have been documented also when cue and target originate from different locations within the same hemifield (e.g. both to the right of the participant), multisensory attention grabbing is maximal when both stimuli are *perceived* as originating from the same location in space (e.g. Frassinetti, Pavani, & Làdavas, 2002; Schmitt, Postma, & de Haan, 2010). Note that encoding the spatial correspondence between the two successive stimuli is not at all trivial when they occur in different sensory channels. Consider for instance the case of vision and hearing. As we discussed in Chapter 7, we perceive visual stimuli with a considerably higher degree of spatial precision compared to auditory events (we typically know much better where the bird is on the foliage of the tree when we see it, compared to when we just hear it). If the irrelevant first stimulus is visual and the target is auditory, the visual stimulus could orient attention to a very confined location in space, which may not necessarily correspond to the broader range of possible locations from which the subsequent auditory target could be perceived. In contrast, if the irrelevant first stimulus is auditory and the target is visual, the sound would orient attention to a larger portion of space, and any visual target falling within that broad region would likely be processed more efficiently. In other words, differences in the spatial properties intrinsic to the various sensory channels can modulate multisensory exogenous attention-orienting effects, resulting sometimes in apparent asymmetries in the cueing phenomenon across the channels (Spence & McDonald, 2004).

More recently, researchers have also started to examine whether a *multisensory irrelevant stimulus* (i.e. an event that combines stimulation in more than one sensory channels, e.g. visual plus auditory) can grab attention more effectively than a unisensory one. Although it would seem quite intuitive that multisensory events are more effective than unisensory ones in grabbing attention, the outcome of the first experiments conducted on this topic did not support this prediction (e.g. Santangelo et al., 2006, 2008). Interestingly, the scenario changed substantially when researchers started to examine the efficacy of salient stimuli in grabbing attention when participants are engaged in another complex perceptual task. This situation is most frequent in real life, and it is therefore a very relevant test bench on which to assess the advantages of multisensory over unisensory stimulation. For instance, returning again to the everyday experience of car driving, it is obvious that any grabbing attention stimulus (e.g. a text message arriving on our mobile, someone asking a question from the back seat, a cyclist pulling into the road from the side street, or the unexpected bump in the road) is an event that competes with the concurrently engaging task of paying attention to the road ahead of us and driving the vehicle.

Among the various attempts to reproduce perceptually engaging tasks in the laboratory, one frequently used approach is to present the participant with a sequence of stimuli that change at a fast pace and occasionally contain a predetermined target. These are known as RSVP or RSAP methods, depending on whether they are a rapid serial visual presentation or a rapid serial auditory presentation. In RSVP, for instance, participants see a sequence of letters presented one after the other at central fixation, and are instructed to detect and report the occasional digit embedded in the sequence. Adding this RSVP (or RSAP) task to the exogenous paradigm, using a unisensory irrelevant stimulus followed by a target in the same or different sensory system, had the unexpected effect of eliminating the (otherwise) robust exogenous grabbing of attention (Santangelo, Olivetti-Belardinelli, & Spence, 2007). However, no such interference between the RSVP (or RSAP) task and exogenous orienting was observed if the irrelevant stimulus was multisensory (Santangelo & Spence, 2007). What this means is that a concurrent demanding perceptual task can override the otherwise powerful effect of exogenous orienting, but not when the cue itself is multisensory. Thus, while multisensory signals do not seem to bring any advantage over unisensory ones under condition of no perceptual load, they are the only ones that seem to retain an attention grabbing effect if the participants are concurrently engaged in a demanding perceptual task (for a review see Spence & Santangelo, 2009) .

As discussed in the previous section, these insights on the rules that govern multisensory attention have very important implications for the design and making of human-machine interfaces, and can, for instance, inform on the best ways of introducing warning signals in cars or cockpits. Importantly for the translational use of these multisensory spatial-orienting effects in real life contexts, beneficial effects of multisensory warning signals have also been documented in cluttered visual scenes—which are admittedly more similar to the everyday environment than the experimental set-ups described above. For instance, search for a visual target among multiple visual distractors can be facilitated by three-dimensional auditory signals coming from the same location as the target (McIntire, Havig, Watamaniuk, & Gilkey, 2010; Perrott, Sadralodabai, Saberi, & Strybel, 1991; Perrot, Cisneros, McKinley, & D'Angelo, 1996). Likewise, tactile signals delivered through an array of vibrotactile stimulators placed at eight evenly spaced locations around the torso of the subject can improve visual search within a visual virtual building (Lindeman, et al., 2005).

Tutorial 9.1 Neural correlates of multisensory attention

Although the interest for the brain correlates of attention predates methodological developments in modern cognitive neuroscience (e.g. Mesulam, 1981), current perspectives on this topic stem primarily from the neuroimaging techniques that became available in the early 1990s (such as PET and fMRI). These techniques were originally applied to attention-orienting tasks in the visual modality (e.g. the spatial-cueing paradigm; Posner et al., 1980).

By the beginning of the present century, two main findings were established. First, a brain network involving frontal and parietal regions—the so-called *FP network*—was observed in association with the orienting of attention, particularly for attention shifts across locations in space (Corbetta, Miezin, Shulman, & Petersen, 1993; Corbetta, et al., 2000; Gitelman et al., 1999). Within the FP network a broad distinction was proposed, attributing different functional specializations to dorsal and ventral components (Corbetta & Shulman, 2002). In neuroanatomy, the term dorsal indicates regions located towards the upper side of the brain, whereas the term ventral indicates regions towards the lower side of the brain. The dorsal FP network (dFP), comprising brain areas such as the frontal eye fields and the intraparietal sulcus, has been associated primarily with the endogenous (i.e. deliberate) orienting of attention. Instead, the ventral FP network (vFP), comprising the inferior frontal gyrus and the temporo-parietal junction, has been linked with the stimulus-driven re-orienting of attention (see Macaluso & Doricchi, 2013 for a critical discussion of this distinction, and a review of the studies that showed that the two systems can interact in a dynamic manner). The second key finding that emerged from neuroimaging studies of attention was the observation that attentional effects can be detected in the activity of early sensory cortices (e.g. the occipital visual cortex, when preparing for a visual target; Kastner, et al., 1999). Research on the neural correlates of multisensory attention mainly grew out these two key findings.

Broadly speaking, the FP network is recruited regardless of which sensory stimulation is chosen for the experiment. It comes into play when participants pay attention to auditory stimuli (e.g., Mayer, Harrington, Adair, & Lee, 2006; Mayer, et al., 2007; Wu, Weissman, Roberts, & Woldorff, 2007), or when they attend to somatosensory events (Macaluso, Frith, & Driver, 2002; Burton, Sinclair, & McLaren, 2008). In addition, the FP network is revealed also in studies using stimuli in more than one sensory channel, while participants attend to single or multiple channels (e.g. Shomstein & Yantis, 2004; Santangelo et al., 2009). For instance, Shomstein and Yantis (2004) observed a transient increase in the activity of the dFP network when participants shifted their attention resources from vision to hearing or vice versa.

Nonetheless, extending the investigation beyond vision alone contributed to challenging the distinction between dFP and vFP and suggested that some of the principles that hold for the unisensory case may actually differ when multisensory stimuli are considered. For instance, in a study (Salmi et al., 2009) participants were instructed to detect occasionally louder tones presented at a specified ear (an endogenous attention orienting). Brain responses while participants were engaged in this auditory task were recorded in both the dFP and vFP network. Furthermore, a largely overlapping FP network came into play also when the target tone was played to the unattended ear (an example of exogenous attention orienting). Thus, when considering the auditory modality the distinction between dFP and vFP network seems to be less pronounced. Even more relevant for showing that a multisensory perspective to attention can challenge notions developed when studying visual stimuli alone is a study by Santangelo and colleagues (2009). An established finding, in relation to the vFP network when using visual stimuli, is that unexpected stimuli activate the temporo-parietal junction (one important node of the vFP network) only when they share some feature with the target, and thus are potentially task-relevant. For instance, unexpected stimuli are less likely to activate the temporo-parietal junction if they are of a different colour with respect to the target (Shulman et al., 2007). This could originate from active 'filtering mechanisms' that have the purpose to limit any interference from events that are not relevant for the task at hand (Corbetta et al., 2008). Santangelo and colleagues (2009) tested whether such a principle holds true also when the unexpected stimulus is a sound. Much to their surprise, when participants were paying attention to visual stimuli, sounds occurring at the unexpected side disrupted performance and intruded in the vFP network, modulating its activation. This suggests that auditory stimuli—unlike visual events—can bypass the filtering mechanism, even when entirely task-irrelevant. Good to know when designing warning signals in applied settings.

Research on the neural correlates of multisensory attention also confirmed the observation that attentional effects can be detected in the activity of early sensory cortices (Kastner et al., 1999). When participants select a single perceptual modality, irrespective of the spatial location of the stimulation, a competition between primary sensory cortices ensues. For instance, Laurienti and colleagues (2002), presented auditory and visual targets from a single central location, and asked participants to pay attention to vision or hearing or to both modalities. The results showed that attention to vision enhanced neural responses in the visual occipital cortex, but reduced activation in the auditory temporal cortex. Conversely, attention to hearing, enhanced responses in the auditory cortex, but suppressed activation in visual cortex. This finding suggests that we can prioritize one sensory modality over the other to some extent. When referring to the notion we introduced in this chapter that multisensory attention resources are 'separable-but-linked' (Spence & Driver, 1996), this observation speaks in favour of the 'separable' side of the formula.

However, if space comes into play things can change substantially and the 'linked' side also emerges. When both the perceptual modality and the spatial location of the targets are relevant for the task (e.g. 'Pay attention only to *visual* stimuli coming from the *left* side'), the separation of labour between sensory cortices begins to blur. If the task entails paying attention to vision, for instance, auditory distractors sharing the same spatial location as the visual targets also modulate the activity of the occipital visual cortex (Ciaramitaro et al., 2007; Santangelo, Fagioli, & Macaluso, 2010; for earlier evidence of this interaction using EEG see also: Hillyard et al., 1984; McDonald & Ward, 2007; see Hillyard et al., 2016 for review). The interpretation of this result is based on the notion that the brain holds some representations of space that are specific for sensory channels, and other representations of space that are multisensory (Santangelo & Macaluso, 2012; see also Chapter 7). When space is relevant, orienting of attention resources calls into play multisensory neuronal populations in the frontal (Graziano, Taylor, Moore, & Cooke, 2002) and parietal (Cohen & Andersen, 2012) cortices that encode space across modalities. This, in turn, enhance *all* sensory signals that originate from the selected spatial location, irrespective of which sensory channel is treating them and—to some extent—irrespective of which perceptual modality the participant is trying to attend. By contrast, when space is not relevant, or when attention for stimuli in different perceptual modalities can be allocated to distinct locations, orienting of attention involves neural populations that encode space more in a sensory-specific fashion (e.g. visual only neurons; Xing & Andersen, 2000). This would allow higher separation of the cascade preparatory signals reaching the primary sensory cortices.

9.4 Non-spatial multisensory facilitation

The results described in the previous sections emphasized spatial coincidence between stimuli to different sensory channels in orienting of spatial attention. Other studies, however, have shown that interactions between sensory channels can influence behaviour, promoting faster and more accurate sensory-motor processes, also when multisensory stimuli originate from different spatial locations. The key requisite is that they approximately co-occur in time. Although it remains to be established to what extent these phenomena can be ascribed to attention mechanisms, we have chosen to discuss them in this chapter because they produce facilitatory effects on perception, as do more classic attention phenomena.

The first empirical reports of non-spatial multisensory facilitation for concurrent stimuli in different sensory channels date back to the 1960s (Bernstein, Clark, & Edelstein, 1969; Hershenson, 1962; Morrell, 1968). The finding was that reaction time to a stimulus in one sensory channel (typically visual) is shortened when an additional stimulus in a different sensory channel (typically auditory) is presented approximately at the same time (Nickerson, 1973). Barry Stein and colleagues showed that visual stimuli presented with white noise bursts are perceived as brighter compared to when they are presented without bursts (Stein, London, Wilkinson, & Price, 1996). Importantly, manifestations of multisensory facilitation have been observed also when stimuli are delivered at different spatial locations. In the brightness study, for instance, increased brightness for multisensory stimuli occurred for a light placed at fixation and sounds delivered to the left or to the right of fixation. Although some of the initial evidence for multisensory facilitation may be interpreted more in terms of response bias rather than genuine perceptual effects (e.g. Odgaard, Arieh, & Marks, 2003), more recent studies have convincingly shown that various aspects of visual processing can be enhanced by concurrent transient sounds (e.g. Andersen & Mamassian, 2008; Noesselt et al., 2008; Olivers & Van der Burg, 2008). Two behavioural effects, described below, illustrate the powerful consequences of non-spatial multisensory attention.

The first effect is known as 'freezing' and was documented by Jean Vroomen and Beatrice de Gelder (Vroomen & Gelder, 2000). In the original version of this paradigm, participants saw four visual displays presented in rapid succession. Each display consisted of four dots arranged at one of the intersections of a 4-by-4 imaginary grid. These dots were hard to see because they lasted only 100 ms and were followed by a mask. In one display, the dots were arranged to form a diamond, and participants were instructed to detect the display with the diamond and respond by indicating the position of the diamond in the display (e.g. the diamond-shape in Figure 9.3 is in the top left corner). Critically, in the experimental condition the target display was paired with a high frequency tone, whereas all other displays were coupled with a low frequency tone. This created an auditory stream of equal sounds in which the deviant tone was clearly perceived. In the control condition, all displays were paired with the same low frequency tone. The striking finding was that at the moment the auditory deviant stood out, also the simultaneous visual display containing the target became more discriminable (i.e. the position of the diamond-shape was easier to determine). In fact, some participant even reported the impression that the duration of the display corresponding to the sound had been prolonged, that the image had been 'frozen'—hence the name of this behavioural effect.

We now know that the effect is not a mere consequence of alertness or preparation, because pairing the deviant tone with the display just before the target does not produce visual facilitation (Vroomen & de Gelder, 2000). We also know that a single high tone presented at the time of the target is sufficient to produce the 'freezing.' In addition, a visual halo around the target, a vibro-tactile stimulation at the wrists, or an audio-tactile stimulus can work just as well (Ngo & Spence, 2010). In fact, the freezing phenomenon has been documented even in the absence of any additional stimulation. If all displays are paired

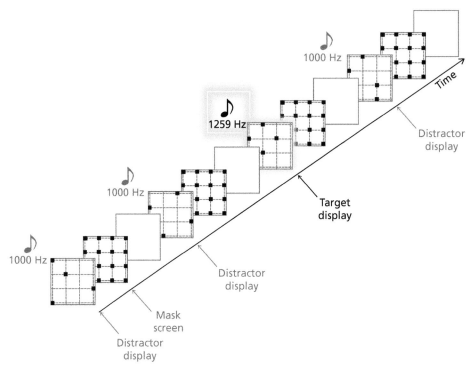

Figure 9.3 Schematics of the stimuli in the study by Vroomen & de Gelder (2000).

Adapted from Vroomen, J. & de Gelder, B. 'Sound enhances visual perception: cross-modal effects of auditory organization on vision' in Journal of Experimental Psychology: Human Perception and Performance, (2000), 26(5), 1583–90.

with a tone of constant frequency and the target display is instead paired with silence, this 'absence' also produces facilitation of target discrimination performance (Ngo & Spence, 2010). What this tells us is that the freezing effect could be the consequence of capture of attention in time. In other words, whenever our perceptual system detects a deviance in the multisensory scene, this has the consequence of focusing attention in a particular point in *time*. This non-spatial mechanism of attention orienting is multisensory in the sense that the deviance need not be produced in the same sensory system as the target, but instead it can be a change in the regularity of sensory streams in other perceptual systems.

A second striking example of non-spatial multisensory attention is the so-called 'pip-pop' phenomenon, documented by Van der Burg and colleagues (Van der Burg, Olivers, Bronkhorst, & Theeuwes, 2008). In the classic version of this paradigm participants see a cluttered visual display, comprising multiple short line segments with different orientations. Hidden in this visual crowd of 24, 36, or 48 elements there is a target: a vertical or horizontal line segment (a demo of the illusion is also available at: www.vupsy.nl/pip-and-pop-effect/). The task for the participant is to find the target as soon as possible and report its orientation. All items in the display are presented in red or green and a random number of them change colour every 50, 100, or 150 ms.

The target too changes colour approximately every second and when this happens it is the only element in the display to change colour. With this procedure, the overall impression is that of staring at a Christmas tree, and the search for the target is typically very difficult! The key manipulation that Van der Burg and colleagues introduced was to run this task either in silence, or with a tone accompanying each change in colour of the target. This tone was delivered through headphones and thus provided no information about the location of the target on the screen. Likewise, it was completely uninformative about the target orientation or colour. It only signalled the moment in time in which the target colour-change occurred. The remarkable consequence of this simple manipulation was that the tone made the target pop-out from the cluttered and flickering scene. In other words, the auditory 'pip' made the visual target 'pop.'

What this implies is that it is possible to influence the competition between multiple visual stimuli by using sounds, even when these are only informative about the moment in time when the relevant information is present. Similar to the freezing effect, the pip-pop is not exclusive to the pairing between vision and hearing. For instance, it has been replicated also when pairing the target colour-change with a vibration delivered to the back of the left hand (Van der Burg, Olivers, Bronkhorst, & Theeuwes, 2009). Unlike the freezing effect, it does not work when a halo of light replaces the tone (Van der Burg et al., 2009).

The freezing effect, the pip-pop effect, and other examples of intersensory facilitation (e.g. Andersen & Mamassian, 2008; Noesselt et al., 2008; Olivers & Van der Burg, 2008) have in common that they emerge in the absence of any spatial correspondence between the multisensory stimulations. This distinguishes these phenomena from the multisensory spatial attention cueing we reported at the beginning of this chapter. Furthermore, it suggests that they do not relate to the mechanisms of multisensory integration occurring at the single neuron level (Stein & Stanford, 2008; see also Tutorial 7.2 in this book). Although there is still debate as to the exact mechanisms that could explain these multisensory phenomena—and, in fact, there could be more than one (Spence & Ngo, 2012)—there is general consensus that they reflect multisensory orienting of attention in time, a process which requires a close temporal correspondence between the multisensory stimuli and has some degree of automaticity.

9.5 The interplay between attention and multisensory processing

In this chapter, we have examined the many ways in which attention, either spatial or non-spatial, can be influenced by multisensory processing. However, it is also important to take the opposite perspective, and ask to what extent multisensory processes are themselves influenced by attention. This question taps into the bigger issue of whether multisensory perception is primarily a *bottom-up* phenomenon, resulting from mandatory interactions between the sensory signals, with little or no influence from previous knowledge, task-demands, availability of processing resources, and attention, or instead if it can be modulated by all of these *top-down* factors. While the answer to this complex question is still incomplete, the available evidence clearly suggests a multifaceted interplay between multisensory processing and attention (Talsma, Senkowski, Soto-Faraco, & Woldorff, 2010, 2012; Talsma, 2015). Again, as we shall see in this section, digging into these issues is not merely a theoretical exercise, because it has implications for taking advantage of multisensory processes in real life situations.

One of the first to address this important topic with an experimental approach was the Belgian psychologist Paul Bertelson, a founding father of the field of multisensory processing and, more generally, of cognitive psychology in Europe. Together with his colleagues he examined to what extent the ventriloquist illusion can be influenced by the deliberate and automatic orienting of visual attention (Bertelson, Vroomen, de Gelder, & Driver, 2000; Vroomen, Bertelson, & de Gelder, 2001). The results of these early studies found no effect of attention orienting on the magnitude of the ventriloquist effect, suggesting that the multisensory interactions subtending this illusion are uninfluenced by this kind of top-down manipulation. In support of this bottom-up account of the ventriloquist illusion, one study conducted in patients with brain lesions showed that visual capture of sound position can occur also towards visual stimuli that have escaped visual awareness (Bertelson, et al., 2000).

Results from EEG studies that have examined the time-course of brain responses to multisensory stimuli have also been considered compatible with a bottom-up account of multisensory processing. One seminal study in this respect, for instance, was conducted by Giard and Peronnet (1999). They measured EEG potentials evoked by auditory and by audio-visual stimuli and noted the brain responses to these two different events start diverging very rapidly, approximately 40 ms after the stimulation. This finding was replicated by other research groups (Molholm et al., 2002; Van der Burg, et al., 2011), and it is of great importance in the multisensory literature because it shows that interactions between the sensory signals can occur at very early stages of sensory processing. For our discussion of the interplay between multisensory processing and attention it is particularly useful to focus on a study that recorded EEG event-related potentials during the pip-pop paradigm (that we described in the section 9.4). Van der Burg and colleagues (2011) found that the sound-induced benefit in visual search that they measured in behaviour was positively correlated with the amplitude of the brain response that characterized the early integration between vision and hearing, recorded between 50 and 60 ms after the stimulation. Critically, they also showed that if a distractor (instead of the target) was paired with the 'pip' tone, the early brain marker of audio-visual integration was still detected, whereas behavioural benefits were obviously absent. Thus, the integration of auditory and visual stimuli occurred *regardless* of whether it was useful for the task or not. If it was useful (i.e. it concerned the target and not the distractor), then it also had positive consequences for behaviour. But the brain clearly followed the path of integration irrespective of this behavioural advantage.

Let's stop for a moment to consider one very important implication of this finding. What it tells us is that multisensory processing can be automatic, at least under certain circumstances. Automatic means that the brain can integrate across sensory signals *irrespective of whether this will be beneficial for behaviour or not.* We can see this as the 'dark side' of multisensory processing and multisensory attention. It is very important to be aware that the same mechanisms that can make multisensory attention advantageous can also be problematic if they automatically divert attention away from our behavioural goals. This can occur, for instance, when we become over-enthusiastic with audio-visual animations in computer slides. It is not infrequent to attend lectures in which the speaker is trying to convey a message with spoken words, while a concurrent stream of computer animations with moving icons and sounds 'enrich' the presentation. In this case, the salient and temporally coincident audio-visual stimuli are very likely to attract the listener's attention, more than the speaker himself. This example may serve as a reminder that any simplistic 'the-more-the-merrier' approach to multisensory stimulation is far from being ideal. We will return to this general concept in the epilogue of this book.

At the same time as researchers found evidence for bottom-up mechanisms in multisensory processing, many other studies revealed that attention and other top-down factors can actually play a key role in modulating multisensory interactions (for review see Talsma, et al., 2010). Several examples of the interplay between attention and multisensory processing have emerged from the study of audio-visual linguistic stimuli (e.g. Alsius et al., 2005, 2007; Fairhall & Macaluso, 2009; Senkowski et al., 2008; Vroomen & Bart, 2009). Here we will focus on two examples that, instead, used audio-visual non-linguistic stimuli, to emphasize that attentional modulations of multisensory processes are not limited to language materials.

The first example is a study conducted by Raymond van Ee and colleagues (van Ee, van Boztel, Parker, & Alais, 2009). They presented participants with two different visual stimuli, one in each eye. One eye would only see a circular object rotating clockwise at fixed speed; the other eye would only see a disc expanding, which appeared as a looming object looming. With this type of presentation, a binocular rivalry phenomenon is observed: participants see alternatively either the stimulus delivered to the left or the right eye, but not both. Paying deliberate attention to one of the two stimuli can make its percept last longer, but does not eliminate the alternation between the two images. The key manipulation that van Ee and colleagues introduced was that on some block of the trials a sound was added to the experiment, concurrent with the presentation of the visual stimulus. The sound was always compatible with one of the two changing images; for instance, it was a looming sound that closely matched the timing of the looming disc. A purely bottom-up account of multisensory perception would predict that this closely matched audio-visual correspondence would direct attention to the looming disc, making its percept more persistent. In fact, this was not the case. The sound changed visual dominance duration for the looming disc only if participants were already attending the visual stimulus (compared to a condition of passive viewing). What this means is that the multisensory binding occurred specifically if the stimulus was attended, and bottom-up correspondence alone was not sufficient.

The second example provides very similar evidence, but studying the EEG response to an auditory stimulus presented concurrently with attended or unattended visual events

(Busse, et al., 2005). Paying attention to a sound determines a distinctive EEG signal that starts at approximately 200 ms after stimulus presentation and peaks over the anterior part of the scalp (fronto-central electrodes; Näätänen, 1982). Busse and colleagues showed that this late negativity can be detected also for a sound that is completely task-irrelevant (i.e. it is never attended) when comparing the trials in which the sound occurred together with an attended visual stimulus and the trials in which same sound was paired with an unattended visual event. Critically, in the study the task-irrelevant sound was always presented centrally, whereas the visual stimuli (either attended or unattended) were delivered to the left or right of fixation. Thus, none of the two visual stimuli match the position of the sound. Yet, the EEG results reveal a spreading of attention from the visual stimulus to the concurrent sound, as if the binding between the auditory and the visual event occurred selectively for the visual stimulus that was relevant for behaviour.

This study shows that a key aspect of the interplay between attention and multisensory processing can actually resolve the seeming conflict discussed in this section. The proposal is that of recursive interactions between top-down and bottom-up processes. When cues to multisensory binding are strong (stimuli co-occur in space and time, and/or are linked by strong previous association), multisensory interaction can occur in a bottom-up fashion and have cascade effects on attention and other high-level cognitive processes. However, when there are not sufficient cues to promote the binding between the multiple sensory signals (stimuli are spatially misaligned, or temporally asynchronous, or loosely/arbitrarily related), bottom-up processes alone do not suffice. In this case, top-down attention to the stimulus that happens to be relevant for behaviour is necessary to promote multisensory binding. This, in turn, could have cascade effects on the automatic mechanisms that rely on spatial or temporal coincidence and lead to merging between the sensory inputs (Talsma et al., 2012).

9.6 From multisensory attention to multisensory learning and memory

Attention is a fundamental prerequisite for learning and memory. Attended events are learned faster, lead to longer lasting memories, and, in general, create stronger associations with other pre-existing notions in our mind. Given that multisensory attention can enhance processing of events in the environment, it would seem obvious to assume that it could also promote learning and memory. This notion that combining multiple information across sensory signals can be optimal for learning environments has been central to several educational approaches. For instance, the twentieth-century Italian pedagogist Maria Montessori postulated that multisensory stimulation is highly advantageous for learning (Montessori, 1912). Her approach to education remains highly influential to this day. However, until recently, there have been very limited attempts to validate the putative advantages of multisensory stimulation for learning and memory with empirical data. In the final section of this chapter, we will turn to this important aspect of multisensory research.

One way to operationalize the question of multisensory learning is to explore how material presented in one modality can promote processing of material in another modality in a *subsequent* moment in time (Shams, Wozny, Kim, & Seitz, 2011; Thelen & Murray, 2013). Note that the key aspect of this research question is not whether people are better at perceiving or remembering multisensory stimuli in comparison to unisensory stimuli. Rather, the question is whether perceptual processing and memory of *unisensory* stimuli can be improved to a greater extent following multisensory training. The answer to this is not at all trivial, as you can appreciate from the following example. Suppose you are studying a new language, and you aim to improve your ability in understanding a conversation over the phone. Strictly speaking this is a unisensory task, pertaining to the auditory channel alone: you need to improve your ability to recognize words perceived only through hearing. Given this aim, which type of training do you think will be most efficient? Do you think it would be better to just listen to as many spoken words as possible, delivered in the absence of any congruent visual information, such as lip movements or written words (a purely *unisensory* learning context)? Or, instead, do you think that it would be best to train your listening ability in a multisensory context, with additional convergent sources of input contributing to word understanding (a *multisensory* learning context)? Which of the two learning approaches will be more effortful and which is most likely to produce long-lasting learning? Recall that your final aim is to improve your ability to understand words over the phone.

For scientists who approached this issue, one obvious starting point was to examine perceptual learning, that is the way in which perceptual functions, e.g. such as detection, discrimination, and identification, can be improved by training. For instance, Seitz, Kim, and Shams examined the effects of multisensory learning on a difficult visual motion task (Seitz, Kim, & Shams, 2006; Kim, Seitz, & Shams, 2008). They trained participants to detect and discriminate the direction of visual motion for 1 hour per day, for 10 consecutive days. In each trial of the training, participants saw two consecutive displays containing dots moving in random directions. In one of the displays, however, a small proportion of the dots were coherently moving towards the left or towards the right. The participant's task was to detect which of the two displays contained the coherent moving stimuli, and report their direction of motion (Figure 9.4). Participants were either trained with visual stimulation alone, or with concurrent sounds in the same temporal interval as the target moving stimulus. When the sound was present it moved either in the same direction as the visual motion (audio-visual congruent) or in the opposite direction (audio-visual incongruent). Importantly, to assess visual learning between conditions all multisensory training sessions included visual only stimuli—in other words, the effects of training were always assessed in a unimodal condition. The effects of multisensory learning on the visual motion task were substantial: congruent sounds increased the rate of unisensory learning by approximately 60 percent, and led to a maximum performance that was about 10 percent bigger compared the one observed in unisensory or in the audio-visual incongruent condition.

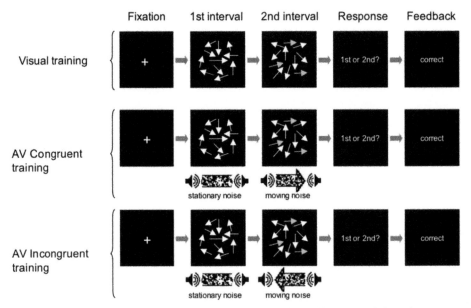

Figure 9.4 Schematics of the perceptual learning study conducted by Kim et al. (2008).

This finding is not isolated, and several other examples of the benefit of multisensory learning on subsequent unisensory performance are now available (e.g. Barakat, Seitz, & Shams, 2015; Strelnikov, Rosito, & Barone, 2011; Von Kriegstein & Giraud, 2006). In fact, a recent study made an observation that at first sight may almost appear paradoxical. Barakat and colleagues trained participants in a visual task that required discrimination of rhythmic temporal sequences (Barakat et al., 2015). Rhythm discrimination in vision is possible, but it is considerably more difficult compared to rhythm discrimination in hearing (or touch). The authors of this study examined whether it was possible to train rhythmic discrimination for temporal sequences through visual, auditory, or audio-visual learning procedures. The striking finding of this experiment was that participants improved in the visual task more when they were trained in the audio-visual or even the auditory only condition, compared to when they were trained only in vision. In other words, they showed that multisensory training or training in a different sensory system can prove—under special conditions—even more beneficial than training occurring within the same sensory channel.

Parallel to this line of studies on multisensory learning, another direction of research explored to what extent exposure to multisensory materials can alter the memory for unisensory materials. In particular, Micah Murray, Antonia Thelen, and collaborators, who have been pioneers in this research domain, addressed this issue within a single-trial approach. What this means is that they examined the effect of single-trial exposure to multisensory (or unisensory) stimuli on their subsequent recognition. The paradigm they adopted in their studies is summarized in Figure 9.5. In each trial they see a line drawing depicting a single, easily recognizable object. The participant's task is to decide whether the image is being presented for the first time ('new' item) or it has been seen before ('old'). Critically, some of the stimuli are delivered in silence, whereas others are delivered with concurrent sounds. Across experiments, Thelen, Murray, and colleagues examined the effects of sounds that were completely unrelated to the visual stimulus (a meaningless pure tone), were semantically related to the stimulus (e.g. a lion's roar, when the picture is a lion), or were semantically unrelated (e.g. the noise of a helicopter when the stimulus is a bell).

The results of this series of experiments revealed that the participants' accuracy in detecting visual object repetition was indeed influenced by the single-trial multisensory experience. In particular, it was improved when the sound and the visual stimulus were congruent. Interestingly, the condition in which the visual stimuli were paired with the meaningless sound impacted on performance more than the condition in which the sound was semantically incongruent (Thelen & Murray, 2013). In fact, a recent study (Thelen, Matusz, & Murray, et al., 2014) has revealed that whether the pairing of the visual image with a meaningless sound hampers or instead facilitate subsequent memory may depend on individual differences at the moment of the stimulus encoding, that can be detected in the EEG response to the multisensory stimulus.

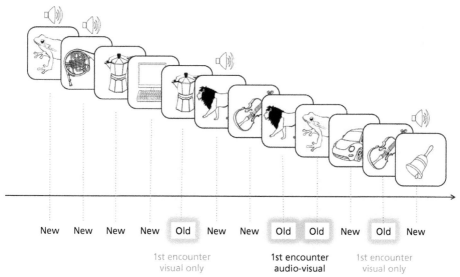

Figure 9.5 Example of stimulus sequence adopted in the studies on single-trial multisensory memory.

Adapted from Antonia Thelen and Micah M. Murray, The efficacy of single-trial multisensory memories, *Multisensory Research*, 26 (5), pp. 483–502, doi: 10.1163/22134808-00002426 Copyright © 2013, Brill.

Although the study of multisensory learning and memory is still in its infancy, it appears that the effects of prioritized processing determined by multisensory stimulation can persist even in unisensory contexts. As explained by Ladan Shams and Robyn Kim, multisensory facilitation of unisensory learning and memory can be simplified as follows: 'training with X + Y results in better performance on Y, relative to training with Y alone' (Shams & Kim, 2012, p.477). From the perspective of brain changes, at least two mechanisms can contribute to these multisensory learning effects (Shams & Kim, 2012; Shams & Seitz, 2008). The first mechanism is linked to the notion that multisensory stimuli can boost activity in unisensory brain areas (see also Tutorial 9.1). Because learning seems to require that neural activation within the brain area processing the relevant stimulus exceeds a certain threshold (Seitz & Dinse, 2007), the activation boost related to multisensory processing and attention could promote learning by early modulation of activity in unisensory regions (e.g. Murray et al., 2005). The other mechanism is linked to the notion of strengthening of functional associations between brain areas dedicated to the processing of different sensory channels. This increased connection between sensory regions could determine the recruitment of wider brain networks, even when the stimulation is unisensory (e.g. von Kriegstein & Giraud, 2006). In addition, more functional accounts could explain the benefit of multisensory learning. For instance, it is possible that multisensory learning promotes faster acquisition of internal models that can be employed for the interpretation of incoming sensory signals. In this respect, multisensory exposure would shape the predictive representations that contribute to the disambiguation of the naturally complex perceptual flow that we constantly receive from the environment (Rao & Ballard, 1999; Friston, 2005).

Whatever the mechanism subtending the enhanced learning related to multisensory processing, the implications for education and, particularly, for rehabilitation are massive. Going back to the example introduced at the beginning of this section, what we have discussed in this section suggests that you may learn more efficiently to understand conversations over the phone if you train yourself in multisensory contexts (spoken words and seen lip movements) than if you struggle with the auditory experience alone. Perhaps you may find this a very counterintuitive notion, and this is precisely why empirical research on these issues is so important.

Chapter 10

Epilogue

10.1 **A paradigm shift?**

For a relatively long time, multisensory work was not fashionable in psychology and cognitive neuroscience. In the year 1990, when the older of us received his PhD, there were only 41 articles indexed as 'multisensory' (or 'cross-modal' or 'polysensory') in the biomedical PubMed database (with a cumulative count of 471 papers published since 1946). By the year 2000, when the younger of us received his, with a count of 87 this number had doubled but remained unimpressive (the cumulative count was 993). At the beginning of the new century, however, things have begun to change. In 2010, when a precursor of this book first appeared in Italian bookstores, the number of PubMed hits for the same keywords that year had risen to 357, an almost nine-fold increase, and in 2015 it has surpassed the 600 threshold. On our last count the cumulative number of papers with these keywords on PubMed was 6878. Still a tiny fraction of the perception literature, no doubt, but strong testimony of the field's growth. In 1999, about 100 delegates spoke at the first International Multisensory Research Forum (IMRF, Figure 10.1) at Oxford. The 2015 Pisa meeting counted almost 350 delegates. In 2012, the monumental *The New Handbook of Multisensory Processes* appeared in print. With a page count close to 1000 and 43 chapters, this may be justly considered the most comprehensive current resource for specialists. In the introductory chapter, editor Barry Stein speculated that the label 'multisensory scientist' will soon replace those that are commonly heard today, such as 'vision scientist', 'auditory scientist', and so on. In 2013, the publishing company Brill launched *Multisensory Research,* the first scholarly journal entirely devoted to studies of multisensory perception. It seems fair to say that multisensory perception has come of age, but is this merely an extension in scope of traditional perception studies, or is it a more radical change in perspective?

For the historian, interest in multisensory perception is not new. For instance, well before the advent of modern science, philosophers were well aware of the importance of multisensory interactions in perception (Polansky, 2007; Gregoric, 2007). As we mentioned in the first chapter of the book, Aristotle believed that humans have five senses, plus an additional common *sense.* He believed that the common sense is the basis of our awareness of having perceptual experiences—a sort of meta-perceptive function, linked to consciousness (*De Somno,* 2, 455 a 13). In addition, he suggested that the common sense was responsible for perceiving distal features that can be accessed through multiple sensory channels, such as size, extension, shape, unity, numerosity, and movement

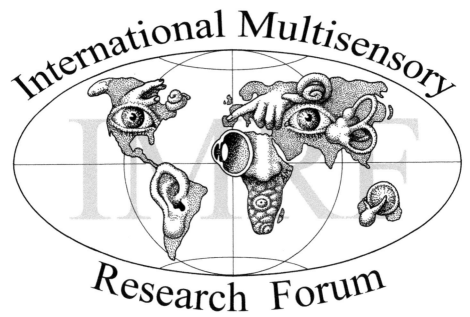

Figure 10.1 The original IMRF logo (variations have been introduced in recent meetings). Started in 1999, the International Multisensory Research Forum has become the main opportunity for multisensory scientists to present and discuss their research. (Updated information on the IMRF meetings, including all conference abstracts, is freely available http://imrf.info/wp_imrf/past-meetings/.)
Courtesy of Alex Meredith

(*De Anima*, III, 1 425 a 14). He called these features *common sensibles*, and distinguished them from unisensory percepts, such as colour or smell, that in his view remained confined to a single channel. This distinction has shaped the philosophy of perception for centuries and can be found in later works by Locke and Galileo. Some of the themes discussed in this book, such as the role of multisensory interactions in the awareness of our own embodied self, or the variety of multisensory interactions in the perception of object features, also echo Aristotle's ideas.

Thus, many of the considerations on the multisensory nature of our minds could be considered as new wine in an old bottle. However, contemporary work suggests that the role of multisensory interactions in perception is much more fundamental than suggested earlier. For instance, empirical results from modern neuroimaging methods and paradigms or from studies using virtual reality technology (allowing full control of multisensory stimulation and extensive recording of behavioural responses) were unconceivable until a few decades ago. These findings, along with sophisticated modelling work, now force us to go beyond the mere conclusion that the mind is multisensory. We suggest, in fact, that contemporary work on multisensory perception could be considered a true paradigm shift in perception science, asking for a radical reconsideration of several empirical and theoretical questions within an entirely new perspective. The key issue here is no longer merely accepting that perception exploits and combines information from multiple sensory channels, but understanding in full all the implications of a multisensory perspective. Consider the history of astronomy. It has always been relatively easy, even with the naked eye, to notice that on the surface of the moon there are dark spots. This observation ran counter the traditional doctrine of the heavenly bodies in the Aristotelian cosmology, which assumed that the moon was perfectly spherical and smooth. However, for a long time the visible spots were explained away with ingenious arguments, such as the great Arab tenth century scientist Alhazen's proposal that the spots were due to variations in the sphere density, causing some regions to absorb more (and therefore reflect less) of the light from the sun. Galileo's observations using newly developed telescopes reopened this old scientific question, showing that the shape of the spots changed with the angle of the illuminating rays from the sun, consistent with the interpretations that they were shadows of mountain and ridges. Galileo's observations thus spurred a rethinking of the dominant theory, at the same time identifying many novel empirical questions such as, for instance, understanding why the outlines of the these mountains were not visible on the border of the moon, which indeed appears round to the naked eye, or why variations in density would not cause the observed changes in the shape of the spots. We believe that the multisensory turn in perception science which we have tried to document in this book should be considered precisely in the above manner.

The conclusion that perception is inherently multisensory is valuable, to the extent that it leads up to consider novel theoretical and empirical implications. In concluding this book, let us therefore consider four of these implications—while at the same time keeping in mind that looking for new answers in science often ends up raising new questions.

10.2 Multisensory perception is the norm, not the exception

As you may recall from reading the first chapter of this book, one of the questions that motivated our choice of topics concerned the scope of multisensory processing in perception. To what extent does our brain exploit the riches of information potentially available to different sensory channels? We hope you will be convinced, after reading the book, that perceptual mechanisms are built to exploit these in full. Multisensory interactions are critical in understanding how we perform several perceptual tasks, such as perceiving our own body, static or moving, or appreciating the flavour of the foods we eat, but they are also pervasive in the perception of the features of all objects in space and time and in the allocation of attention to those features. Most features of our perceived world are, in fact, the product of multisensory interactions, even in many instances when our phenomenal awareness is confined to a single perceptual modality. According to the traditional model of perception, the 'senses' operate as independent modules and their inputs are combined only at later, 'integration' stages of cognition. This was, in a nutshell, the modular model of the mind proposed by Fodor (1983), which was discussed in the first chapter. However, similar ideas about the relationship between perception and cognition have been proposed by many other great psychology theorists, such as for instance Jean Piaget (Piaget & Inhelder, 1966). The complexity and the extent of the multisensory interactions documented in this book, however, suggest that the traditional model is fundamentally wrong, or at least incomplete. In ordinary perception, multisensory perception is the norm, not the exception.

To some, our plea for the primacy of multisensory perception may sound overstated. One of the colleagues that kindly read preliminary chapters of this book, for instance, pointed out that there is nothing inherently multisensory in detecting a small spot of light or comparing the colours of two adjacent fields. Tasks such as these have been used extensively to study contrast and colour perception in psychophysics laboratories, and much has been understood about the visual systems from data collected in this way. Our answer is that these tasks are indeed unisensory because they were designed to address certain, specific, empirical questions at a certain level of analysis. For instance, precise colour reproduction require basic information on the spectral sensitivity of retinal cone photoreceptors to determine, using a colourimetric model, whether a given mixture of lights on, say, a computer monitor will stimulate the retina in the same way as the light reflected by the surface of the reproduced object under certain conditions of illumination. If one is interested in this type of question a unisensory approach is not only appropriate but also desirable. We suggest, however, that studying a visual function at this level of analysis is not studying perception as a general cognitive process. Understanding perception as a way of knowing things about the environment and about ourselves requires a more global level of analysis, and this, we claim, is always multisensory. Two arguments in support of this claim should be apparent from the content of this book, the first of these already from reading its index: some domains of our perceptual experience cannot be understood at all without a multisensory perspective. One obvious example discussed in the book is perceived food flavour, which remains completely unexplained if one disregards multisensory interactions. The second argument follows from the first, and is that in many of these multisensory cases percepts emerge that cannot be reduced to the mere juxtaposition of the unisensory inputs. This happens again with food flavours, but also in many other cases documented in the chapters of this book.

Finally, a third argument stems from the key role of motor behaviours in perception, which we have also documented throughout the book. Motor behaviours are multisensory by definition, as they involve monitoring proprioceptive information from muscles and joints, but also from vision, and combining it with information about the external environment that could come in principle from any channel. And this is true not only for performatory actions, which aim at modifying some feature of the external environment, but also for exploratory actions. Consider eye movements, a form of perceptual exploration that we all engage in at all times. Whenever we move our eyes, the proximal projections of the distal environment are displaced on our retinas, but the environment remains perceptually stable. How our brains achieve this is a classic question in vision science, and we now know that visual stability is achieved by multisensory-motor interactions: Predictive motor models and proprioceptive signals about the motion of the eye are combined with the changing visual signal from the eye's retina through several mechanisms (for a review of this fascinating field, see Melcher & Colby, 2008).

10.3 At least some multisensory interactions take place early in processing

According to the traditional model, sensory channels process sensory-specific information independently and the outcome of this process is merged only later in higher-order brain centres. This view is reflected in the traditional distinction between *primary sensory areas*, responsible for sensory-specific processing, and *association areas* that combine outputs from sensory channels. As we have seen in several places in this book, however, there is evidence that the so-called primary sensory areas can be activated after stimulation in sensory channels outside their putative sensory specificity. This change in perspective started at the end of the twentieth century. Studies using EEG were among the first to suggest that at least some multisensory interactions can take place at the level of the so-called primary sensory areas. In one such study, the French researchers Marie-Helene Giard and Franck Peronnet recorded event-related electrophysiological potentials (ERP) from electrodes distributed over the scalp while participants indicated which of two objects was presented (Giard & Peronnet, 1999). In one condition, the objects were defined by a combination of auditory and visual features, marking trials that required audio-visual integration. Evidence that this integration occurred was also provided by reaction times, which were reliably lower in multisensory trials in comparison to visual or auditory only conditions. From the electrophysiology, Giard and Peronnet were able to time-stamp modulations of visual and of auditory EEG components (that is, measured from electrodes over the corresponding sensory areas) in multisensory conditions, in comparison to the corresponding unisensory conditions. These modulations occurred very early (as early as 40 ms after the multisensory stimulus in the visual area, and around 100 ms in auditory areas). Critically, activity in fronto-temporal areas occurred only later (about 150 ms post-stimulus). These data were therefore suggestive of multisensory interactions occurring not only in sensory-aspecific 'association' areas (e.g. the frontal cortices), but early on also in 'primary sensory' areas (the visual and auditory cortices).

Around the same time, another seminal work in the field of multisensory processes in early sensory cortices appeared in the journal *Science* (Macaluso, Frith, & Driver, 2000). This study reported that the hemodynamic response to a light flash, as measured in primary visual cortex using fMRI, is amplified by the simultaneous presentation of a tactile stimulus in the proximity of the visual stimulus. Functional magnetic resonance imaging, however, does not have the same temporal precision as EEG, and unlike the study by Giard and Perronet (1999) the authors could not determine how early the modulation in the primary visual cortex started. Instead, taking advantage of a statistical model of the cortico-cortical connections between occipital and parietal areas, Emiliano Macaluso and collaborators proposed that visual and tactile signals were merged in multisensory regions of the parietal lobe, and that these regions then issue a re-entrant signal back to primary visual areas. Feedback connections in cortico-cortical networks are well-established, and a possible role for these connections could be that of implementing multisensory interactions. However, if multisensory interactions are fundamental rather than accessory for perception, it would be reasonable to expect that a great deal of them take place at the initial steps of perception, that is, even before cortical feedback from higher-order centres. This coexistence of early and late multisensory interaction was later documented by several studies in human and non-human animals (for reviews, see Ghanzafar & Schroeder, 2006; Macaluso, 2006). Now, more than 15 years after these original studies, several general principles of early multisensory interactions are starting to emerge, particularly in relation to the primary visual cortex (Murray et al., 2016). First, it has now been established that multisensory processes in the primary visual cortex do not just entail convergence of multiple sensory inputs, but also integration. Second, it has been established that primary visual cortex is involved in multisensory processes during early post-stimulus stages, thus consolidating the original Giard and Peronnet's finding. Third, it has become apparent that multisensory processes in primary visual cortex directly impact behaviour and influence perceptual processes, revealing their functional role in cognition.

In addition, it should not be forgotten that multisensory interactions might take place even before cortical processing. Specifically, there are at least two subcortical brain structures that collect information from multiple sensory channels: the superior colliculus (SC) and the thalamus. We have already discussed multisensory processing in the SC in Tutorial 7.2, in the chapter on the space perception. The SC is a region of the brainstem which contains multisensory space-aligned maps, including a neural layer involved in the control of eye movements. The thalamus is, in contrast, the main intermediate processing station in the stream of signals from sensory receptors to the cortex. As reported in all physiology and psychology textbooks, all sensory signals reach the thalamus before being redirected to cortical areas. The only exception to this general rule is represented by olfactory signals, which reach the cortex via the indirect thalamic route but also through a direct route. Thus, in the thalamus are neural populations that code signals from all sensory channels. In the thalamic structure known as the *geniculate nucleus,* for instance, it is well documented that the lateral portion (lateral geniculate nucleus, or LGN) receives signals from the retina, whereas the medial portion (medial geniculate nucleus or MGN) receives signals from the cochlea. Although standard textbook accounts of the thalamus emphasize the segregation of these neural populations as a function of the sensory input, it seems plausible that the central nervous system would take advantage of an opportunity for multisensory interactions also within the thalamus (Cappe et al., 2009).

10.4 Multisensory interactions come in different kinds

The fMRI and EEG evidence discussed in the preceding section is consistent with the idea that multisensory interactions can occur in higher-order 'association' areas but also in brain centres that perform earlier steps of perceptual processing, such as the so-called primary sensory areas and the SC. Recent studies indicate that the difference may not be merely one of brain localization, but may correspond also to different computational strategies. Multisensory modulations of activity within early areas may involve automatic, mandatory processes that are governed by relatively simple and fixed rules. Higher-order interactions, in contrast, may reflect more flexible and context-sensitive processes. Intriguing evidence that this may indeed be the case was provided very recently in a paper by Tim Rohe and Uta Noppeney, working at the German Max Planck Institute in Tübingen and at the University of Birmingham in the UK, respectively (Rohe & Noppeney, 2016). Using synchronous audio-visual signals and combining behavioural and fMRI measures within a task that involved reporting the perceived location of either the visual or the auditory stimulus, Rohe and Noppeney were able to document distinct multisensory effects in the primary visual cortex and parietal cortex. Localization responses encoded in the primary visual cortex were modulated by auditory signals, but only when the signals were in spatial register and without taking into account their relative reliability. In higher-order parietal areas, conversely, responses reflected audio-visual integration of signals, weighted by their relative reliability. In addition, the relative weights changed depending on the perceptual modality that was selected for the response, while also taking into account the spatial disparity of the signals. Thus, when the signals were not in spatial register, the data were consistent with greater weights being assigned to the attended modality. This led to behaviourally distinct responses to the same audio-visual stimuli depending on whether participants reported the auditory and visual perceived locations.

The results of the Rohe and Noppeney study echo many considerations that we have presented in earlier chapters of this book. For instance, Tutorial 7.2 discussed multisensory integration by single neurons at the level of the SC (Stein & Meredith, 1993). The response of these neurons is strongly modulated by spatial proximity or temporal coincidence, and may well be part of a neural network that implements relatively fixed, automatic processes. In contrast, in Chapter 4 on multisensory object perception we discussed the notion of optimal multisensory integration, which represents a more flexible integration scheme taking into account the relative reliability of the multisensory signals. In that context, we introduced Bayesian models that combine sensory information with a-priori expectations to take into account more global constraints on multisensory interactions. One of the fundamental challenges posed by these more complex situations is that the brain must be able to flexibly determine if integration should indeed be performed or if the signals should be kept separate. Within the Bayesian framework, this is conceptualized as the problem of estimating the environmental cause of the incoming signals: a single object or event (implying that the signals should be integrated) or separate objects (implying instead segregation of the signals). This estimation may again exploit a spatial coding of the stimulus sources, as in the Rohe and Noppeney study, or it may exploit even more abstract, semantic information acquired through experience.

10.5 **Unisensory processing retains a place even in a multisensory world**

Finally, one of the main tenets of the current perspective is that multisensory interactions make perception more precise and accurate. In this book, we have reported several observations that are consistent with this general idea. With regard to precision, you may recall that after merging redundant visual and tactile signals about an object's size or location, the resulting integrated percepts are often more precise than any of the percepts based on visual or tactile signals alone. As discussed in Chapter 4, this is the key finding supporting the notion of 'optimal' integration of multisensory signals when perceiving object features. With regard with accuracy, you may recall that when judging the distance between two touched points on the skin surface, we tend to overestimate distances on some body parts (for instance, on the fingertips) and to underestimate them on others (for instance, on the forearm). As discussed in Chapter 2, the consequence is that the same distance appears larger on the finger and shorter on the forearm, an observation known as Weber's illusion. Qualitatively, the pattern of Weber's illusion is consistent with the differences in mechanoreceptor density between body parts, and with the corresponding differences in the corresponding cortical areas in primary somatosensory cortex. Quantitatively, however, our estimates are still much more accurate than the distortions one would expect based on relative cortical areas. This suggests that other sources of information are taken into account in our estimates of distances on the skin, and Chapter 2 presented intriguing evidence that a key role in 'correcting' the somatosensory distortion is played by visual signals about the body. But to affirm that multisensory processing can make perception more precise and accurate does not entail that it would *always* have this effect. We have encountered this problem in several chapters of the book: even though multisensory interactions are pervasive in natural perception, there are many cases in which multisensory interactions can in fact lead to *less* accurate perception in comparison to keeping the unisensory signals distinct.

Thus, in some cases, it would make sense for the brain to retain the ability of accessing the information in single sensory channels. An interesting observation with this regard comes from a study published some years ago by the group of Khalafalla Bushara at the National Institute of Health in Bethesda, USA (Bushara et al., 2003). This study used a version of the stream-bounce motion display, which has proved extremely useful to study multisensory interactions in many domains (for instance, multisensory grouping as discussed in Chapter 4, or the temporal window of multisensory integration in Chapter 8). Participants saw an animation with two vertical bars moving horizontally towards each other to meet at a central point and then continue until they reached the end of the screen. This is an ambiguous visual display, and participants tend to alternate streaming (the bars cross paths) or bouncing (the bars collide and bounce back) interpretations. You will recall that if a sound is added to the animation at the point in time when the bars meet, the frequency of a bouncing interpretation rises substantially in comparison to the version without a sound. Although bouncing becomes more likely in the multisensory version, however, there are still several trials whereby participants report the streaming interpretation. Reasoning that the outcome of these trials should reflect brain activations that privilege unisensory processing over multisensory processing, Bushara and collaborators exploited this fact to compare fMRI haemodynamic responses in these two conditions. They observed that, in trials leading to a bouncing interpretation, the strongest brain activations were in areas that are classically associated with multisensory processing, such as the SC and the posterior parietal cortex. In contrast, in trials retaining the streaming interpretation, the strongest activations were in the traditional primary sensory areas, such as the occipital cortex for the visual signals and the superior temporal gyrus for the auditory signals. These findings support the idea that the brain can access unisensory information even in conditions that tend to favour multisensory integration, provided that the integration did not occur. In addition, they suggest that unisensory processing and multisensory integration of the very same stimulus material lead to two distinct patterns of brain activation.

Results such as those of Bushara and collaborators pose the problem of understanding what is the 'switch' that activates the integration option, that is, how does the brain decide that multisensory signals should be combined rather than kept separate. We already encountered this problem and some of the solutions currently being explored in Chapter 4 when we discussed integration priors in Bayesian models. When considering the broader implications of a multisensory perspective, we can now appreciate that this approach may be misleading at least in part. If we take multisensory perception as a sort of 'added value' that is activated on top of unisensory processing, we are still outside a truly multisensory perspective on perception. Unisensory perception is still considered as a sort of benchmark for normal perceptual operation, and multisensory processes remain something that is added on top. If multisensory processing is the norm rather than the exception, however, we should be asking a different question. We should consider multisensory interactions as the normal perceptual operation implemented by the brain, and strive to understand what is the switch that turns it off in certain conditions. On this specific problem, however, empirical data are still very limited.

10.6 **What next?**

Multisensory research has grown considerably over the last decades, as we have tried to document in this book. Having reached its conclusion, it is only natural to wonder about future directions. What will come next for multisensory research? Foreseeing future directions for a research field is a challenge. However, hints are found in the topics that dominate specialized meetings (such as the International Multisensory Research Forum), and in other things like the overall trend of publications, the priorities of funding agencies, and the activity of leading laboratories.

Our impression is that one key issue in the next decade will be the inter-individual variability of multisensory processes, especially in relation to changes across the lifespan from infancy to senility. Interest in development is not entirely new in multisensory perception (see, for instance, the book edited by Andrew Bremner in 2012). We know that the neural circuits that support multisensory processing mature during postnatal life. Early exposure seems to be important for this maturation (Putzar et al., 2010; Nava et al., 2014) and seems to work by progressively narrowing the range of multisensory signals that are processed. For instance, until about 6 months of age human babies will look longer at a monkey face coupled with a congruent monkey call (such as 'coo' or 'grunt'), in comparison to a monkey face that did not match the current auditory call. This preferential looking behaviour is consistent with cross-modal matching of the visual and auditory signals. Surprisingly, older babies no longer do, suggesting that a narrowing mechanism restricts detectable cross-modal matches to *human* voicings and faces at that age (Lewkowicz & Ghazanfar, 2006). This narrowing of cross-modal matching seems to correlate with the ability to perceive more sophisticated and complex multisensory associations, and to experience the McGurk effect (Murray et al., 2016). In addition, we now have data suggesting that the integration of redundant multisensory signals (see Chapter 4) develops surprisingly late in life, around 8 years of age (Burr & Gori, 2011). David Burr and Monica Gori speculated that integration may not occur early in development because developing organisms need to continuously recalibrate sensory channels. Receptor systems, sense organs, and body limbs all grow at their own rates (Gottlieb, 1971), and coding of sensory signals needs to take into account these changes for successful perception. For instance, as the relative distance of the ears change, so must the coding of binaural cues for localization; and as the size, shape, and relative distance of the eyes changes, so must the coding of visual cues to depth. One possible mechanism for recalibrating signals in one sensory channel during development is to use signals from another channel. For instance, somatosensation could provide such calibration signals for spatial vision in peripersonal space. For this to occur, however, vision and somatosensation should not be integrated but kept separated—at least until this specific calibration is no longer needed.

These, however, are just pieces of the complex puzzle of multisensory changes across the life-span. What happens to multisensory processes from infants to toddlers, and from toddlers to adults is still largely unexplored. Only few studies have examined multisensory interactions in adolescence for instance (Brandwein et al., 2011). Likewise, our understanding of multisensory processes in the elderly remains scattered and incomplete. In the last decade, several research groups have started to examine this issue, in line with the general trend to study cognition in healthy and pathological ageing, spurred by the increasing proportion of individuals in this age range. The emerging finding is that older adults may be more adept at multisensory interactions than younger adults (for a review, see Mozolic et al., 2011). Furthermore, effective multisensory processing may be a key component of successful ageing, promoting independence in daily life activities (de Dieuleveult et al., 2017). However, the mechanisms that govern multisensory processes in ageing are far from clear, and their full understanding is made particularly difficult by the concurrent changes in unisensory processing and top-down control that occur in old age. In addition, attempts to explore multisensory processing across the life span are complicated by the problem of individual differences. Recent evidence has started to reveal the inter-individual variability in multisensory integration (Thelen et al., 2014), but very likely this is also the tip of a scientific iceberg.

A second final question concerns the possibility of translating the many findings and general principles of multisensory research into socially useful applications. The use of 'multisensory' as an adjective is already common practice in marketing. Products, activities, or approaches are regularly advertised as 'multisensory' in education, clinical rehabilitation, telecommunication, architecture, toy industry, event management, and in the food and cosmetics industry, to name just a few. Multisensory workshops are offered with relaxation and therapeutic intents, multisensory delights are promised in relation to vine and food tasting, multisensory bubble baths are advertised as the ultimate self-indulgent and cuddling experience for children and adults, and so forth. Although some of these approaches are scientifically grounded, for the most part they build loosely on the notion that the external world is multisensory, hence activating more than one sensory channel ought to be beneficial. We call this perspective 'the more the merrier' approach to multisensory perception. This way of promoting multisensory is questionable and will probably be short lived. Multisensory processes can indeed make our perceptual interpretation of the world more accurate, stable, and informative. However, as we have shown in all chapters of this book, multisensory contexts can also lead perception astray.

Multisensory conflicts can produce biased estimates (as in the ventriloquist illusion, or in the rubber hand phenomenon), can alter the actual stimulation (as in the McGurk phenomenon), or can divert our attention from the relevant information (as we have in multisensory attention capture phenomena). Negative effects of multisensory perception can also occur in the memory domain. Although memories for objects can be better if they are learned in multisensory than unisensory contexts, this typically happens if the multisensory stimuli are semantically related (e.g. the picture of a dog paired with a barking sound; Thelen & Murray, 2013). When the relation is weaker (e.g. the picture of a dog paired with a cat's meow) or when there is none altogether (e.g. the picture of a dog paired with a white noise burst) recalling in multisensory conditions can actually become worse in comparison to unisensory conditions (Thelen, Cappe, & Murray, 2012; Thelen, Talsma, & Murray, 2015). Concurrent stimulation within different sensory channels can thus prove ineffective or, worse, counterproductive. In brief, next to the bright side of multisensory processing, there is also a non-negligible dark side. Whether multisensory approaches to daily life problems lie on the positive or negative side largely depend on paying attention to the various rules that govern the interactions between multisensory processing and behaviour. We believe the only way forward for introducing multisensory based practices in society is an empirically grounded and evidence-based approach. The outreach beyond the laboratory contexts, however, is largely a responsibility of multisensory scientists. Translating the complexity of the evidence into concepts that can be accessible by professionals from other domains, must become a skill of the multisensory researcher of the future. Perhaps this book will serve as a step in this direction.

References

Adams, W.J., Graf, E.W., & Ernst, M.O. 2004. Experience can change the "light-from-above" prior. *Nat Neurosci*, **7**(10), 1057–8.

Aglioti, S., Bonazzi, A., & Cortese, F. 1994. Phantom lower limb as a perceptual marker of neural plasticity in the mature human brain. *Proc Biol Sci*, **255**(1344), 273–8.

Aitken, S. & Bower, G.R. 1983. Developmental aspects of sensory substitution. *Int J Neurosci*, **19**(1–4), 13–19.

Alais, D. & Burr, D. 2004. The ventriloquist effect results from near-optimal bimodal integration. *Curr Biol*, **14**(3), 257–62.

Alais, D., Newell, F.N., & Mamassian, P., 2010. Multisensory processing in review: from physiology to behaviour. *Seeing Perceiving*, **23**, 3–38.

Allan, L.G., 1979. The perception of time. *Percept Psychophys* **26**, 340–54.

Allen, P.G. & Kolers, P.A., 1981. Sensory specificity of apparent motion. *J Exp Psychol Hum Percept Perform*, **7**(6), 1318–28.

Alsius, A., Navarra, J., Campbell, R., & Soto-Faraco, S. 2005. Audiovisual integration of speech falters under high attention demands. *Curr Biol*, **15**(9), 839–43.

Alsius, A., Navarra, J., & Soto-Faraco, S., 2007. Attention to touch weakens audiovisual speech integration. *Exp Brain Res*, **183**(3), 399–404.

Altschuler, E.L., Vankov. A., Hubbard, E.M., Roberts, E., Ramachandran, V.S., & Pineda, J.A. 2000. Mu wave blocking by observation of movement and its possible use as a tool to study theory of other minds. Abstract 67.23, *30th Annual Meeting of the Society For Neuroscience (New Orleans, 4–9 November 2000)*.

Amedi, A., Stern, W. M., Camprodon, J. A., Bermpohl, F., Merabet, L., Rotman, S., et al., 2007. Shape conveyed by visual-to-auditory sensory substitution activates the lateral occipital complex. *Nat Neurosci*, **10**(6), 687–9.

Ammon, K. & Gandevia, S.C., 1990. Transcranial magnetic stimulation can influence the selection of motor programmes. *J Neurol Neurosurg Psychiatry*, **53**(8), 705–7.

Ammon, K.H., Moerman, C., & Guleac, J.D., 1977. Aphasics' defective perception of connotative meaning of verbal items which have no denotative meaning. *Cortex*, **13**(4), 453–7.

Andersen, T.S. & Mamassian, P., 2008. Audiovisual integration of stimulus transients. *Vision Res*, **48**(25), 44–51.

Andersen, R.A., Snyder, L.H., Bradley, D.C., & Xing, J., 1997. Multimodal representation of space in the posterior parietal cortex and its use in planning movements. *Ann Review Neurosci*, **20**, 303–30.

Ansuini, C., Santello, M., Tubaldi, F., Massaccesi, S., & Castiello, U., 2007. Control of hand shaping in response to object shape perturbation. *Exp Brain Res*, **180**(1), 85–96.

Armel, K.C. & Ramachandran, V.S., 2003. Projecting sensations to external objects: evidence from skin conductance response. *Proc Biol Sci*, **270**(1523), 1499–1506.

Arno, P., Capelle, C., Wanet-Defalque, M. C., Catalan-Ahumada, M., & Veraart, C., 1999. Auditory coding of visual patterns for the blind. *Perception*, **28**(8), 1013–29.

Arzy, S., Overney, L.S., Landis, T., & Blanke, O., 2006. Neural mechanisms of embodiment: asomatognosia due to premotor cortex damage. *Arch Neurol*, **63**(7), 1022–5.

Aspell, J.E., Heydrich, L., Marillier, G., Lavanchy, T., Herbelin, B., & Blanke, O., 2013. Turning body and self inside out: visualized heartbeats alter bodily self-consciousness and tactile perception. *Psychol Sci*, **24**(12), 2445–53.

Auvray, M. & Spence, C., 2008. The multisensory perception of flavor. *Conscious Cogn*, **17**(3), 1016–31.

Auvray, M., Gallace, A., Tan, H.Z., & Spence, C., 2007. Crossmodal change blindness between vision and touch. *Acta Psychol*, **126**(2), 79–97.

Auvray, M., Hanneton, S., & O'Regan, J.K., 2007. Learning to perceive with a visuo—auditory substitution system: localisation and object recognition with 'the vOICe'. *Perception*, **36**, 416–30.

Azañón, E. & Soto-Faraco, S., 2008. Changing reference frames during the encoding of tactile events. *Curr Biol,* **18**(14), 1044–9.

Baccarini, M., Martel, M., Cardinali, L., Sillan, O., Farnè, A, & Roy A.C., 2014. Tool use imagery triggers tool incorporation in the body schema. *Front Psychol* **5**, 492.

Bach-y-Rita, P., 1967. Sensory plasticity. Applications to a vision substitution system. *Acta Neurol Scand*, **43**(4), 417–26.

Bach-Y-Rita, P., 1972. *Brain Mechanisms in Sensory Substitution System*. New York: Academic Press.

Bach-y-Rita, P., 2004. Tactile sensory substitution studies. *Ann N Y Acad Sci*, **1013**, 83–91.

Bach-y-Rita, P. & Kercel, S.W., 2003. Sensory substitution and the human-machine interface. *Trends Cogn Sci*, **7**, 541–6.

Baizer, J.S., Kralj-Hans, I., & Glickstein, M., 1999. Cerebellar lesions and prism adaptation in macaque monkeys. *J Neurophysiol*, **81**(4), 1960–5.

Ballester, J., Abdi, H., Langlois, J., Peyron, D., & Valentin, D., 2009. The odor of colors: can wine experts and novices distinguish the odors of white, red, and rose wines? *Chem Percept*, **2**, 203–13.

Banakou, D., Groten, R., & Slater, M., 2013. Illusory ownership of a virtual child body causes overestimation of object sizes and implicit attitude changes. *Proc Natl Acad Sci USA*, **110**(31), 12846–51.

Baraduc, P. & Wolpert, D.M., 2002. Adaptation to a visuomotor shift depends on the starting posture. *J Neurophysiol*, **88**(2), 973–81.

Barakat, B., Seitz, A.R., & Shams, L., 2015. Visual rhythm perception improves through auditory but not visual training. *Curr Biol*, **25**(2), R60–1.

Bard, C., Turrell, Y., Fleury, M., Teasdale, N., Lamarre, Y., & Mart, O., 1999. Deafferentation and pointing with visual double-step perturbations. *Exp Brain Res*, **125** (4), 410–6.

Barnett-Cowan, M., 2010. An illusion you can sink your teeth into: haptic cues modulate the perceived freshness and crispness of pretzels. *Perception*, **39**, 1684–6.

Baron-Cohen, S., Burt, L., Smith-Laittan, F., Harrison, J., & Bolton, P., 1996. Synaesthesia: prevalence and familiality. *Perception*, **25**(9), 1073–9.

Baron-Cohen, S., Harrison, J., Goldstein, L.H., & Wyke, M., 1993. Coloured speech perception: is synesthesia what happens when modularity breaks down? *Perception*, **22**(4), 419–26.

Bassolino, M., Serino, A., Ubaldi, S., & Làdavas E., 2010. Everyday use of the computer mouse extends peripersonal space representation. *Neuropsychologia*, **48**(3), 803–11.

Bays, P.M., Wolpert, D.M., & Flanagan, J.R., 2005. Perception of the consequences of self-action is temporally tuned and event driven. *Curr Biol*, **15**(12), 1125–8.

Beeli, G., Esslen, M., & Jancke, L., 2008. Time course of neural activity correlated with colored-hearing synesthesia. *Cereb Cortex*, **18**(2), 379–85.

Benedetti, F., 1986. Tactile diplopia (diplesthesia) on the human fingers. *Perception*, **15**(1), 83–91.

Benedetti, F., 1988. Exploration of a rod with crossed fingers. *Percept Psychophys*, **44**(3), 281–4.

Benton, A.L., 1956. Jacques Loeb and the method of double stimulation. *J Hist Med Allied Sci*, **11**, 47–53.

Bergenheim, M., Johansson, H., Granlund, B., & Pedersen, J., 1996. Experimental evidence for a sensory synchronization of sensory information to conscious experience, in S.R. Hameroff, A.W. Kaszniak, & A.C. Scott (Eds.), *Toward a Science of Consciousness: The first Tuscon discussions and debates*, Cambridge, Mass., MIT Press, pp. 303–10.

Berlucchi, G. & Aglioti, S., 1997. The body in the brain: neural bases of corporeal awareness. *Trends Neurosci*, **20**(12), 560–4.

Bernstein, I.H., Clark, M.H., & Edelstein, B.A., 1969. Effects of an auditory signal on visual reaction time. *J Exper Psychol*, **80**(3), 567–9.

Bernstein, I. H., & Edelstein, B. A., 1971. Effects of some variations in auditory input upon visual choice reaction time. *J Exper Psychol*, **87**, 241–7.

Bertalannfy von, K.L., 1968. *General System Theory. Foundations, Development, Applications*. New York: Braziller.

Bertamini, M., Masala, L., Meyer, G., & Bruno, N., 2010. Vision, haptics, and attention: new data from a multisensory Necker cube. *Perception*, **39**(2), 195–207.

Bertelson, P. & Aschersleben, G., 2003. Temporal ventriloquism: crossmodal interaction on the time dimension. 1. Evidence from auditory-visual temporal order judgment. *Int J Psychophysiol*, **50**(1-2), 147–55.

Bertelson, P., Pavani F, Ladavas E, Vroomen J, & de Gelder B. 2000. Ventriloquism in patients with unilateral visual neglect. *Neuropsychologia*, **38**(12), 1634–42.

Bertelson, P. & Radeau, M. 1981. Cross-modal bias and perceptual fusion with auditory-visual spatial discordance radeau. *Percept Psychophys* **29**, 578.

Bertelson, P., Vroomen, J., de Gelder., B., & Driver, J., 2000. The ventriloquist effect does not depend on the direction of deliberate visual attention. *Percept Psychophys*, **62**(2), 321–32.

Bertenthal, B.I., Banton, T., & Bradbury, A., 1993. Directional bias in the perception of translating patterns. *Perception*, **22**(2), 193–207.

Berti, A. & Frassinetti, F., 2000. When far becomes near: remapping of space by tool use. *J Cognitive Neurosci*, **12**(3), 415–20.

Biederman, I., 1987. Recognition-by-components: a theory of human image understanding. *Psychol Rev*, **94**(2), 115–47.

Biederman, I. & Gerhardstein, P.C., 1993. Recognizing depth-rotated objects: evidence and conditions for three-dimensional viewpoint invariance. *J Exp Psychol Hum Percept Perform*, **19**(6), 1162–82.

Bien, N., ten Oever, S., Goebel, R., & Sack, A.T., 2012. The sound of size: crossmodal binding in pitch-size synesthesia: a combined TMS, EEG and psychophysics study. *Neuroimage*, **59**(1), 663–72.

Binkofski, F., Dohle, C., Posse, S., Stephan, K.M., Hefter, H., Seitz, R.J., & Freund, H.J., 1998. Human anterior intraparietal area subserves prehension. *Neurology*, **50**(5), 1253–9.

Bisiach, E., Rusconi, M.L., & Vallar, G., 1991. Remission of somatoparaphrenic delusion through vestibular stimulation. *Neuropsychologia*, **29**(10), 1029–31.

Blakemore, S.J., Wolpert, D.M., & Frith, C.D., 1998. Central cancellation of self-produced tickle sensation. *Nat Neurosci*, **1**(7), 635–40.

Blakemore, S.J., Wolpert, D., & Frith, C., 2000. Why can't you tickle yourself? *Neuroreport*, **11**(11), R11–16.

Blanke, O., 2012. Multisensory brain mechanisms of bodily self-consciousness. *Nature Rev Neurosci*, **13**(8), 556–71.

Blanke, O. & Metzinger, T., 2009. Full-body illusions and minimal phenomenal selfhood. *Trends Cogn Sci*, **13**(1), 7–13.

Blanke, O. & Mohr, C., 2005. Out-of-body experience, heautoscopy, and autoscopic hallucination of neurological origin Implications for neurocognitive mechanisms of corporeal awareness and self-consciousness. *Brain Res. Brain Res Rev*, **50**(1), 184–99.

Blanke, O., Ortigue, S., Landis, T., & Seeck, M., 2002. Stimulating illusory own-body perceptions. *Nature*, **419**(6904), 269–70.

Blanke, O., Slater, M., & Serino, A., 2015. Behavioral, neural, and computational principles of bodily self-consciousness. *Neuron*, **88**(1), 145–66.

Blauert, J., 1997. *Spatial Hearing*, Cambridge (MA): MIT Press.

Block, R.A. & Gruber, R.P., 2014. Time perception, attention, and memory: a selective review. *Acta Psychol*, **149**, 129–33.

Blom, R.M., Hennekam, R.C., & Denys, D., 2012. Body integrity identity disorder. *PLoS ONE*, **7**(4), p.e34702.

Bola, Ł., Zimmermann, M., Mostowski, P., Jednoróg, K., Marchewka, A., Rutkowski, P., & Szwed, M., 2017. Task-specific reorganization of the auditory cortex in deaf humans. *Proc Natl Acad Sci USA*, **114**(4), E600–9.

Bolognini, N., Cecchetto, C., Geraci, C., Maravita, A., Pascual-Leone, A., & Papagno, C., 2012. Hearing shapes our perception of time: temporal discrimination of tactile stimuli in deaf people. *J Cogn Neurosci*, **24**(2), 276–86.

Bolognini, N., Papagno, C., Moroni, D., & Maravita, A., 2010. Tactile temporal processing in the auditory cortex. *J Cogn Neurosci*, **22**(6), 1201–11.

Bolton, T.L., 1894. Rhythm. *Am J Psychol*, **6**(2), 145–238.

Bonnier, P., 1905. L' Aschématie [Aschematia]. *Rev Neurol*, **12**, 605–9.

Booth, D.A., 2013. Configuring of extero- and interoceptive senses in actions on food. *Multisens Res*, **26**(1-2), 123–42.

Boring, E.G., 1950. *A History of Experimental Psychology*. New York: Appleton-Century-Crofts.

Botvinick, M. & Cohen, J., 1998. Rubber hands 'feel' touch that eyes see. *Nature*, **391**(6669), 756.

Bradshaw, M. F., Elliott, K. M., Watt, S. J., Hibbard, P. B., Davies, I. R., & Simpson, P. J. 2004. Binocular cues and the control of prehension. *Spat Vis*, **17**(1-2), 95–110.

Brandwein, A.B., Foxe, J.J., Russo, N.N., Altschuler, T.S., Gomes, H., & Molholm, S., 2011. The development of audiovisual multisensory integration across childhood and early adolescence: a high-density electrical mapping study. *Cereb Cortex*, **21**(5), 1042–55.

Brang, D., Hubbard, E.M., Coulson, S., Huang, M., & Ramachandran, V.S., 2010. Magnetoencephalography reveals early activation of V4 in grapheme-color synesthesia. *Neuroimage*, **53**(1), 268–74.

Brang, D., McGeoch, P.D., & Ramachandran, V.S., 2008. Apotemnophilia: a neurological disorder. *Neuroreport*, **19**(13), 1305–6.

Brang, D. & Ramachandran, V.S., 2011. Survival of the synesthesia gene: why do people hear colors and taste words? *PLoS Biol*, **9**(11), e1001205.

Brasil-Neto, J. P., Pascual-Leone, A., Valls-Sole, J., Cohen, L. G., & Hallett, M., 1992. Focal transcranial magnetic stimulation and response bias in a forced-choice task. *J Neurol Neurosurg Psychiatry*, **55**(10), 964–6.

Brass, M. & Haggard, P. 2007. To do or not to do: the neural signature of self-control. *J Neurosci*, **27**(34), 9141–5.

Bratzke, D., Schröter, H., & Ulrich, R., 2014. The role of consolidation for perceptual learning in temporal discrimination within and across modalities. *Acta Psychol*, **147**, 75–9.

Bratzke, D., Seifried, T., & Ulrich, R., 2012. Perceptual learning in temporal discrimination: asymmetric cross-modal transfer from audition to vision. *Exper Brain Res*, **221**(2), 205–10.

Bregman, A. S., 1990. *Auditory Scene Analysis*. Cambridge (MA): MIT Press.

Bremmer, F., 2011. Multisensory space: from eye-movements to self-motion. *J Physiol*, **589**, 815–23.

Bremner, A.J., Caparos, S., Davidoff, J., de Fockert, J., Linnell, K.J., & Spence, C., 2013. "Bouba" and "Kiki" in Namibia? A remote culture make similar shape-sound matches, but different shape-taste matches to Westerners. *Cognition*, **126**(2), 165–72.

Bremner, A.J., Lewkowicz, D.J., & Spence, C., 2012. *Multisensory Development*, Oxford University Press, Oxford.

Brewer, A.A. & Barton, B., 2016. Maps of the auditory cortex. *Ann Rev Neurosci*, **39**(1), 385–407.

Bridgeman, B., 2010. How the brain makes the world appear stable. *i-Perception*, **1**, 69–72.

Britten, K. H. & van Wezel, R. J., 1998. Electrical microstimulation of cortical area MST biases heading perception in monkeys. *Nat Neurosci*, **1**(1), 59–63.

Broadbent, D.E., 1958. *Perception and Communication*, Oxford: Pergamon.

Brochard, R., Abecasis, D., Potter, D., Rago, R., & Drake C., 2003. The "ticktock" of our internal clock. *Psychol Sci*, **14**(4), 362–6.

Brodie, E.E., Whyte, A., & Niven, C.A., 2007. Analgesia through the looking-glass? A randomized controlled trial investigating the effect of viewing a "virtual" limb upon phantom limb pain, sensation and movement. *European J Pain*, **11**(4), 428–36.

Brotchie, P.R., Andersen, R.A., Snyder, L.H., & Goodman, S.J., 1995. Head position signals used by parietal neurons to encode locations of visual stimuli. *Nature*, **375**(6528), 232–5.

Brozzoli, C., Ehrsson, H.H., & Farnè, A., 2014. Multisensory representation of the space near the hand: from perception to action and interindividual interactions. *Neuroscientist*, **20**(2), 122–35.

Brozzoli, C., Gentile, G. Bergouignan, L., & Ehrsson, H.H., 2013. A shared representation of the space near oneself and others in the human premotor cortex. *Curr Biol*, **23**(18), 1764–8.

Brozzoli, C., Gentile, G., & Ehrsson, H.H., 2012. That's near my hand! Parietal and premotor coding of hand-centered space contributes to localization and self-attribution of the hand. *J Neurosci*, **32**(42), 14573–82.

Brozzoli, C., Gentile, G., Petkova, V.I., & Ehrsson, H.H., 2011. FMRI adaptation reveals a cortical mechanism for the coding of space near the hand. *J Neurosci*, **31**(24), 9023–31.

Brozzoli, C. Pavani, F., Urquizar, C., Cardinali, L., & Farnè, A., 2009. Grasping actions remap peripersonal space. *Neuroreport*, **20**(10), 913–7.

Bruce, V., Green, P.R., & Georgeson, M.A., 2003. *Visual Perception*. Hove (UK) : Psychology Press.

Bruggeman, H., Zosh, W., & Warren, W. H., 2007. Optic flow drives human visuo-locomotor adaptation. *Curr Biol*, **17**(23), 2035–40.

Brugger, P. & Lenggenhager, B., 2014. The bodily self and its disorders: neurological, psychological and social aspects. *Curr Opinion Neurol*, **27**(6), 644–652.

Brugger, P., Regard, M., & Landis, T., 1997. Illusory reduplication of one's own body: phenomenology and classification of autoscopic phenomena. *Cogn Neuropsychiatry*, **2**(1), 19–38.

Bruno, N., 2017. The three-dimensional Necker cube, in A. Shapiro & D. Todorovic, D. (Eds.), *The Oxford Compendium on Visual Illusions*. Oxford: Oxford University Press, pp. 787–790.

Bruno, N. & Bertamini, M., 2010. Haptic perception after a change in hand size. *Neuropsychologia*, **48**(6), 1853–6.

Bruno, N. & Cutting, J.E., 1988. Minimodularity and the perception of layout. *J Exp Psychol Gen*, **117**(2), 161–70.

Bruno, N., Dell'Anna, A., & Jacomuzzi, A., 2006. Ames's window in proprioception. *Perception,* **35**(1), 25–30.

Bruno, N., Jacomuzzi, A., Bertamini, M., & Meyer, G., 2007. A visual-haptic Necker cube reveals temporal constraints on intersensory merging during perceptual exploration. *Neuropsychologia,* **45**(3), 469–75.

Bruno, N., Martani, M., Corsini, C., & Oleari, C., 2013. The effect of the color red on consuming food does not depend on achromatic (Michelson) contrast and extends to rubbing cream on the skin. *Appetite,* **71**, 307–13.

Bruno, N., Pavani, F., & Zampini, M., 2010. *La percezione multisensoriale.* Bologna (I): Il Mulino.

Buccino, G., Binkofski, F., Fink, G.R., Fadiga, L., Fogassi, L., Gallese, V., et al., 2001. Action observation activates premotor and parietal areas in a somatotopic manner: an fMRI study. *Eur J Neurosci,* **13**(2), 400–4.

Buchholz, V.N., Jensen, O., & Medendorp, W.P., 2011. Multiple reference frames in cortical oscillatory activity during tactile remapping for saccades. *J Neurosci,* **31**(46), 16864–71.

Buck, L.B., 1996. Information coding in the vertebrate olfactory system. *Annu Rev Neurosci,* **19**, 517–44.

Bueti, D., 2011. The sensory representation of time. *Front Integr Neurosci,* **5**, 34.

Buhusi, C.V. & Meck, W.H., 2005. What makes us tick? Functional and neural mechanisms of interval timing. *Nature Rev Neurosci,* **6**(10), 755–65.

Bülthoff, H.H., Edelman, S.Y., & Tarr, M.J., 1995. How are three-dimensional objects represented in the brain. *Cereb Cortex,* **5**(3), 247–60.

Burnett, C.T., 1904. Studies in the influence of abnormal position upon the motor impulse. *Psychological Rev,* **11**, 371–94.

Burr, D. & Gori, M., 2011. Multisensory integration develops late in humans, in M. M. Murray & M. T. Wallace (Eds.), *The Neural Bases of Multisensory Processes.* Frontiers in Neuroscience. Boca Raton (FL): CRC Press, pp. 345–62.

Burton, H., Sinclair, R.J., & McLaren, D.G., 2008. Cortical network for vibrotactile attention: a fMRI study. *Human Brain Mapp,* **29**(2), 207–21.

Bushara, K.O., Hanakawa, T., Immisch, I., Toma, K., Kansaku, K., & Hallet, M. 2003. Neural correlates of cross-modal binding. *Nature Neurosci,* **6**(2), 190–5.

Busse, L., Roberts, K.C., Crist, R.E., Weissman, D.H., & Woldorff. M.G., 2005. The spread of attention across modalities and space in a multisensory object. *Proc Natl Acad Sci USA ,* **102**(51), 18751–6.

Caggiano, V., Fogassi, L., Rizzolatti, G., Thier, P., & Casile, A., 2009. Mirror neurons differentially encode the peripersonal and extrapersonal space of monkeys. *Science,* **324**(5925), 403–6.

Calvert, G.A., Bullmore, E.T., Brammer, M.J., Campbell, R., Williams, S.C., McGuire, P. K., et al., 1997. Activation of auditory cortex during silent lipreading. *Science,* **276**, 593–6.

Calvert, G., Spence, C., & Stein, B. E. (Eds.) 2004. *The Handbook of Multisensory Processing.* Cambridge, MA: MIT Press.

Canny, J., 1986. A computational approach to edge detection. *IEEE Trans. Pattern Analysis Machine Intell,* **8**(6):679–98.

Capelle, C., Trullemans, C., Arno, P., & Veraart, C., 1998. A real-time experimental prototype for enhancement of vision rehabilitation using auditory substitution. *IEEE Trans Biomed Eng,* **45**(10), 1279–93.

Cappe, C., Morel, A., Barone, P., & Rouiller, E. M., 2009. The thalamocortical projection systems in primate: an anatomical support for multisensory and sensorimotor interplay. *Cereb Cortex,* **19**(9), 2025–37.

Cardinali, L. Frassinetti, F., Brozzoli, C., Urquizar, C., Roy, A.C., & Farnè A., 2009. Tool-use induces morphological updating of the body schema. *Curr Biol,* **19**(12), R478–9.

Carello, C., Grosofsky, A., Reichel, F.D., Solomon, H.Y. & Turvey, M.T., 1989. Visually perceiving what is reachable. *Ecol Psychol*, **1**(1), 27–54.

Carlsson, K., Petrovic, P., Skare, S., Petersson, K.M., & Ingvar, M., 2000. Tickling expectations: neural processing in anticipation of a sensory stimulus. *J Cogn Neurosci*, **12**(4), 691–703.

Casale, R., Damiani, C., & Rosati, V., 2009. Mirror therapy in the rehabilitation of lower-limb amputation: are there any contraindications? *Am J Phys Med Rehabil*, **88**(10), 837–42.

Castelli, L., Vanzetto, K., Sherman, J., & Arcuri, L. 2001. The explicit and implicit perception of in-group members who use stereotypes: Blatant rejection but subtle conformity. *J Exp Soc Psychol*, **37**, 419–26.

Castiello, U., 1997. Arm and mouth coordination during the eating action in humans: a kinematic analysis. *Exp Brain Res*, **115**(3), 552–6.

Castiello, U., Giordano, B. L., Begliomini, C., Ansuini, C., & Grassi, M. 2010. When ears drive hands: the influence of contact sound on reaching to grasp. *PLoS One*, **5**(8), e12240.

Castiello, U., Zucco, G. M., Parma, V., Ansuini, C., & Tirindelli, R. 2006. Cross-modal interactions between olfaction and vision when grasping. *Chem Senses*, **31**(7), 665–71.

Cavina-Pratesi, C., Monaco, S., Fattori, P., Galletti, C., McAdam, T.D., Quinlan, D.J., et al., 2010. Functional magnetic resonance imaging reveals the neural substrates of arm transport and grip formation in reach-to-grasp actions in humans. *J Neurosci*, **30**(31), 10306–23.

Caviness, JA, 1964. *Visual and Tactual Perception of Solid Shape*. Unpublished doctoral dissertation, Cornell University (NY).

Chan, B.L., Witt, R., Charrow, A.P., Magee, A., Howard, R., Pasquina, P.F., et al., 2007. Mirror therapy for phantom limb pain. *New Engl J Med*, **357**(21), 2206–7.

Chapman, H.L., Eramudugolla, R., Gavrilescu, M., Strudwick, M.W., Loftus, A., Cunnington, R., & Mattingley, J.B., 2010. Neural mechanisms underlying spatial realignment during adaptation to optical wedge prisms. *Neuropsychologia*, **48**(9), 2595–601.

Charpentier, A., 1891. Analyse experimentale: De quelques elements de la sensation de poids. *Arch Physiolo Norm Pathol*, **3**, 122–35.

Cherry, E.C., 1953. Some experiments on the recognition of speech, with one and with two ears. *J Acoust Soc Am*, **25**, 975–9.

Choe, C.S. & Welch, R.B., 1974. Variables affecting the intermanual transfer and decay of prism adaptation. *J Exp Psychol*, **102**(6), 1076–84.

Chong, T.T., Cunnington, R., Williams, M.A., Kanwisher, N., & Mattingley, J.B., 2008. fMRI adaptation reveals mirror neurons in human inferior parietal cortex. *Curr Biol*, **18**(20), 1576–80.

Christensen, C. 1983. Effects of color on aroma, flavor and texture judgments of foods. *J Food Sci*, **48**, 787–90.

Chronicle, E.P. & Glover, J., 2003. A ticklish question: does magnetic stimulation of the primary motor cortex give rise to an "efference copy"? *Cortex*, **39**(1), 105–10.

Ciaramitaro, V.M., Buracas, G.T., & Boynton, G.M., 2007. Spatial and cross-modal attention alter responses to unattended sensory information in early visual and auditory human cortex. *J Neurophysiol*, **98**(4), 2399–413.

Clydesdale, F.M., 1993. Color as a factor in food choice. *Crit Rev Food Sci Nutr*, **33**(1), 83–101.

Cochin, S., Barthelemy, C., Roux, S., & Martineau, J., 1999. Observation and execution of movement: similarities demonstrated by quantified electroencephalography. *Eur J Neurosci*, **11**(5), 1839–42.

Cohen, Y.E. & Andersen, R.A., 2002. A common reference frame for movement plans in the posterior parietal cortex. *Nature Rev Neurosci*, **3**(7), 553–62.

Cohen, Y.E. & Andersen, R.A., 2012. Multisensory representations of space in the posterior parietal cortex, in B.E. Stein (Ed.), *The New Handbook of Multisensory Processes*. Cambridge (MA): MIT Press, pp. 463–79.

Cole, J. (1995). *Pride and a Daily Marathon*. Cambridge (MA): MIT Press.

Cole, J., Crowle, S., Austwick, G., & Slater, D.H., 2009. Exploratory findings with virtual reality for phantom limb pain; from stump motion to agency and analgesia. *Disabil Rehabil*, **31**(10), 846–54.

Collignon, O., Dormal, G., Albouy, G., Vandewalle, G., Voss, P., Phillips, C., & Lepore, F. 2013. Impact of blindness onset on the functional organization and the connectivity of the occipital cortex. *Brain*, **136**(Pt 9), 2769–83.

Collings, V. B., 1974. Human taste response as a function of location of stimulation on the tongue and soft palate. *Percep Psychophys*, **16**, 169–74.

Connolly, J.D., Andersen, R.A., & Goodale, M.A., 2003. FMRI evidence for a "parietal reach region" in the human brain. *Exp Brain Res*, **153**(2), 140–5.

Connolly, K., 2013. How to test Molyneux's question empirically. *i-Perception*, **4**(8), 508–10.

Conway, C.M., Pisoni, D.B., & Kronenberger, W.G., 2009. The importance of sound for cognitive sequencing abilities: the auditory scaffolding hypothesis. *Curr Dir Psychol Sci.*, **18**(5), 275–9.

Corbetta, M., Kincade, J.M., Ollinger, J.M., McAvoy, M.P., & Shulman, G.L., 2000. Voluntary orienting is dissociated from target detection in human posterior parietal cortex. *Nature Neurosci*, **3**(3), 292–7.

Corbetta, M., Miezin, F.M., Shulm, G.L., & Petersen, S.E., 1993. A PET study of visuospatial attention. *J Neurosci*, **13**(3), 1202–26.

Corbetta, M., Patel, G., & Shulman, G. L. 2008. The reorienting system of the human brain: from environment to theory of mind. *Neuron*, **58**(3), 306–24.

Corbetta, M. & Shulman, G.L., 2002. Control of goal-directed and stimulus-driven attention in the brain. *Nature Rev Neurosci*, **3**(3), 201–15.

Coull, J.T., Vidal, F., Nazarian, B., & Macar, F., 2004. Functional anatomy of the attentional modulation of time estimation. *Science*, **303**(5663), 1506–8.

Craig, A.D., 2002. How do you feel? Interoception: the sense of the physiological condition of the body. *Nature Rev Neurosci*, **3**(8), 655–66.

Critchley, H. & Seth, A., 2012. Will studies of macaque insula reveal the neural mechanisms of self-awareness? *Neuron*, **74**(3), 423–6.

Critchley, H.D., Wiens, S., Rotshtein, P., Ohman, A., & Dolan, R.J. , 2004. Neural systems supporting interoceptive awareness. *Nature Neurosci*, **7**(2), 189–95.

Critchley, M., 1953. *The Parietal Lobes*, London: Edward Arnold.

Cronly-Dillon, J., Persaud, K., & Gregory, R.P., 1999. The perception of visual images encoded in musical form: a study in cross-modality information transfer. *Proc Biol Sci.*, **266**(1436), 2427–33.

Cruz, A. & Green, B.G., 2000. Thermal stimulation of taste. *Nature*, **403**, 889–91.

Cui, Q. N., Bachus, L., Knoth, E., O'Neill, W. E., & Paige, G. D. 2008. Eye position and cross-sensory learning both contribute to prism adaptation of auditory space. *Prog Brain Res*, **171**, 265–70.

Cunningham, D.W., Billock, V.A., & Tsou, B.H., 2001. Sensorimotor adaptation to violations of temporal contiguity. *Psychol Sci*, **12**(6), 532–5.

Cutting, J.E., 1986. *Perception with an Eye for Motion*. Cambridge (MA): MIT Press.

Cutting, J.E. & Vishton, P.M., 1995. Perceiving layout and knowing distances, in W. Epstein & S. Rogers, (Eds.), *Handbook of Perception and Cognition. Vol 5: Perception of Space and Motion*. NewYork: Academic Press, pp. 69–117.

Cytowic, R.E., 2002. *The Man Who Tasted Shapes*. Cambridge (MA): MIT Press.

Cytowic, R.E. & Wood, F.B., 1982. Synesthesia. I. A review of major theories and their brain basis. *Brain Cogn*, **1**(1), 23–35.

D'Alonzo, M., Clemente, F., & Cipriani, C., 2015. Vibrotactile stimulation promotes embodiment of an alien hand in amputees with phantom sensations. *IEEE TransNeural SystRehabil Eng*, **23**(3), 450–7.

Dalton, P., Doolittle, N., Nagata, H., & Breslin, P.A., 2000. The merging of the senses: integration of subthreshold taste and smell. *Nat Neurosci*, **3**(5), 431–2.

Danilov, Y. P., Tyler, M. E., Skinner, K. L., & Bach-y-Rita, P., 2006. Efficacy of electrotactile vestibular substitution in patients with bilateral vestibular and central balance loss. *Conf Proc IEEE Eng Med Biol Soc, Suppl*, 6605–9.

Danquah, A.N., Farrell, M.J., & O'Boyle, D.J., 2008. Biases in the subjective timing of perceptual events: Libet et al. (1983) revisited. *Conscious Cogn*, **17**(3), 616–27.

Darwin, C., 1871. *The Descent of Man, and Selection in Relation to Sex*. London: John Murray.

Day, B.L. & Fitzpatrick, R.C., 2005. The vestibular system. *Curr Biol,* , **15**(15), R583–6.

de Bruin, N., Sacrey, L. A., Brown, L. A., Doan, J., & Whishaw, I. Q., 2008. Visual guidance for hand advance but not hand withdrawal in a reach-to-eat task in adult humans: reaching is a composite movement. *J Mot Behav*, **40**(4), 337–46.

de Dieuleveult, A.L., Siemonsma, P.C., van Erp. J.B. & Brouwer AM., 2017. Effects of aging in multisensory integration: a systematic review. *Front Aging Neurosci*, **9**, 80.

de Vignemont, F., 2007. How many representations of the body? *Behav Brain Sci*, **30**, 204–5.

de Vignemont, F., 2010. Body schema and body image–pros and cons. *Neuropsychologia*, **48**(3), 669–80.

Degenaar, M., 1996. *Molyneux's Problem: Three Centuries of Discussion on the Perception*, London: Kluwer Academic Publishers.

Dekle, D.J., Fowler, C.A., & Funnell, M.G., 1992. Audiovisual integration in perception of real words. *Percept Psychophys*, **51**(4), 355–62.

Delwiche, J.F., 2012. You eat with your eyes first. *Physiol Behav*, **107**(4), 502–4.

Delwiche, J.F., Lera, M.F., & Breslin, P.A., 2000. Selective removal of a target stimulus localized by taste in humans. *Chem Senses*, **25**(2), 181–7.

Dennett, D.C., 2006. The self as a responding—and responsible—artifact. *Ann N Y Acad Sci.*, **10001**, 39–50.

Deroy, O. & Auvray, M., 2012. Reading the world through the skin and ears: a new perspective on sensory substitution. *Front Psychol*, **3**, 457.

Deroy, O. & Spence, C., 2013. Why we are not all synesthetes (not even weakly so). *Psychon Bull Rev*, **20**(4), 643–64.

Desmurget, M. & Grafton, S., 2000. Forward modeling allows feedback control for fast reaching movements. *TICS*, **4**(11), 423–31.

Di Luca, M., Machulla, T.-K., & Ernst, M.O., 2009. Recalibration of multisensory simultaneity: cross-modal transfer coincides with a change in perceptual latency. *J Vision*, **9**(12), 7.1–16.

di Pellegrino, G., Fadiga, L., Fogassi, L., Gallese, V., & Rizzolatti, G. 1992. Understanding motor events: a neurophysiological study. *Exp Brain Res*, **91**(1), 176–80.

di Pellegrino, G., Làdavas, E., & Farne, A., 1997. Seeing where your hands are. *Nature*, **388**(6644), 730.

Dichgans, J. & Brandt, T., 1978. Visual-vestibular interaction: effects on self-motion perception and postural control, in R. Held, H.W. Leibowitz, & H.L. Tueber (Eds.), *Perception*. Berlin: Springer, pp. 755–804.

Dickinson, M. H., Farley, C. T., Full, R. J., Koehl, M. A., Kram, R., & Lehman, S. 2000. How animals move: an integrative view. *Science*, **288**(5463), 100–6.

Dijker, A.J., 2014. The role of expectancies in the size-weight illusion: a review of theoretical and empirical arguments and a new explanation. *Psychon Bull Rev*, **21**(6), 1404–14.

Dijkerman, H.C. & de Haan, E.H.F., 2007. Somatosensory processes subserving perception and action. *Behav Brain Sci*, **30**(2), 189–201, discussion 201–39.

Dinstein, I., Gardner, J.L., Jazayeri, M., & Heeger, D.J., 2008. Executed and observed movements have different distributed representations in human aIPS. *J Neurosci*, **28**(44), 11231–9.

Dinstein, I., Hasson, U., Rubin, N., & Heeger, D.J., 2007. Brain areas selective for both observed and executed movements. *J Neurophysiol*, **98**(3), 1415–27.

Dixon, M.J., Smilek, D., & Merikle, P.M., 2004. Not all synaesthetes are created equal: Projector versus associator synaesthetes. *Cogn Affect Behav Neurosci. Neurosci,* **4**(3), 335–43.

Dixon, M.J., Smilek, D., Cudahy, C., & Merikle, P.M., 2000. Five plus two equals yellow. *Nature*, **406**(6794), 365.

Dixon, N.F., & Spitz, L., 1980. The detection of auditory visual desynchrony. *Perception*, **9**(6), 719–21.

Dohle, C., Püllen, J., Nakaten, A., Küst, J., Rietz, C., & Karbe H., 2009. Mirror therapy promotes recovery from severe hemiparesis: a randomized controlled trial. *Neurorehabil Neural Repair.*, **23**(3), 209–17.

Domino, G., 1989. Synaesthesia and creativity in fine arts students: An empirical look., *Creativity Res J*, **2** (1–2), 17–29.

Driver, J. & Noesselt, T. 2008. Multisensory interplay reveals crossmodal influences on 'sensory-specific' brain regions, neural responses, and judgments. *Neuron*, **57**(1):11–23.

Driver, J. & Spence, C., 1994. Spatial synergies between auditory and visual attention, in C. Umiltà & M. Moscovitch (Eds.), *Attention and Performance XV*. Cambridge, MA: MIT Press, pp. 311–31.

Driver, J. & Spence, C., 2000. Multisensory perception: Beyond modularity and convergence. *Curr Biol*, **10**, R731–5.

DuBose, C.N., Cardello, A.V., & Maller, O., 1980. Effects of colorants and flavorants on identification, perceived flavor intensity, and hedonic quality of fruit-flavored beverages and cake. *J Food Sci*, **45**(5), 1393–9.

Duhamel, J.-R., Colby, C.L., & Goldberg, M.E., 1991. Congruent representations of visual and somatosensory space in single neurons of monkey ventral intraparietal cortex (area VIP), in J. Paillard (Ed.), *Brain and Space*. Oxford: Oxford University Press, pp. 223–36.

Duncan, J., Martens, S., & Ward, R., 1997. Restricted attentional capacity within but not between sensory modalities. *Nature*, **387**(6635), 808–10.

Durkheim, E., 1915. *The Elementary Forms of the Religious Life, London:* George Allen & Unwin Ltd.

Eagleman, D.M., Kagan, A.D., Nelson, S.S., Sagaram, D., & Sarma, A.K., 2007. A standardized test battery for the study of synesthesia. *J Neurosci Methods,* **159**(1), 139–45.

Easton, R.D. & Basala, M., 1982. Perceptual dominance during lipreading. *Percept Psychophys*, **32**(6), 562–70.

Easton, R.D., Greene, A.J., & Srinivas, K., 1997. Transfer between vision and haptics: Memory for 2-D patterns and 3-D objects. *Psychon Bull Rev*, **4**, 403–10.

Ebisch, S.J.H., Ferri, F., Salone, A., Perrucci, M.G., D'Amico, L., Ferro, F.M., et al., 2011. Differential involvement of somatosensory and interoceptive cortices during the observation of affective touch. *J Cogn Neurosci*, **23**(7), 1808–22.

Egeth, M., 2008. Two new illusions of the tongue. *Perception*, **37**(8), 1305–7.

Ehrsson, H.H., 2007. The experimental induction of out-of-body experiences. *Science*, **317**(5841), 1048.

Ehrsson, H.H., Kito, T., Sadato, N., Passingham, R.E., & Naito, E., 2005. Neural substrate of body size: illusory feeling of shrinking of the waist. *PLoS Biol*, **3**(12), p.e412.

Ehrsson, H.H., Spence, C., & Passingham, R.E., 2004. That's my hand! Activity in premotor cortex reflects feeling of ownership of a limb. *Science*, **305**(5685), 875–7.

Ehrsson, H.H., Wiech, K., Weiskopf, N., Dolan, R.J., & Passingham, R.E., 2007. Threatening a rubber hand that you feel is yours elicits a cortical anxiety response. *Proc Natl Acad Sci USA*, **104**(23), 9828–33.

Ekroll, V., Sayim, B., Van der Hallen, R., & Wagemans, J., 2016. Illusory visual completion of an object's invisible backside can make your finger feel shorter. *Curr Biol*, **26**(8), 1029–33.

Elliott, D., Helsen, W.F., & Chua, R., 2001. A century later: Woodworth's (1899) two-component model of goal-directed aiming. *Psychol Bull*, **127**(3), 342–57.

Engbert, K., Wohlschläger, A., & Haggard, P. 2008. Who is causing what? The sense of agency is relational and efferent-triggered. *Cognition*, **107**(2), 693–704.

Enns, J. T. & Di Lollo, V., 1997. Object substitution: A new form of masking in unattended visual locations. *Psychol Sci*, **8**, 135–9.

Eramudugolla, R., Irvine, D.R., McAnally, K.I., Martin, R.L., & Mattingley, J.B., 2005. Directed attention eliminates "change deafness" in complex auditory scenes. *Curr Biol*, **15**(12), 1108–13.

Ernst, M.O. & Banks, M.S., 2002. Humans integrate visual and haptic information in a statistically optimal fashion. *Nature*, **415**(6870), 429–33.

Ernst, M.O. & Bülthoff, H.H., 2004. Merging the senses into a robust percept. *Trends Cogn Sci*, **8**(4), 162–9.

Ernst, M.O., Banks, M.S., & Bülthoff, H.H., 2000. Touch can change visual slant perception. *Nat Neurosci*, **3**(1), 69–73.

Eshkevari, E., Rieger, E., Longo, M.R., Haggard, P., & Treasure, J., 2012. Increased plasticity of the bodily self in eating disorders. *Psychol Med*, **42**(4), 819–28.

Evans, K.K. & Treisman, A., 2010. Natural cross-modal mappings between visual and auditory features. *J Vision*, **10**(1), 1–12.

Fabre-Thorpe, M., Richard, G., & Thorpe, S.J., 1998. Rapid categorization of natural images by rhesus monkeys. *Neuroreport*, **9**(2), 303–8.

Fadiga, L., Fogassi, L., Pavesi, G., & Rizzolatti, G., 1995. Motor facilitation during action observation: a magnetic stimulation study. *J Neurophysiol*, **73**(6), 2608–11.

Fairhall, S.L. & Macaluso, E., 2009. Spatial attention can modulate audiovisual integration at multiple cortical and subcortical sites. *European J Neurosci*, **29**(6), 1247–57.

Farah, M.J., Wong, A.B., Monheit, M.A., & Morrow, L.A., 1989. Parietal lobe mechanisms of spatial attention: modality-specific or supramodal? *Neuropsychologia*, **27**(4), 461–70.

Farmer, H., Tajadura-Jiménez, A., & Tsakiris, M., 2012. Beyond the colour of my skin: how skin colour affects the sense of body-ownership. *Consc Cogn*, **21**(3), 1242–56.

Farnè, A., Bonifazi, S., & Làdavas, E., 2005. The role played by tool-use and tool-length on the plastic elongation of peri-hand space: a single case study. *Cogn Neuropsychol*, **22**(3), 408–18.

Farnè, A., Demattè, M.L., & Làdavas, E., 2003. Beyond the window: multisensory representation of peripersonal space across a transparent barrier. *Int J Psychophysiol*, **50**(1–2), 51–61.

Farnè, A., Iriki, A., & Làdavas, E., 2005. Shaping multisensory action-space with tools: evidence from patients with cross-modal extinction. *Neuropsychologia*, **43**(2), 238–48.

Farnè, A. & Làdavas, E., 2000. Dynamic size-change of hand peripersonal space following tool use. *Neuroreport*, **11**(8), 1645–9.

Fattori, P., Breveglieri, R., Bosco, A., Gamberini, M., & Galletti. C. 2017. Vision for prehension in the medial parietal cortex. *Cereb Cortex*, **27**(2), 1149–63.

Fedina, A. & Glasman, K. 2006. Lip-sync: the evaluation of audio-to-video timing errors over shot intervals, *ISCE '06. 2006 IEEE Tenth International Symposium on Consumer Electronics 2006*, *pp. 1–7.*

Feldman, J., 2013. Tuning your priors to the world. *Top Cogn Sci*, **5**(1), 13–34.

Ferrè, E.R., Lopez, C. & Haggard, P., 2014. Anchoring the self to the body: vestibular contribution to the sense of self. *Psychol Sci*, **25**(11), 2106–8.

Ferrari, V., Mastria, S., & Bruno, N., 2014. Crossomodal interactions during affective picture processing. *PLoS ONE*, **2**, 45–58.

Finger, R. & Davis A.W., 2001. *Measuring Video Quality in Videoconferencing Systems*. Technical Report SN187D. Los Gatos, CA: Pixel Instrument Corporation.

Finisguerra, A., Canzoneri, E., Serino, A., Pozzo, T., & Bassolino, M., 2015. Moving sounds within the peripersonal space modulate the motor system. *Neuropsychologia*, **70**, 421–8.

First, M.B., 2005. Desire for amputation of a limb: paraphilia, psychosis, or a new type of identity disorder. *Psychol Med*, **35**(6), 919–28.

Fisher, S., 1976. Body perception upon awakening. *Percept Motor skills*, **43**(1), 275–8.

Fiske, A.P., 2004. Four modes of constituting relationships: Consubstantial assimilation; space, magnitude, time and force; concrete procedures; abstract symbolism, in N. Haslam (Ed.) *Relational Models Theory: A Contemporary Overview*. Mahwah, (NJ): Erlbaum, pp. 61–146.

Flanagan, J.R. & Bandomir, C.A., 2000. Coming to grips with weight perception: effects of grasp configuration on perceived heaviness. *Percept Psychophys*, **62**(6), 1204–19.

Flanagan, J.R. & Beltzner, M.A., 2000. Independence of perceptual and sensorimotor predictions in the size-weight illusion. *Nat Neurosci*, **3**(7), 737–41.

Flanagan, J.R., Bittner, J.P., & Johansson, R.S., 2008. Experience can change distinct size-weight priors engaged in lifting objects and judging their weights. *Curr Biol*, **18**(22), 1742–7.

Fleury, M., Bard, C., Teasdale, N., Paillard, J., Cole, J., Lajoie, Y., & Lamarre, Y., 1995. Weight judgment. The discrimination capacity of a deafferented subject. *Brain*, **118**(5), 1149–56.

Fodor, J. A., 1983. *The Modularity of Mind*. Cambridge (MA): MIT Press, Bradford books.

Fogassi, L. & Gallese, V. 2004. Action as a binding key to multisensory integration, in B.E. Stein (Eds.), *Handbook of Multisensory Processes*. Cambridge (MA): MIT Press, pp. 425–44.

Fogassi, L., Ferrari, P.F., Gesierich, B., Rozzi, S., Chersi, F., & Rizzolatti, G., 2005. Parietal lobe: from action organization to intention understanding. *Science*, **308**(5722), 662–7.

Fontana, F., Fusiello, A., Gobbi, M., Murino, V., Rocchesso, D., Sartor, L., & Panuccio, A., 2002. A cross-modal electronic travel aid device, in F. Paternò (Ed.), *Human Computer Interaction with Mobile Devices*. Berlin: Springer-Verlag Berlin Heidelberg, pp. 393–7.

Fowler, C.A. & Dekle, D.J., 1991. Listening with eye and hand: cross-modal contributions to speech perception. *J Exp Psychol Hum Percept Perform*, **17**(3), 816–28.

Fraisse, P., 1964. *The Psychology of Time*, London: Eyre & Spottiswoode.

Frank, S., Kullmann, S., & Veit, R., 2013. Food related processes in the insular cortex. *Front Hum Neurosci*, **7**, 499.

Frassinetti, F., Pavani, F., & Làdavas, E., 2002. Acoustical vision of neglected stimuli: interaction among spatially converging audiovisual inputs in neglect patients. *J Cogn Neurosci*, **14**(1), 62–9.

Freeman, E. & Driver, J., 2008. Direction of visual apparent motion driven solely by timing of a static sound. *Curr Biol*, **18**(16), 1262–6.

Freeman, E.D., Ipser, A., Palmbaha, A., Paunoiu, D., Brown, P., Lambert, C., et al., 2013. Sight and sound out of synch: fragmentation and renormalisation of audiovisual integration and subjective timing. *Cortex*, **49**(10), 2875–87.

Friston, K., 2005. A theory of cortical responses. *Philos Trans R Soc Lond B Biol Sci.*, **360**(1456), 815–36.

Fryer, L., Freeman, J., & Pring, L., 2014. Touching words is not enough: how visual experience influences haptic-auditory associations in the "Bouba-Kiki" effect. *Cognition*, **132**(2), 164–73.

Fujisaki, W., Shimojo, S., Kashino, M., & Nishida, S., 2004. Recalibration of audiovisual simultaneity. *Nature Neurosci*, **7**(7), 773–8.

Gallace, A., Auvray, M., Tan, H.Z., & Spence C., 2006. When visual transients impair tactile change detection: a novel case of crossmodal change blindness? *Neurosci Lett*, **398**(3), 280–5.

Gallace, A., Boschin, E., & Spence, C., 2011. On the taste of "Bouba" and "Kiki": An exploration of word-food associations in neurologically normal participants. *Cogn Neurosci*, **2**(1), 34–46.

Gallace, A. & Spence, C., 2006. Multisensory synesthetic inter- actions in the speeded classification of visual size. *Percept Psychophys*, **68**, 1191–203.

Gallace, A., Tan, H.Z., & Spence, C., 2007. Do "mudsplashes" induce tactile change blindness? *Percept Psychophys*, **69**(4), 477–86.

Gallagher, S., 1986. Body image and body schema: a conceptual clarification, *J Mind and Behavior*, 7, 541–54.

Gallagher, S. 2005. *How the Body Shapes the Mind*. Oxford University Press.

Gallese, V., Fadiga, L., Fogassi, L., & Rizzolatti, G., 1996. Action recognition in the premotor cortex. *Brain*, 119 (Pt 2), 593–609.

Gallese, V., Gernsbacher, M.A., Heyes, C., Hickok, G., & Iacoboni, M., 2011. Mirror neuron forum. *Perspect Psychol Sci*, **6**(4), 369–407.

Galton, F., 1883. *Inquiries into Human Faculty and its Development*. New York: MacMillan.

Gandevia, S.C. & Phegan, C.M., 1999. Perceptual distortions of the human body image produced by local anaesthesia, pain and cutaneous stimulation. *J Physiol*, **514**(Pt 2), 609–16.

Garavaldi, A., Pacchioli, M.T., & Vecchia, P., 2009. L'analisi sensoriale per caratterizzare il parmigiano reggiano. Opuscolo C.R.P.A (Centro ricerche produzioni animali), **6**, 1–6.

Garbarini, F., Fossataro, C., Berti, A., Gindri, P., Romano, D., Pia, L., et al., 2015. When your arm becomes mine—pathological embodiment of alien limbs using tools modulates own body representation. *Neuropsychologia*, **70**(C), 402–13.

Gaspar, J.G., Street, W.N., Windsor, M.B., Carbonari, R., Kaczmarski, H., Kramer, A.F., & Mathewson, K.E., 2014. Providing views of the driving scene to drivers' conversation partners mitigates cell-phone-related distraction. *Psychol Sci*, **25**(12), 2136–46.

Gastaut, H.J. & Bert, J., 1954. EEG changes during cinematographic presentation; moving picture activation of the EEG. *Electroencephalogr Clin Neurophysiol*, **6**(3), 433–44.

Genschow, O., Reutner, L., & Wänke, M., 2012. The color red reduces snack food and soft drink intake. *Appetite*, **58**, 699–702.

Gentilucci, M., 2003. Grasp observation influences speech production. *Eur J Neurosci*, **17**(1), 179–84.

Gentilucci, M., Benuzzi, F., Gangitano, M., & Grimaldi, S. 2001. Grasp with hand and mouth: a kinematic study on healthy subjects. *J Neurophysiol*, **86**(4), 1685–99.

Gentilucci, M. & Cattaneo, L., 2005. Automatic audiovisual integration in speech perception. *Exp Brain Res*, **167**(1), 66–75.

Gentilucci, M. & Corballis, M.C., 2006. From manual gesture to speech: a gradual transition. *Neurosci Biobehav Rev*, **30**(7), 949–60.

Gentilucci, M., Toni, I., Chieffi, S., & Pavesi, G., 1994. The role of proprioception in the control of prehension movements: a kinematic study in a peripherally deafferented patient and in normal subjects. *Exp Brain Res*, **99**(3), 483–500.

Gepshtein, S. & Banks, M.S., 2003. Viewing geometry determines how vision and haptics combine in size perception. *Curr Biol*, **13**(6), 483–8.

Gepshtein, S., Burge, J., Ernst, M.O., & Banks, M.S., 2005. The combination of vision and touch depends on spatial proximity. *J Vis*, **5**(11), 1013–23.

Gerstmann, J. 1942. Problem of imperception of disease and of impaired body territories with organic lesions relation to body scheme and its disorders. *Arch Neur Psych*, **48**(6), 890–913

Ghazanfar, A.A. & Schroeder, C.E., 2006. Is neocortex essentially multisensory? *Trends Cogn Sci*, **10**(6), 278–85.

Ghazanfar, A. A. & Turesson, H. K. 2008. Speech production: how does a word feel? *Curr Biol*, **18**(24), R1142–4.

Ghulyan-Bedikian, V., Paolino, M., & Paolino, F., 2013. Short-term retention effect of rehabilitation using head position-based electrotactile feedback to the tongue: influence of vestibular loss and old-age. *Gait Posture*, **38**(4), 777–83.

Giard, M.H. & Peronnet, F., 1999. Auditory-visual integration during multimodal object recognition in humans: a behavioral and electrophysiological study. *J Cogn Neurosci*, **11**(5), 473–90.

Gibbon, J., Church, R.M., & Meck, W.H., 1984. Scalar timing in memory. *Ann N Y Acad Sci*, **423**, 52–77.

Gibson, J.J., 1979. *The Ecological Approach to Visual Perception*. Boston (MA): Houghton Mifflin.

Gibson, J.J., 1962. Observations on active touch. *Psychol Rev*, **69**(6), 477–91.

Gibson, J.J., 1966. *The Senses Considered as Perceptual Systems*. Boston (MA): Houghton Mifflin.

Gick, B. & Derrick, D., 2009. Aero-tactile integration in speech perception. *Nature*, **462**(7272), 502–4.

Girgus, J.J., Rock, I., & Egatz, R., 1977. The effect of knowledge of reversibility on the reversibility of ambiguous figures. *Percept Psychophys*, **22**(6), 550–6.

Gitelman, D.R., Nobre, A.C., Parrish, T.B., LaBar, K.S., Kim, Y.H., Meyer, J.R., & Mesulam, M., 1999. A large-scale distributed network for covert spatial attention: further anatomical delineation based on stringent behavioural and cognitive controls. *Brain*, **122** (6), 1093–106.

Goldstone, S. & Lhamon, W.T., 1974. Studies of auditory-visual differences in human time judgment. 1. Sounds are judged longer than lights. *Percept Mot Skills*, **39**(1), 63–82.

Goller, A.I., Richards, K., Novak, S., & Ward, J., 2013. Mirror-touch synaesthesia in the phantom limbs of amputees. *Cortex*, **49**(1), 243–51.

Gottlieb, G., 1971. Ontogenesis of sensory function in birds and mammals, in E. Tobach, L.R. Aronson, & E. Shaw (Eds.), *The Biopsychology of Development*. Academic Press, New York, pp. 67–128.

Grafton, S.T., Arbib, M.A., Fadiga, L., & Rizzolatti, G., 1996. Localization of grasp representations in humans by positron emission tomography. 2. Observation compared with imagination. *Exp Brain Res*, **112**(1), 103–11.

Grahn, J.A., Henry, M.J., & McAuley, J.D., 2011. FMRI investigation of cross-modal interactions in beat perception: audition primes vision, but not vice versa. *NeuroImage*, **54**(2), 1231–43.

Grassi, M. & Casco, C., 2009. Audiovisual bounce-inducing effect: attention alone does not explain why the discs are bouncing. *J Exp Psychol Hum Percept Perform*, **35**(1), 235–43.

Gravina, S.A., Yep, G.L., & Khan, M., 2013. Human biology of taste. *Ann Saudi Med*, **33**(3), 217–22.

Gray, R., 2008. Multisensory information in the control of complex motor actions. *Curr Dir Psychol Sci*, **17**(4), 244–8.

Graziano, M.S.A. & Cooke, D.F., 2006. Parieto-frontal interactions, personal space, and defensive behavior. *Neuropsychologia*, **44**(13), 2621–35.

Graziano, M.S. & Gross, C.G., 1993. A bimodal map of space: somatosensory receptive fields in the macaque putamen with corresponding visual receptive fields. *Exp Brain Res*, **97**(1), 96–109.

Graziano, M. & Gross, C.G., 1995. The representation of extrapersonal space: a possible role for bimodal, visual-tactile neurons, in M. Gazzaniga (Ed.), *The Cognitive Neurosciences*. Cambridge (MA): MIT Press, pp. 1021–34.

Graziano, M.S.A., Taylor, C.S., Moore, T., & Cooke, D.F., 2002. The cortical control of movement revisited. *Neuron*, **36**(3), 349–62.

Graziano, M.S.A., Taylor, C.S.R., & Moore, T., 2002. Probing cortical function with electrical stimulation. *Nature Neurosci*, **5**(10), 921.

Green, B.G. 1982. The perception of distance and location for dual tactile pressures, *Percept Psychophys* **31**, 315.

Green, B.G., 2002. Studying taste as a cutaneous sense. *Food Qual Prefer,* **14**, 99–109.

Green, K.P. & Gerdeman, A., 1995. Cross-modal discrepancies in coarticulation and the integration of speech information: the McGurk effect with mismatched vowels. *J Exp Psychol Hum Percept Perform*, **21**(6), 1409–26.

Green, K.P., Kuhl, P.K., Meltzoff, A.N., & Stevens, E.B., 1991. Integrating speech information across talkers, gender, and sensory modality: female faces and male voices in the McGurk effect. *Percept Psychophys*, **50**(6), 524–36.

Green, B.G. & Lawless, H.T., 1991. The psychophysics of somatosensory chemoreception in the nose and mouth, in T.V. Getchell, R.L. Doty, L.M. Bartoshuk, & J.B. Snow (Eds.), *Smell and Taste in Health and Disease*. New York: Raven Press, pp. 235–54.

Greenwald, A.G., McGhee, D.E., & Schwartz, J.L., 1998. Measuring individual differences in implicit cognition: the implicit association test. *J Pers Soc Psychol*, **74**(6), 1464–80.

Gregersen, P.K., Kowalsky, E., Lee, A., Baron-Cohen, S., Fisher, S.E., Asher, J.E., et al., 2013. Absolute pitch exhibits phenotypic and genetic overlap with synesthesia. *Hum Mol Genet,* **22**(10), 2097–104.

Gregoric, P., 2007. *Aristotle on the Common Sense*. Oxford: Oxford University Press (UK).

Gregory, R. L., 1986. *Odd Perceptions*. London: Methuen & Co.

Grèzes, J., Armony, J.L., Rowe, J., & Passingham, R.E., 2003. Activations related to "mirror" and "canonical" neurones in the human brain: an fMRI study. *Neuroimage*, **18**(4), 928–37.

Grillner, S., 1975. Locomotion in vertebrates: central mechanisms and reflex interaction. *Physiol Rev*, **55**(2), 247–304.

Grimes, J., 1996. On the failure to detect changes in scenes across saccades. In K. Akins (Ed.), *Vancouver Studies in Cognitive Science: Vol. 5. Perception*. New York: Oxford University Press, pp. 89–109.

Grivaz, P., Blanke, O., & Serino, A., 2017. Common and distinct brain regions processing multisensory bodily signals for peripersonal space and body ownership. *NeuroImage*, **147**, 602–18.

Groh, J.M., 2014. *Making Space: How the Brain Knows Where Things Are*. Cambridge, MA: Harvard University Press.

Grondin, S. & Ulrich, R., 2011. Duration discrimination performance: No cross-modal transfer from audition to vision even after massive perceptual learning, in A. Vatakis, A. Esposito, M. Giagkou, M. F. Cummins, & G. Papadelis (Eds.), *Multidisciplinary Aspects of Time and Time Perception*. Berlin: Springer, pp. 92–100.

Grossenbacher, P.G. & Lovelace, C.T., 2001. Mechanisms of synesthesia: cognitive and physiological constraints. *Trends Cogn Sci*, **5**(1), 36–41.

Guarniero, G., 1974. Experience of tactile vision. *Perception*, **3**(1), 101–4.

Guterstam, A., Björnsdotter, M., Gentile, G., & Ehrsson, H.H., 2015. Posterior cingulate cortex integrates the senses of self-location and body ownership. *Curr Biol*, **25**(11),1416–25.

Guterstam, A. & Ehrsson, H.H., 2012. Disowning one's seen real body during an out-of-body illusion. *Conscious Cogn*, **21**(2), 1037–42.

Guttman, S.E., Gilroy, L.A., & Blake, R., 2005. Hearing what the eyes see: auditory encoding of visual temporal sequences. *Psychol Sci*, **16**(3), 228–35.

Haggard, P. & Clark, S. 2003. Intentional action: conscious experience and neural prediction. *Conscious Cogn*, **12**(4), 695–707.

Haggard, P. & Eimer, M., 1999. On the relation between brain potentials and the awareness of voluntary movements. *Exp Brain Res*, **126**(1), 128–33.

Haggard, P. & Jundi, S., 2009. Rubber hand illusions and size-weight illusions: self-representation modulates representation of external objects. *Perception*, **38**(12), 1796–803.

Haggard, P., Clark, S., & Kalogeras, J., 2002. Voluntary action and conscious awareness. *Nat Neurosci*, **5**(4), 382–5.

Haggard, P. & Wolpert, D.M., 2005. Disorders of body schema, in H.J. Freund, M. Jeannerod, M. Hallett, & R. Leiguarda (Eds.), *Higher-order Motor Disorders: from Neuroanatomy and Neurobiology to Clinical Neurology*. Oxford: Oxford University Press.

Hall, E.T., 1966. *The Hidden Dimension*, New York: Doubleday.

Halper, F., 1997. The illusion of The Future. *Perception*, **26**(10), 1321–2.

Hanggi, J., Wotruba, D., & Jancke, L., 2011. Globally altered structural brain network topology in grapheme-color synesthesia. *J Neurosci*, **31**(15), 5816–28.

Hanig, D. P., 1901. Zur psychophysik des geschmacksinnes. *Philosophische Studien*, **17**, 576–623.

Hanneton, S., Auvray, M., & Durette, B., 2010. The Vibe: a versatile vision-to-audition sensory substitution device. *Appl Bionics Biomechan*, **4**, 269–76.

Hanson-Vaux, G., Crisinel, A.S., & Spence, C., 2013. Smelling shapes: crossmodal correspondences between odors and shapes. *Chem Senses*, **38**(2), 161–6.

Hanson, J.V.M., Heron, J., & Whitaker, D., 2008. Recalibration of perceived time across sensory modalities. *Exp Brain Res*, **185**(2), 347–52.

Harnad, S., 1990. The symbol grounding problem. *Physica D: Nonlin Phenom*, **42**, 335–46.

Harrar, V. & Harris, L.R., 2007. Multimodal Ternus: visual, tactile, and visuo-tactile grouping in apparent motion. *Perception*, **36**(10), 1455–64.

Harrar, V. & Harris, L.R., 2008. The effect of exposure to asynchronous audio, visual, and tactile stimulus combinations on the perception of simultaneity. *Exp Brain Res*, **186**(4), 517–24.

Harrar, V., Piqueras-Fiszman, B., & Spence, C., 2011. There's more to taste in a coloured bowl. *Perception*, **40**(7), 880–2.

Harrar, V., Winter, R., & Harris, L.R., 2008. Visuotactile apparent motion. *Percept Psychophys*, **70**(5), 807–17.

Harré, R., 1981. *Great Scientific Experiments. Twenty Experiments that Changed our View of the World*. Oxford: Oxford University Press.

Harris, C., 1999. The mystery of ticklish laughter: pleasure or pain? Social response or reflex? Tickling and the laughter it induces are an enigmatic aspect of our primate heritage. *Am Sci*, **87**(4), 344–51.

Harris, C.R., & Christenfeld, N., 1999. Can a machine tickle? *Psychon Bull Rev*, **6**(3), 504–10.

Hayward, W.G. & Tarr, M.J., 1997. Testing conditions for viewpoint invariance in object recognition. *J Exp Psychol Hum Percept Perform*, **23**(5), 1511–21.

Head, H. & Holmes, G., 1911. Sensory disturbances in cerebral lesions. *Brain*, **34**, 102–254.

Hediger, H., 1955. *Studies of the Psychology and Behaviour of Captive Animals in Zoos and Circuses*. London: Butterworths Scientific Publications

Heed, T. & Azañón, E., 2014. Using time to investigate space: a review of tactile temporal order judgments as a window onto spatial processing in touch. *Front Psychol*, **5**, p.76.

Heed, T. & Röder, B., 2011. The body in a multisensory world, in M. M. Murray & M. T. Wallace (Eds.), *The Neural Bases of Multisensory Processes*. Boca Raton (FL): CRC Press.

Heed, T., Buchholz, V.N., Engel, A.K., & Röder, B., 2015. Tactile remapping: from coordinate transformation to integration in sensorimotor processing. *Trends Cogn Sci*, **19**(5), 251–8.

Helbig, H.B. & Ernst, M.O., 2007. Knowledge about a common source can promote visual-haptic integration. *Perception*, **36**(10), 1523–33.

Helbig, H.B. & Ernst, M.O., 2007. Optimal integration of shape information from vision and touch. *Exp Brain Res*, **179**(4), 595–606.

Helbig, H.B. & Ernst, M.O., 2008. Visual-haptic cue weighting is independent of modality-specific attention. *J Vis*, **8**(1), 21.1–16.

Held, R., Ostrovsky, Y., de Gelder, B., Gandhi, T., Ganesh, S., Mathur, U., & Sinha, P., 2011. The newly sighted fail to match seen with felt. *Nat Neurosci*, **14**(5), 551–3.

Heller, M.A., Calcaterra, J.A., Green, S.L., & Brown, L., 1999. Intersensory conflict between vision and touch: the response modality dominates when precise, attention-riveting judgments are required. *Percept Psychophys*, **61**(7), 1384–98.

Helmholtz, H. von, 1867. *Handbuch der physiologischen Optik*. Leipzig: L. Voss (D).

Herbert, B.M., Muth, E.R., Pollatos, O., & Herbert, C., 2012. Interoception across modalities: on the relationship between cardiac awareness and the sensitivity for gastric functions. *PLoS ONE,* **7**(5), p.e36646.

Hermosillo, R., Ritterband-Rosenbaum, A., & van Donkelaar, P., 2011. Predicting future sensorimotor states influences current temporal decision making. *J Neurosci*, **31**(27), 10019–22.

Hershberger, W.A. & Misceo, G.F., 1996. Touch dominates haptic estimates of discordant visual-haptic size. *Percept Psychophys,* **58**(7), 1124–32.

Hershenson, M., 1962. Reaction time as a measure of intersensory facilitation. *J Exp Psychol*, **63**, 289–93.

Hillyard, S.A., Simpson, G.V., Woods, D.L., VanVoorhis, S., & Münte, T.F., 1984. Event-related brain potentials and selective attention to different modalities, in F. Reinoso-Suarez & C. Aimone-Marsan (Eds.), *Cortical Integration*. New York: Raven, pp. 295–314.

Hillyard, S.A., Störmer, V.S., Feng, W., Martinez, A., & McDonald, J.J., 2016. Cross-modal orienting of visual attention. *Neuropsychologia*, **83**, 170–8.

Hilti, L.M., Hänggi, J., Vitacco, D.A., Kraemer, B., Palla, A., Luechinger, R., et al., 2013. The desire for healthy limb amputation: structural brain correlates and clinical features of xenomelia. *Brain*, **136**(Pt 1), 318–29.

Hluštík, P., Solodkin, A., Gullapalli, R.P., Noll, D.C., & Small, S.L. , 2001. Somatotopy in human primary motor and somatosensory hand representations revisited. *Cereb Cortex*, **11**(4), 312–21.

Ho, C. & Spence, C. 2017. *The Multisensory Driver: Implications For Ergonomic Car Interface Design*. Boca Raton (FL): CRC Press.

Hogan, J.A., 1994. The concept of cause in the study of behavior, in J.A. Hogan & J.J. Bolhuis (Eds.), *Causal Mechanisms of Behavioural Development*. Cambridge: Cambridge University Press, pp. 3–15.

Holle, H., Banissy, M.J., & Ward, J., 2013. Functional and structural brain differences associated with mirror-touch synaesthesia. *Neuroimage*, **83**, 1041–50.

Holmes, N.P., 2012. Does tool use extend peripersonal space? A review and re-analysis. *Exp Brain Res*, **218**(2), 273–82.

Holmes, N.P., Crozier, G., & Spence, C., 2004. When mirrors lie: "visual capture" of arm position impairs reaching performance. *Cogn Affect Behav Neurosci*, **4**(2), 193–200.

Holst, E.V., 1954. Relations between the central nervous system and the peripheral organs. *Br J Animal Behaviour*, **2**(3), 89–94.

Horn, G. & Hill, R.M., 1966. Responsiveness to sensory stimulation of units in the superior colliculus and subjacent tectotegmental regions of the rabbit. *Exp Neurol*, **14**(2), 199–223.

Hornbostel, E.M. von, 1927. Die Einheit der Sinne. *Melos, Zeitschrift für Musik*, **4**, 290–7.

Howard, I.P. & Templeton, W.B., 1966. *Human Spatial Orientation*. New York: Wiley.

Huang, J., Gamble, D., Sarnlertsophon, K., Wang, X., & Hsiao, S., 2012. Feeling music: integration of auditory and tactile inputs in musical meter perception. *PLoS ONE*, **7**(10), p.e48496.

Hubbard, T.L., 1996. Synesthesia-like mappings of lightness, pitch, and melodic interval. *Am J Psychol*, **109**(2), 219–38.

Hubbard, E.M., Arman, A.C., Ramachandran, V.S., & Boynton, G.M., 2005. Individual differences among grapheme-color synesthetes: brain-behavior correlations. *Neuron*, **45**(6), 975–85.

Hubbard, E.M., Brang, D., & Ramachandran, V.S., 2011. The cross-activation theory at 10. *J Neuropsychol*, **5**(2), 152–77.

Hubel, D.H. & Wiesel, T.N. 1968. Receptive fields and functional architecture of monkey striate cortex. *J Physiol*, **195**(1), 215–43.

Huddleston, W.E., Lewis, J.W., Phinney, R.E., & DeYoe, E.A., 2008. Auditory and visual attention-based apparent motion share functional parallels. *Percept Psychophys,* **70**(7), 1207–16.

Hummel, T., Knecht, M., & Kobal, G.,1996. Peripherally obtained electro- physiological responses to olfactory stimulation in man: Electro-olfactograms exhibit a smaller degree of desensitization compared with subjective intensity estimates. *Brain Research*, **117**(1-2), 160–4.

Humphreys, G.W. & Riddoch, M.J., 1984. Routes to object constancy: Implications from neurological impairments of object constancy. *Q J Exp Psychol A*, **J36**(3), 385–415.

Hyvärinen, J., 1982. Posterior parietal lobe of the primate brain. *Physiol Rev*, **62**(3), 1060–129.

Hyvärinen, J. & Poranen, A., 1974. Function of the parietal associative area 7 as revealed from cellular discharges in alert monkeys. *Brain*, **97**(4), 673–92.

Ipser, A., Agolli, V., Bajraktari, V., Al-Alawi, F., Djaafara, N., & Freeman, E.D., 2017. Sight and sound persistently out of synch: stable individual differences in audiovisual synchronisation revealed by implicit measures of lip-voice integration. *Sci Rep*, **7**, p.46413.

Ionta, S., Heydrich, L., Lenggenhager, B., Mouthon, M., Fornari, E., Chapuis, D., et al., 2011. Multisensory mechanisms in temporo-parietal cortex support self-location and first-person perspective. *Neuron*, **70**(2), 363–74.

Iriki, A., Tanaka, M., & Iwamura, Y., 1996. Coding of modified body schema during tool use by macaque postcentral neurones. *Neuroreport*, **7**(14), 2325–30.

Irmak, C., Vallen, B., & Robinson, S. R. 2011. The impact of product name on dieter's and nondieter's food evaluations and consumption. *J Consumer Res*, **38**(2), 390.

Iversen, J.R., Patel, A.D., Nicodemus, B., & Emmorey, K.., 2015. Synchronization to auditory and visual rhythms in hearing and deaf individuals. *Cognition*, **134**(C), 232–44.

Jackson, C.V., 1953. Visual factors in auditory localization. *Q J Exp Psychol*, **5**, 52–65.

Jackson, F., 1982. Epiphenomenal qualia. *Philosoph Q*, **32**, 127–36.

Jackson, J.H., 1931. *Selected Writings of John Hughlings Jackson: On Epilepsy and epileptiform convulsions*, London: Hodder and Stoughton.

Jacob, P. & Jeannerod, M., 2003. *Ways of Seeing: The Scope and Limits of Visual Cognition*. Oxford University Press (UK).

Jacomuzzi, A., Kobau, P., & Bruno, N., 2003. Molyneux's question redux. *Phenomenol Cogn Sci*, **2**, 255–80.

Jäkel, F., Singh, M., Wichmann, F.A., & Herzog, M.H., 2016. An overview of quantitative approaches in Gestalt perception. *Vision Res*, **126**, 3–8.

James, W., 1890. *The Principles of Psychology*, New York: Henry Holt & Co.

James, T. W., Humphrey, G. K., Gati, J. S., Servos, P., Menon, R. S., & Goodale, M. A. 2002. Haptic study of three-dimensional objects activates extrastriate visual areas. *Neuropsychologia*, **40**(10), 1706–14.

Jancke, L. & Langer, N., 2011. A strong parietal hub in the small-world network of coloured-hearing synaesthetes during resting state EEG. *J Neuropsychol*, **5**(2), 178–202.

Jay, M.F. & Sparks, D.L., 1987. Sensorimotor integration in the primate superior colliculus. I. Motor convergence. *J Neurophysiol*, **57**(1), 22–34.

Jeannerod, M., 1981. Intrasegmental coordination during reaching at natural visual objects, in J. Long & A. Baddeley (Eds.), *Attention and Performance*, **IX**, Erlbaum (NJ), pp. 153–69.

Jeannerod, M., 2006. *Motor Cognition: What Actions Tell the Self.* Oxford: Oxford University Press.

Jeannerod, M., Arbib, M.A., Rizzolatti, G., & Sakata, H., 1995. Grasping objects: the cortical mechanisms of visuomotor transformation. *Trends Neurosci*, **18**(7), 314–20.

Jensen, T.S. & Nikolajsen, L., 1999, *Phantom Pain and Other Phenomena after Amputation*. Edinburgh: Churchill Livingstone.

Johnson, M.H., Dziurawiec, S., Ellis, H., & Morton, J. 1991. Newborns' preferential tracking of face-like stimuli and its subsequent decline. *Cognition*, **40**(1-2), 1–19

Jones, J.A. & Jarick, M., 2006. Multisensory integration of speech signals: the relationship between space and time. *Exp Brain Res*, **174**(3), 588–94.

Joordens, S., van Duijn, M., & Spalek, T. M., 2002. When timing the mind one should also mind the timing: biases in the measurement of voluntary actions. *Conscious Cogn*, **11**(2), 231–40.

Jousmäki, V. & Hari, R., 1998. Parchment-skin illusion: Sound-biased touch. *Curr Biol*, **8**, 869–72.

Kabbaligere, R., Lee, B.C., & Layne, C.S., 2017. Balancing sensory inputs: Sensory reweighting of ankle proprioception and vision during a bipedal posture task. *Gait Posture*, **52**, 244–50.

Kalckert, A. & Ehrsson, H.H., 2014. The spatial distance rule in the moving and classical rubber hand illusions. *Conscious Cogn*, **30**, 118–32.

Kamm, K., Thelen, E., & Jensen, J.L., 1990. A dynamical systems approach to motor development. *Phys Ther*, **70**(12), 763–75.

Kanai, R., Lloyd, H., Bueti, D., & Walsh, V., 2011. Modality-independent role of the primary auditory cortex in time estimation. *Exp Brain Res*, **209**(3), 465–71.

Kanayama, N., Morandi, A., Hiraki, K., & Pavani, F., 2017. Causal dynamics of scalp electroencephalography oscillation during the rubber hand illusion. *Brain Topog*, **30**(1), 122–35.

Kandel, E. R. & Schwartz, J.H., 1985. *Principles of Neural Science, 2nd Ed*. New York: McGraw-Hill.

Kanizsa, G. 1979. *Organization in Vision: Essays on Gestalt Perception*. New York: Praeger.

Kanizsa, G., 1955. Margini quasi-percettivi in campi con stimolazione omogenea. *Rivista di psicologia*, **49**(1), 7–30.

Kant, I. ([1787] 2003). *Critique of Pure Reason*. Translated by N. Kemp Smith. New York: Palgrave MacMillan.

Karmarkar, A. & Lieberman, I., 2006. Mirror box therapy for complex regional pain syndrome. *Anaesthesia*, **61**(4), 412–13.

Kastner, S. Pinsk, M.A., De Weerd, P., Desimone, R., & Ungerleider, L.G., 1999. Increased activity in human visual cortex during directed attention in the absence of visual stimulation. *Neuron*, **22**(4), 751–61.

Kawachi, Y. & Gyoba, J., 2006. Presentation of a visual nearby moving object alters stream/bounce event perception. *Perception*, **35**(9), 1289–94.

Kawamura, Y. & Kare, M.R., 1987. *Umami: a Basic Taste*. New York: Marcel Dekker (NY).

Keeley, B.L., 2013. What exactly is a sense, in J. Simner & E. Hubbard (Eds.), *Oxford Handbook of Synesthesia*. Oxford: Oxford University Press, pp. 1–4.

Keetels, M. & Vroomen, J., 2005. The role of spatial disparity and hemifields in audio-visual temporal order judgments. *Exp Brain Res*, **167**(4), 635–40.

Keetels, M. & Vroomen, J., 2008. Temporal recalibration to tactile-visual asynchronous stimuli. *Neurosci Letters*, **430**(2), 130–4.

Keetels, M. & Vroomen, J., 2012. Perception of synchrony between the senses, in M. M. Murray & M. T. Wallace (Eds.), *The Neural Bases of Multisensory Processes*. Frontiers in Neuroscience. Boca Raton (FL): CRC Press, pp. 147–78.

Kennett, S., Taylor-Clarke, M., & Haggard, P., 2001. Noninformative vision improves the spatial resolution of touch in humans. *Curr Biol*, **11**(15), 1188–91.

Kersten, D. & Yuille, A., 2003. Bayesian models of object perception. *Curr Opin Neurobiol,* **13**(2), 150–8.

Keysers, C., Kohler, E., Umiltà, M.A., Nanetti, L., Fogassi, L., & Gallese, V., 2003. Audiovisual mirror neurons and action recognition. *Exp Brain Res,* **153**(4), 628–36.

Kilteni, K., Maselli, A., Kording, K.P., & Slater, M. , 2015. Over my fake body: body ownership illusions for studying the multisensory basis of own-body perception. *Front Human Neurosci,* **9**(703), p.141.

Kim, R.S., Seitz, A.R., & Shams, L., 2008. Benefits of stimulus congruency for multisensory facilitation of visual learning. *PLoS ONE,* **3**(1), p.e1532.

King, A.J. & Palmer, A.R., 1985. Integration of visual and auditory information in bimodal neurones in the guinea-pig superior colliculus. *Exp Brain Res,* **60**(3), 492–500.

King, A.J., Schnupp, J.W.H., & Doubell, T.P., 2001. The shape of ears to come: dynamic coding of auditory space. *Trends Cogn Sci,* **5**(6), 261–70.

Kitazawa, S., Kimura, T., & Uka, T., 1997. Prism adaptation of reaching movements: specificity for the velocity of reaching. *J Neurosci,* **17**(4), 1481–92.

Klemen, J., & Chambers, C.D., 2012. Current perspectives and methods in studying neural mechanisms of multisensory interactions. *Neurosci Biobeh Rev,* **36**(1), 111–33.

Klingner, C. M., Axer, H., Brodoehl, S., & Witte, O. W. 2016. Vertigo and the processing of vestibular information: A review in the context of predictive coding. *Neurosci Biobehav Rev,* **71**, 379–87.

Koelewijn, T., Bronkhorst, A., & Theeuwes, J., 2009. Auditory and visual capture during focused visual attention. *J Exp Psychol: Hum Percep Perf,* **35**(5), 1303–15.

Koffka, K. 1935. *Principles of Gestalt Psychology.* London, UK: Lund Humphries.

Kohler, E., Keysers, C., Umiltà, M.A., Fogassi, L., Gallese, V., & Rizzolatti, G., 2002. Hearing sounds, understanding actions: action representation in mirror neurons. *Science,* **297**(5582), 846–8.

Kohler, I., 1962. The formation and transformation of the perceptual world. *Psychological Issues, Monograph 12,* **3**(4), 1–173.

Köhler, W., 1947. *Gestalt Psychology: An introduction to New Concepts in Modern Psychology.* New York: Liveright Publication.

Komura, Y., Tamura, R., Uwano, T., Nishijo, H., & Ono, T. 2005. Auditory thalamus integrates visual inputs into behavioral gains. *Nat Neurosci,* **8**(9), 1203–9.

Körding, K.P., Beierholm, U., Ma, W.J., Quartz, S., Tenenbaum, J.B., & Shams, L., 2007. Causal inference in multisensory perception. *PLoS One,* **2**(9), e943.

Kowalska, J. & Szelag, E., 2006. The effect of congenital deafness on duration judgment. *J Child Psychol Psychiatry,* **47**(9), 946–53.

Kramer, J., 1988. *The Time Of Music.* New York: Schirmer.

Kriegstein, von, K. & Giraud, A.-L., 2006. Implicit multisensory associations influence voice recognition. *PLoS biology,* **4**(10), p.e326.

Krishna, A., Cian, L., & Aydınoğlu, N.Z. 2017. Sensory aspects of package design. *J Retailing,* **93**, 43–54.

Krüger, H.M., Collins, T., Englitz, B., & Cavanagh, P., 2016. Saccades create similar mislocalizations in visual and auditory space. *J Neurophysiol,* **115**(4), 2237–45.

Kubovy, M. & Minhong, Y., 2014. Multistability, cross-modal binding and the additivity of conjoined grouping principles. *Philos Trans R Soc Lond B Biol Sci.,* **367**, 954–64.

Kubovy, M. & Wagemans, J., 1995. Grouping by proximity and multistability in dot lattices: A quantitative Gestalt theory. *Psychol Sci,* **6**(4), 225–34.

Kunar, M.A., Carter, R., Cohen, M., & Horowitz, T.S., 2008. Telephone conversation impairs sustained visual attention via a central bottleneck. *Psychon Bull Rev,* **15**(6), 1135–40.

Kurata, K. & Hoshi, E., 1999. Reacquisition deficits in prism adaptation after muscimol microinjection into the ventral premotor cortex of monkeys. *J Neurophysiol*, **81**(4), 1927–1938.

La Mettrie, J. 1745. L'histoire naturelle de l'âme, in *Oeuvres philosophiques* (Trad., M. Charp). Olms Verlag, 1970.

Lackner, J. R. & DiZio, P. A., 2000. Aspects of body self-calibration. *Trends Cogn Sci*, **4**(7), 279–88.

Lackner, J.R., 1988. Some proprioceptive influences on the perceptual representation of body shape and orientation. *Brain*, **111** (Pt 2), 281–97.

Làdavas, E., di Pellegrino, G., Farnè, A., & Zeloni, G., 1998a. Neuropsychological evidence of an integrated visuotactile representation of peripersonal space in humans. *J Cogn Neurosci*, **10**(5), 581–9.

Làdavas, E., Farnè, A., Zeloni, G., & di Pellegrino, G., 2000. Seeing or not seeing where your hands are. *Exp Brain Res*, **131**(4), 458–467.

Làdavas, E., Zeloni, G., & Farne, A., 1998b. Visual peripersonal space centred on the face in humans. *Brain*, **121** (12), 2317–26.

Lafargue, G. & Duffau, H., 2008. Awareness of intending to act following parietal cortex resection. *Neuropsychologia*, **46**(11), 2662–7.

Lamont, K., Chin, M., & Kogan, M., 2011. Mirror box therapy: seeing is believing. *Explore*, 7(6), 369–72.

Lapid, E., Ulrich, R., & Rammsayer, T., 2009. Perceptual learning in auditory temporal discrimination: No evidence for a cross-modal transfer to the visual modality. *Psychon Bull Rev*, **16**, 382–9.

Laurienti, P.J., Burdette, J.H., Wallace, M.T., Yen, Y.F., Field, A.S., & Stein, B.E., 2002. Deactivation of sensory-specific cortex by cross-modal stimuli. *J Cogn Neurosci*, **14**(3), 420–9.

Lawson, R., 1999. Achieving visual object constancy across plane rotation and depth rotation. *Acta Psychol*, **102**, 221–45.

Lederman, S.J. & Klatzky, R.L., 2009. Haptic perception: A tutorial. *Atten Percept Psychophys*, **71**(7), 1439–59.

Lee, D. N. & Lishman, J. R., 1975. Visual proprioceptive control of stance. *J Hum Movement Stud*, **1**, 87–95.

Leibniz, G. 1765. *Nouveaux essais sur l'entendement humain*. Presses Universitaires de France (F), 1961.

Lenay, C., Gapenne, O., Hanneton, S., Marque, C., & Genouëlle, C. 2003. Sensory substitution: Limits and perspectives, in Y. Hatwell, A. Streri, & E. Gentaz (Eds.), *Touching for Knowing: Cognitive Psychology of Haptic Manual Perception*. New York: John Benjamins, pp. 275–92.

Lenggenhager, B., Halje, P., & Blanke, O., 2011. Alpha band oscillations correlate with illusory self-location induced by virtual reality. *European J Neurosci*, **33**(10), 1935–43.

Lenggenhager, B. & Lopez, C., 2015. Vestibular contributions to the sense of body, self, and others. In T. Metzinger & J. M. Windt (Eds). *Open MIND*. Frankfurt am Main: MIND Group.

Lenggenhager, B., Tadi, T., Metzinger, T., & Blanke, O., 2007. Video ergo sum: manipulating bodily self-consciousness. *Science*, **317**(5841), 1096–9.

Levin, J., 2008. Molyneux's question and the individuation of perceptual concepts. *Philosoph Stud*, **139**(1), 1–28.

Lewis, C.I., 1929. *Mind and the world order*. New York: Scribner Sons.

Lewkowicz, D.J. & Ghazanfar, A.A., 2006. The decline of cross-species intersensory perception in human infants. *Proc Natl Acad Sci USA*, **103**(17), 6771–4.

Lhermitte, J. & Tchehrazi, E., 1937. L'image du moi corporel et ses déformations pathologiques. *L'Encéphale*, **32**, 1–24.

Liberman, A.M., Cooper, F.S., Shankweiler, D.P., & Studdert-Kennedy, M. , 1967. Perception of the speech code. *Psychol Rev*, **74**(6), 431–61.

Libet, B., Gleason, C. A., Wright, E. W., & Pearl, D. K. 1983. Time of conscious intention to act in relation to onset of cerebral activity (readiness-potential). The unconscious initiation of a freely voluntary act. *Brain*, **106**(Pt 3), 623–42.

Liman, E.R., Zhang, Y.V., & Montell, C., 2014. Peripheral coding of taste. *Neuron*, **81**(5), 984–1000.

Lindeman, R.W., Page, R., Sibert, J.L., & Templeman, J.N., 2005. Using vibrotactile cues for virtual contact and data display in tandem, *Proc. of the 11th Int Conference on Human-Computer Interaction* (HCII 2005), Jul. 22-27, 2005, Las Vegas, Nevada, USA.

Lingnau, A., Gesierich, B., & Caramazza, A., 2009. Asymmetric fMRI adaptation reveals no evidence for mirror neurons in humans. *Proc Natl Acad Sci USA*, **106**(24), 9925–30.

Livingstone, M. S. & Hubel, D. H., 1987. Psychophysical evidence for separate channels for the perception of form, color, movement, and depth. *J Neurosci*, **7**, 3416–68.

Lloyd, D.M., 2007. Spatial limits on referred touch to an alien limb may reflect boundaries of visuo-tactile peripersonal space surrounding the hand. *Brain Cogn*, **64**(1), 104–9.

Lloyd, D.M., Merat, N., McGlone, F., & Spence, C., 2003. Crossmodal links between audition and touch in covert endogenous spatial attention. *Percept Psychophys*, **65**(6), 901–24.

Lloyd, J. & Mitchinson, J., 2006. *The Book of General Ignorance*. London: Faber and Faber.

Logothetis, N.K., 2008. What we can do and what we cannot do with fMRI. *Nature*, **453**, 869–78.

Longo, M.R., Pernigo, S., & Haggard, P., 2011. Vision of the body modulates processing in primary somatosensory cortex. *Neurosci Lett*, **489**(3), 159–63.

Longo, M.R., Schüür, F., Kammers, M.P., Tsakiris, M., & Haggard P., 2009. Self awareness and the body image. *Acta Psycholo*, **132**(2), 166–72.

Loomis, J. M., Beall, A. C., Macuga, K. L., Kelly, J. W., & Smith, R. S., 2006. Visual control of action without retinal optic flow. *Psychol Sci*, **17**(3), 214–221.

Lopez, C., 2013. A neuroscientific account of how vestibular disorders impair bodily self-consciousness. *Front Integr Neurosci*, **7**, p.91.

Lopez, C., Lenggenhager, B., & Blanke, O., 2010. How vestibular stimulation interacts with illusory hand ownership. *Conscious Cogn*, **19**(1), 33–47.

Lopez, C., Schreyer, H.M., Preuss, N., & Mast, F.W., 2012. Vestibular stimulation modifies the body schema. *Neuropsychologia*, **50**(8), 1830–7.

Lukos, J., Ansuini, C., & Santello, M., 2007. Choice of contact points during multidigit grasping: effect of predictability of object center of mass location. *J Neurosci*, **27**(14), 3894–903.

Luria, A., 1968. *The Mind of a Mnemonist: A Little Book About a Vast Memory*. Harvard University Press (MA).

Lyons, G., Sanabria, D., Vatakis, A., & Spence, C., 2006. The modulation of crossmodal integration by unimodal perceptual grouping: a visuotactile apparent motion study. *Exp Brain Res*, **174**(3), 510–16.

Macaluso, E., 2006. Multisensory processing in sensory-specific cortical areas. *The Neuroscientist* **12**, 327–38.

Macaluso, E. & Doricchi, F., 2013. Attention and predictions: control of spatial attention beyond the endogenous-exogenous dichotomy. *Front Hum Neurosci*, **7**, p.685.

Macaluso, E., Frith, C.D., & Driver, J., 2002. Supramodal effects of covert spatial orienting triggered by visual or tactile events. *J Cogn Neurosci*, **14**(3), 389–401.

Mack, A. & Rock, I., 1998. *Inattentional Blindness*. Cambridge, MA: MIT Press.

MacKay, W.A. & Crammond, D.J., 1987. Neuronal correlates in posterior parietal lobe of the expectation of events. *Behav Brain Res*, **24**(3), 167–79.

Maidenbaum, S., Abboud, S., & Amedi, A. 2014. Sensory substitution: closing the gap between basic research and widespread practical visual rehabilitation. *Neurosci Biobehav Rev*, **41**, 3–15.

Maister, L., Sebanz, N., Knoblich, G., & Tsakiris M., 2013. Experiencing ownership over a dark-skinned body reduces implicit racial bias. *Cognition*, **128**(2), 170–8.

Maister, L., Slater, M., Sanchez-Vives, M.V., & Tsakiris M., 2015. Changing bodies changes minds: owning another body affects social cognition. *Trends Cogn Sci*, **19**(1), 6–12.

Maister, L., Tsiakkas, E., & Tsakiris, M., 2013. I feel your fear: shared touch between faces facilitates recognition of fearful facial expressions. *Emotion*, **13**(1), 7–13.

Makin, T.R., Holmes, N.P., Brozzoli, C., Rossetti, Y., & Farnè, A., 2009. Coding of visual space during motor preparation: Approaching objects rapidly modulate corticospinal excitability in hand-centered coordinates. *J Neurosci*, **29**(38), 11841–51.

Makin, T.R., Holmes, N.P., & Ehrsson, H.H., 2008. On the other hand: dummy hands and peripersonal space. *Behav Brain Res*, **191**(1), 1–10.

Makin, T.R., Holmes, N.P., & Zohary, E., 2007. Is that near my hand? Multisensory representation of peripersonal space in human intraparietal sulcus. *J Neurosci*, **27**(4), 731–40.

Mamassian, P., 2006. Bayesian inference of form and shape, in S. Martinez-Conde, S. Macknick, L. Martinez, J.-M. Alonso & P.U. Tse (Eds.), *Progress in Brain Research*, Vol.158, Elsevier (NL), pp. 265–70.

Mamassian, P., Landy, M., & Maloney, L.T. 2002. Bayesian modelling of visual perception, in R.P.N. Rao, B.A. Olhausen, & M.S. Lewicki (Eds.), *Probabilistic Models of the Brain: Perception and Neural Function*, pp. 13–36.

Maravita, A., Spence, C., Kennett, S., & Driver, J., 2002. Tool-use changes multimodal spatial interactions between vision and touch in normal humans. *Cognition*, **83**(2), B25–34.

Marder, E. & Calabrese, R. L., 1996. Principles of rhythmic motor pattern generation. *Physiol Rev*, **76**(3), 687–717.

Marinetti, F.T. & Fillia, 1932. *La cucina futurista*. Milano (I): Sonzogno.

Marks, L., 1978. *The Unity of the Senses: Interrelations among the Modalities*. New York: Academic Press.

Marks, L.E., 1983. Similarities and differences among the senses. *Int J Neurosci*, **19**(14), 1–11.

Marks, L.E. 1991. Metaphor and the unity of the senses, in H.T. Lawless & B.P. Klein (Eds.), *Sensory Science Theory and Applications in Foods*. New York: Marcel Dekker, pp. 185–205.

Marks, L.E., 2004. Cross-modal interactions in speeded classification, in G.A. Calvert, C. Spence, & B.E. Stein (Eds.), *Handbook of Multisensory Processing*. Cambridge (MA): MIT Press, pp. 85–105.

Marks, L.E., Elgart, B.Z., Burger, K., & Chakwin, E.M., 2007. Human flavor perception: Application of information integration theory. *Teor Model*, **1**(2), 121–32.

Marks, L.E. & Mulvenna, C.M., 2013. Synesthesia, at and near its borders. *Front Psychol*, **4**, 651.

Marr, D., 1982. *Vision*. New York: Freeman.

Marr, D. & Hildreth, E., 1980. Theory of edge detection. *Proc R Soc London, B*, **207**(1167), 187–217.

Marr, D. & Nishihara, H.K., 1978. Representation and recognition of the spatial organization of three-dimensional shapes. *Proc R Soc London, B*, **200**(1140), 269–94.

Martel, M., Cardinali, L., Roy, A.C., & Farnè, A., 2016. Tool-use: An open window into body representation and its plasticity. *Cogn Neuropsychol*, **33**(1-2), 82–101.

Marteniuk, R. G., Leavitt, C. L., MacKenzie, C. L., & Athenes, S. 1990. Functional relationship between grasp and transport components in a prehension task. *Hum Mov Sci*, **9**, 149–76.

Marteniuk, R.G., MacKenzie, C.L., Jeannerod, M., Athenes, S., & Dugas, C., 1987. Constraints on human arm movement trajectories. *Can J Psychol*, **41**(3), 365–78.

Martin, T.A., Keating, J.G., Goodkin, H.P., Bastian, A.J., & Thach, W.T., 1996. Throwing while looking through prisms. I. Focal olivocerebellar lesions impair adaptation. *Brain*, **119**(Pt 4), 1183–98.

Martino, G. & Marks, L.E., 2001. Synesthesia: strong and weak. *Curr Direct Psychol Sci*, **10**(2), 61–5.

Massaro, D., 1987. *Speech Perception by Ear and Eye: A Paradigm for Psychological Inquiry*. Hillsdale (NJ): Erlbaum.

Massaro, D.W. & Cohen, M.M., 1993. Perceiving asynchronous bimodal speech in consonant vowel and vowel syllables. *Speech Commun*, **13**, 127–34.

Massaro, D.W. & Friedman, D., 1990. Models of integration given multiple sources of information. *Psychol Rev*, **97**(2), 225–52.

Maurer, D., 1993. Neonatal synesthesia: implications for the processing of speech and faces, in B. de Boysson-Bardies, S. de Schonen, P. Jusczyk, P. McNeilage, & J. Morton (Eds.), *Developmental Neurocognition: Speech and Face Processing in the First Year of Life*. Kluwer Academic Publishers (NL).

Maurer, D., Pathman, T., & Mondloch, C.J., 2006. The shape of boubas: sound-shape correspondences in toddlers and adults. *Dev Sci*, **9**(3), 316–22.

Mayer, A.R., Harrington, D., Adair, J.C., & Lee, R., 2006. The neural networks underlying endogenous auditory covert orienting and reorienting. *NeuroImage*, **30**(3), 938–49.

Mayer, A.R., Harrington, D.L., Stephen, J., Adair, J.C., & Lee, R.R., 2007. An event-related fMRI Study of exogenous facilitation and inhibition of return in the auditory modality. *J Cogn Neurosci*, **19**(3), 455–67.

Mazzurega, M., Pavani, F., Paladino, M.P, & Schubert, T.W., 2011. Self-other bodily merging in the context of synchronous but arbitrary-related multisensory inputs. *Exp Brain Res*, **213**(2-3), 213–21.

McAuley, J.D. & Henry, M.J., 2010. Modality effects in rhythm processing: Auditory encoding of visual rhythms is neither obligatory nor automatic. *Atten Percep Psychophys*, **72**(5), 1377–89.

McCormick, D. & Mamassian, P., 2008. What does the illusory-flash look like? *Vision Res*, **48**(1), 63–9.

McDonald, J.J., Teder-Sälejärvi, W.A., Di Russo, F., & Hillyard, S.A., 2005. Neural basis of auditory-induced shifts in visual time-order perception. *Nature Neurosci*, **8**(9), 1197–202.

McDonald, J.J., Teder-Sälejärvi, W.A., & Hillyard, S.A., 2000. Involuntary orienting to sound improves visual perception. *Nature*, **407**(6806), 906–8.

McGeoch, P.D., Brang, D., Song, T., Lee, R.R., Huang, M., & Ramachandran, V.S., 2011. Xenomelia: a new right parietal lobe syndrome. *J Neurol Neurosurg Psychiatr*, **82**(12), 1314–19.

McGurk, H. & MacDonald, J., 1976. Hearing lips and seeing voices. *Nature*, **264**(5588), 746–8.

McIntosh, R.D. & Lashley, G., 2008. Matching boxes: familiar size influences action programming. *Neuropsychologia*, **46**(9), 2441–4.

McIntire, J.P., Havig, P.R., Watamaniuk, S.N., & Gilkey, R.H., 2010. Visual search performance with 3-D auditory cues: effects of motion, target location, and practice. *Hum Fact*, **52**(1), 41–53.

Meijer, P., 1992. An experimental system for auditory image representations. *IEEE Trans Biomed Eng*, **39**, 112–21.

Melcher, D. & Colby, C. L. 2008. Trans-saccadic perception. *Trends Cogn Sci*, **12**(12), 466–73.

Melmoth, D. R. & Grant, S. 2006. Advantages of binocular vision for the control of reaching and grasping. *Exp Brain Res*, **171**(3), 371–88.

Melzack, R., 1990. Phantom limbs and the concept of a neuromatrix. *Trends Neurosci*, **13**(3), 88–92.

Merabet, L.B. & Pascual-Leone, A., 2010. Neural reorganization following sensory loss: the opportunity of change. *Nat Rev Neurosci*, **11**(1), 44–52.

Meredith, M.A., Allman, B.L., Keniston, L.P., & Clemo, H.R., 2012. Are bimodal neurons the same throughout the brain? in M.M., Murray, M.T., Wallace (Eds.), *The Neural Bases of Multisensory Processes*. Boca Raton (FL): CRC Press, pp. 51–64.

Merzenich, M.M., Nelson, R.J., Stryker, M.P., Cynader, M.S., Schoppmann, A., & Zook, J.M., 1984. Somatosensory cortical map changes following digit amputation in adult monkeys. *J Compar Neurol*, **224**, 591–605.

Mesulam, M.M., 1981. A cortical network for directed attention and unilateral neglect. *Ann Neurol*, **10**(4), 309–25.

Metzger, W., 1934. Beobachtungen über phänomenale Identität. *Psychologische Forschung*, **19**, 1–60.

Metzger, W., 1941. *Psychologie. Die Entwicklung ihrer Grundannahmen seit der Einführung des Experiments*. Steinkoppfs Verlag (Germany).

Meule, A. & Vögele, C., 2013. The psychology of eating. *Front Psychol*, **4**(215), 1–2.

Michel, C., Velasco, C., Gatti, E., & Spence, C., 2014. A taste of Kandinsky: assessing the influce of the artistic visual presentation of food on the dining experience. *Flavour*, **3**(7), 1–10.

Michel, C., Vernet, P., Courtine, G., Ballay, Y., & Pozzo, T., 2008. Asymmetrical after-effects of prism adaptation during goal oriented locomotion. *Exp Brain Res*, **185**(2), 259–68.

Michotte, A., Thinès, G., & Crabbé, G., 1964. *Les Compléments amodaux des structures perceptives*. Louvain publications universitaires.

Milner, D. & Goodale, M.A., 1995. *The Visual Brain in Action*. Oxford: Oxford University Press.

Mishra, J., Martinez, A., & Hillyard, S.A., 2013. Audition influences color processing in the sound-induced visual flash illusion. *Vision Res*, **93**, 74–9.

Mitchell, S.W., 1871. Phantom limbs. *Lippincott Mag*, **8**, 563–9.

Molholm, S., Ritter, W., Murray, M.M., Javitt, D.C., Schroeder, C.E., & Foxe, J.J., 2002. Multisensory auditory-visual interactions during early sensory processing in humans: a high-density electrical mapping study. *Brain Res Cogn Brain Res*, **14**(1), 115–28.

Mollon, J.D. & Perkins, A.J., 1996. Errors of judgement at Greenwich in 1796. *Nature*, **380**(6570), 101–2.

Montale, E., 1993. *Cuttlefish Bones (1920–1927)*, Translated by William Arrowsmith, New York: W.W. Norton & Company.

Montessori, M., 1912. *The Montessori Method*. New York: Frederick A. Stokes Company

Morein-Zamir, S., Soto-Faraco, S., & Kingstone, A., 2003. Auditory capture of vision: examining temporal ventriloquism. *Brain Res. Cogn Brain Res*, **17**(1), 154–63.

Morrell, L. K., 1968. Temporal characteristics of sensory integration in choice reaction times. *J Exp Psychol*, **77**, 14–18.

Morrone, M. C., Tosetti, M., Montanaro, D., Fiorentini, A., Cioni, G., & Burr, D. C., 2000. A cortical area that responds specifically to optic flow, revealed by fMRI. *Nat Neurosci*, **3**(12), 1322–8.

Morrot, G., Brochet, F., & Dubourdieu, D., 2001. The color of odors. *Brain Lang*, **79**, 309–20.

Morton, S.M. & Bastian, A.J., 2004. Prism adaptation during walking generalizes to reaching and requires the cerebellum. *J Neurophysiol*, **92**(4), 2497–509.

Mostafa, A.A., Salomonczyk, D., Cressman, E.K., & Henriques, D.Y., 2014. Intermanual transfer and proprioceptive recalibration following training with translated visual feedback of the hand. *Exp Brain Res*, **232**(6), 1639–51.

Mountcastle, V.B., Lynch, J.C., Georgopoulos, A., Sakata, H., & Acuna, C., 1975. Posterior parietal association cortex of the monkey: command functions for operations within extrapersonal space. *J Neurophysiol*, **38**(4), 871–908.

Mozolic, J.L., Hugenschmidt, C.E., Peiffer, A.M., & Laurienti, P.J., 2011. Multisensory integration and aging, in M. M. Murray & M. T. Wallace (Eds.), *The Neural Bases of Multisensory Processes*. Boca Raton (FL): CRC Press, pp. 381–92.

Muggleton, N., Tsakanikos, E., Walsh, V., & Ward, J., 2007. Disruption of synaesthesia following TMS of the right posterior parietal cortex. *Neuropsychologia*, **45**(7), 1582–5.

Mukamel, R., Ekstrom, A.D., Kaplan, J., Iacoboni, M., & Fried, I., 2010. Single-neuron responses in humans durgin execution and observation of actions. *Curr Biol*, **20**, 750–6.

Müller, H.J. & Rabbitt, P.M., 1989. Reflexive and voluntary orienting of visual attention: time course of activation and resistance to interruption. *J Exp Psychol Hum Percept Perform*, **15**(2), 315–30.

Murphy, C.L., Cain, W.S., & Bartoshuck, L.M. 1977. Mutual action of taste and olfaction. *Sens Proc*, **1**, 204–11.

Murray, M.M. & Wallace, M.T. (Eds.) 2012. *The Neural Bases of the Multisensory Processes*. Boca Raton (FL): CRC Press.

Murray, C.D., Patchick, E.L., Caillette, F., Howard, T., & Pettifer, S. 2006. Can immersive virtual reality reduce phantom limb pain? *Stud Health Technol Informatics*, **119**, 407–12.

Murray, M.M., Lewkowicz, D.J., Amedi, A., & Wallace, M.T., 2016. Multisensory processes: a balancing act across the lifespan. *Trends Neurosci*, **39**(8), 567–79.

Murray, M.M., Molholm, S., Michel, C.M., Heslenfeld, D.J., Ritter, W., & Javitt, D.C., 2005. Grabbing your ear: rapid auditory-somatosensory multisensory interactions in low-level sensory cortices are not constrained by stimulus alignment. *Cereb Cortex*, **15**(7), 963–74.

Mussap, A.J. & Salton, N., 2006. A "rubber-hand" illusion reveals a relationship between perceptual body image and unhealthy body change. *J Health Psychol*, **11**(4), 627–39.

Näätänen, R., 1982. Processing negativity: an evoked-potential reflection of selective attention. *Psychol Bull*, **92**(3), 605–40.

Nagarajan, S.S., Blake, D.T., Wright, B.A., Byl, N., & Merzenich, M.M., 1998. Practice-related improvements in somatosensory interval discrimination are temporally specific but generalize across skin location, hemisphere, and modality. *J Neurosci*, **18**(4), 1559–70.

Nagel, T., 1974. What Is It Like to Be a Bat? *The Philosophical Review*, **83**(4), 435–50.

Nashner, L. M., 1976. Adapting reflexes controlling the human posture. *Exp Brain Res*, **26**(1), 59–72.

Natsoulas, T. & Dubanoski, R.A., 1964. Inferring the locus and orientation of the perceiver from responses to stimulation of the skin. *Am J Psychol*, **77**, 281–5.

Nava, E., Bottari, D., Villwock, A., Fengler, I., Büchner, A., Lenarz, T., & Röder, B., 2014. Audio-tactile integration in congenitally and late deaf cochlear implant users. *PLoS ONE*, **9**(6), p.e99606.

Nava, E. & Pavani, F., 2013. Changes in sensory dominance during childhood: converging evidence from the colavita effect and the sound-induced flash illusion. *Child Develop*, **84**(2), 604–16.

Navarra, J., Vatakis, A., Zampini, M., Soto-Faraco, S., Humphreys, W., & Spence C., 2005. Exposure to asynchronous audiovisual speech extends the temporal window for audiovisual integration. *Brain Res. Cogn Brain Res*, **25**(2), 499–507.

Necker, L.A. 1832. Observations on some remarkable phenomena seen in Switzerland: And on an optical phenomenon which occurs on viewing a crystal or geometrical solid. *The London and Edinburgh Philosophical Magazine and Journal of Science*, **1**, 329–37.

Neisser, U., 1976. *Cognition and Reality*. New York: Freeman.

Neisser U., 1979. The control of information pickup in selective looking, in A.D. Pick (Ed.) *Perception and its Development: A Tribute to Eleanor J Gibson*. Hillsdale (NJ): Lawrence Erlbaum Associates, pp. 201–9.

Newell, F.N., Ernst, M.O., Tjan, B.S., & Bülthoff, H.H., 2001. Viewpoint dependence in visual and haptic object recognition. *Psychol Sci*, **12**(1), 37–42.

Newport, R., Brown, L., Husain, M., Mort, D., & Jackson, S.R., 2006. The role of the posterior parietal lobe in prism adaptation: Failure to adapt to optical prisms in a patient with bilateral damage to posterior parietal cortex. *Cortex*, **42**(5), 720–9.

Ngo, M.K. & Spence, C., 2010. Auditory, tactile, and multisensory cues facilitate search for dynamic visual stimuli. *Atten Percept Psychophys*, **72**(6), 1654–65.

Nickerson, R.S., 1973. Intersensory facilitation of reaction time: Energy summation or preparation enhancement. *Psychol Rev*, **80**, 489–509.

Nielsen, J.M., 1938. Gerstmann syndrome: Finger agnosia, agraphia, confusion of right and left and acalculia. *Arch Neurol Psychiatry*, **39**, 536–59

Nikolic, D., 2009. Is synaesthesia actually ideaestesia? An inquiry into the nature of the phenomenon. *Proceedings of the Third Int Congress on Synaesthesia, Science & Art*, Granada, Spain, April 26–29, 2009.

Nikolic, D., Jurgens, U. M., Rothen, N., Meier, B., & Mroczko, A. 2011. Swimming-style synesthesia. *Cortex*, **47**(7), 874–9.

Nishijo, H., Ono, T., & Nishino, H. 1988. Single neuron responses in amygdala of alert monkey during complex sensory stimulation with affective significance. *J Neurosci*, **8**(10), 3570–83.

Nobre, A.C. & Kastner, S., 2014. *The Oxford Handbook of Attention*. Oxford: Oxford University Press.

Nöe, A., 2004. *Action in Perception*. Cambridge (MA): MIT Press.

Noesselt, T., Bergmann D, Hake M, Heinze HJ, Fendrich R., 2008. Sound increases the saliency of visual events. *Brain Res*, **1220**, 157–63.

Nordin, M., 1990. Low-threshold mechanoreceptive and nociceptive units with unmyelinated (C) fibres in the human supraorbital nerve. *J Physiol*, **426**, 229–40.

Norman, J.F., Clayton, A.M., Norman, H.F., & Crabtree, C.E., 2008. Learning to perceive differences in solid shape through vision and touch. *Perception*, **37**(2), 185–96.

Nunn, J.A., Gregory, L.J., Brammer, M., Williams, S.C., Parslow, D.M., Morgan, M.J., et al., 2002. Functional magnetic resonance imaging of synesthesia: activation of V4/V8 by spoken words. *Nat Neurosci*, **5**(4), 371–5.

Oakley, B., 1985. Taste responses of human chorda tympani nerve. *Chem Senses,* **10**, 469–81.

Oberman, L.M. & Ramachandran, V.S., 2008. Preliminary evidence for deficits in multisensory integration in autism spectrum disorders: the mirror neuron hypothesis. *Soc Neurosci*, **3**(3-4), 348–55.

Obhi, S. S. & Haggard, P. 2004. Free will and free won't. *American Sci*, July-August, 358–65.

Odgaard, E.C., Arieh, Y., & Marks, L.E., 2003. Cross-modal enhancement of perceived brightness: sensory interaction versus response bias. *Percept Psychophys*, **65**(1), 123–32.

Oesterbauer, R.A., Matthews, P.M., Jenkinson, M., Beckmann, C.F., Hansen, P.C., & Calvert, G.A., 2005. Color of scents: chromatic stimuli modulate odor responses in the human brain. *J Neurophysiol,* **93**, 3434–41.

Oestrum, K.M., Catalanotto, F.A., Gent, J.F., & Bartoshuk, L.M., 1985. Effect of oral sensory field loss on taste scaling ability. *Chem Sens,* **10**, 459.

Olausson, H., Wessberg, J., Morrison, I., McGlone, F., & Vallbo, A., 2010. The neurophysiology of unmyelinated tactile afferents. *Neurosci Biobehav Rev*, **34**(2), 185–91.

Olivers, C.N.L. & Van der Burg, E., 2008. Bleeping you out of the blink: sound saves vision from oblivion. *Brain Res*, **1242**, 191–9.

Overvliet, K.E., Azañón, E., & Soto-Faraco, S., 2011. Somatosensory saccades reveal the timing of tactile spatial remapping. *Neuropsychologia*, **49**(11), 3046–3052.

Packard, V. 1957. *The Hidden Persuaders*. Harmondsworth (UK): Penguin Books.

Paillard, J., 1999. Body schema and body image: A double dissociation in deafferented patients, in G.N. Gantchev, S. Mori, & J. Massion (Eds.), *Motor Control, Today and Tomorrow*, Sofia, Bulgaria: Academic Publishing House, pp. 197–214.

Paladino, M.P., Mazzurega, M., Pavani, F., & Schubert, T.W., 2010. Synchronous multisensory stimulation blurs self-other boundaries. *Psychol Sci*, **21**(9), 1202–7.

Palmer, S. & Rock, I., 1994. Rethinking perceptual organization: The role of uniform connectedness. *Psychon Bull Rev*, **1**, 29–55.

Palmer, S., Rosch, E., & Chase, P., 1981. Canonical perspective and the perception of objects. *Atten Perf*, **IX**, 131–51.

Palmeri, T.J., Blake, R., Marois, R., Flanery, M.A., & Whetsell, W.J., 2002. The perceptual reality of synesthetic colors. *Proc Natl Acad Sci USA*, **99**(6), 4127–31.

Parise, C.V. & Pavani, F., 2011. Evidence of sound symbolism in simple vocalizations. *Exp Brain Res*, **214**(3), 373–80.

Parise, C.V. & Spence, C., 2009. "When birds of a feather flock together": synesthetic correspondences modulate audiovisual integration in non-synesthetes. *PLoS One*, **4**(5), e5664.

Parma, V., Ghirardello, D., Tirindelli, R., & Castiello, U. 2011a. Grasping a fruit. Hands do what flavour says. *Appetite*, **56**(2), 249–54.

Parma, V., Roverato, R., Ghirardello, D., Bulgheroni, M., Tirindelli, R., & Castiello, U. 2011b. When flavor guides motor control: an effector independence study. *Exp Brain Res*, **212**(3), 339–46.

Pascolo, P.B. & Budai, R., 2013. Just how consistent is the mirron neuron system paradigm? *Progress Neurosci*, **1**(1-4), 29–43.

Patané, I., Iachini, T., Farnè, A., & Frassinetti, F., 2016. Disentangling action from social space: tool-use differently shapes the space around us. *PLoS ONE*, **11**(5), p.e0154247.

Patel, A.D. & Iversen, J.R., 2014. The evolutionary neuroscience of musical beat perception: the Action Simulation for Auditory Prediction (ASAP) hypothesis. *Front Syst Neurosci*, **8**(183), 57.

Patel, A.D., Iversen, J.R., Chen, Y., & Repp, B.H., 2005. The influence of metricality and modality on synchronization with a beat. *Exp Brain Res*, **163**(2), 226–38.

Patel, A.D., Iversen, J.R., Bregman, M.R., & Schulz, I., 2009. Experimental evidence for synchronization to a musical beat in a nonhuman animal. *Curr Biol* **19**(10), 827–30.

Paulesu, E., Harrison, J., Baron-Cohen, S., Watson, J.D., Goldstein, L., Heather, J., et al., 1995. The physiology of coloured hearing. A PET activation study of colour-word synaesthesia. *Brain*, **118** (Pt 3), 661–76.

Pavani, F. & Turatto, M., 2008. Change perception in complex auditory scenes. *Perception & Psychophysics*, **70**(4), 619–29.

Pavani, F. & Zampini, M., 2007. The role of hand size in the fake-hand illusion paradigm. *Perception*, **36**(10), 1547–54.

Pavani, F., Husain, M., & Driver, J., 2008. Eye-movements intervening between two successive sounds disrupt comparisons of auditory location. *Exp Brain Res*, **189**(4), 435–49.

Pavani, F., Spence, C., & Driver, J., 2000. Visual capture of touch: out-of-the-body experiences with rubber gloves. *Psychol Sci*, **11**(5), 353–9.

Peck, T.C., Seinfeld, S., Aglioti, S.M., & Slater, M.., 2013. Putting yourself in the skin of a black avatar reduces implicit racial bias. *Conscious Cogn*, **22**(3), 779–87.

Penfield, W. & Boldrey, E., 1937. Somatic motor and sensory representation in the cerebral cortex of man as studied by electrical stimulation. *Brain*, **60**(4), 389–443.

Penfield, W. & Rasmussen, T., 1950. *The Cerebral Cortex of Man; a Clinical Study of Localization of Function*, New York: Macmillan.

Perrault, T. Jr, Rowland, B.A., & Stein, B.E., 2012, in M.M. Murray & M.T. Wallace (Eds.), *The Neural Bases of Multisensory Processes*. Boca Raton (FL): CRC Press, pp. 279–300.

Perrault, T.J., Vaughan, J.W., Stein, B.E., & Wallace, M.T., 2005. Superior colliculus neurons use distinct operational modes in the integration of multisensory stimuli. *J Neurophysiol*, **93**(5), 2575–86.

Perrott, D.R., Cisneros, J., McKinley, R.L., & D'Angelo, W.R., 1996. Aurally aided visual search under virtual and free-field listening conditions. *Hum Fact*, **38**(4), 702–15.

Perrott, D.R. & Saberi, K., 1990. Minimum audible angle thresholds for sources varying in both elevation and azimuth. *J Acoust Soc Am*, **87**(4), 1728–31.

Perrott, D.R., Sadralodabai, T., Saberi, K., & Strybel, T.Z., 1991. Aurally aided visual search in the central visual field: effects of visual load and visual enhancement of the target. *Hum Fact*, **33**(4), 389–400.

Peters, M.A., Balzer, J., & Shams, L., 2015. Smaller = denser, and the brain knows it: natural statistics of object density shape weight expectations. *PLoS One*, **10**(3), e0119794.)

Peters, M.A., Ma, W.J., & Shams, L., 2016. The size-weight illusion is not anti-Bayesian after all: a unifying Bayesian account. *PeerJ*, **4**, e2124.

Peterson, M.A., 2001. Object perception, in E.B. Goldstein (Ed.), *Blackwell Handbook of Sensation and Perception*. Oxford: Blackwell Publishing, pp. 168–203.

Petkova, V.I., Björnsdotter, M., Gentile, G., Jonsson, T., Li, T.Q., & Ehrsson, H.H., 2011. From part- to whole-body ownership in the multisensory brain. *Curr Biol*, , **21**(13), 1118–22.

Petkova, V.I. & Ehrsson, H.H., 2008. If I were you: perceptual illusion of body swapping. *PLoS ONE*, **3**(12), p.e3832.

Phillips-Silver, J. & Trainor, L.J., 2005. Feeling the beat: movement influences infant rhythm perception. *Science*, **308**(5727), 1430.

Phillips-Silver, J. & Trainor, L.J., 2008. Vestibular influence on auditory metrical interpretation. *Brain and Cognition*, **67**(1), 94–102.

Piaget, J. & Inhelder, B. 1966. *The Psychology of the Child*. 2nd English Edition 2000. New York: Basic Books.

Piéron, H., 1952. *The Sensations: Their Functions, Processes and Mechanisms*, London: Muller.

Piqueras-Fiszman, B., Alcaide, J., Roura, E., & Spence, C., 2012. Is it the plate or is it the food? Assessing the influence of the color (black or white) and shape of the plate on the perception of the food placed on it. *Food Qual Preference*, **24**, 205–8.

Piqueras-Fiszman, B., Laughlin, Z., Miodownik, M., & Spence, C., 2012. Tasting spoons: Assessing how the material of a spoon affects the taste of food. *Food Qual Preference*, **24**, 24–9.

Polanksy, R., 2007. *Aristotle's De anima*. Cambridge: Cambridge University Press.

Pöppel, E., 1997. A hierarchical model of temporal perception. *Trends Cogn Sci*, **1**(2), 56–61.

Posner, M.I., 1980. Orienting of attention. *Q J Exp Psychol*, **32**(1), 3–25.

Pouget, A., Deneve, S., & Duhamel, J.-R., 2004. A computational neural theory of multisensory spatial representations, in C. Spence & J. Driver (Eds.), *Crossmodal Space and Crossmodal Attention*. Oxford: Oxford University Press, pp. 123–40.

Power, R.P., 1980. The dominance of touch by vision: sometimes incomplete. *Perception*, **9**(4), 457–66.

Prescott, J., 1999. Flavour as a psychological construct: implications for perceiving and measuring the sensory qualities of foods. *Food Qual Preference*, **10**, 349–56.

Press, C. Taylor-Clarke, M., Kennett, S., & Haggard, P. , 2004. Visual enhancement of touch in spatial body representation. *Exp Brain Res*, **154**(2), 238–45.

Previc, F. H., 1998. The neuropsychology of 3-D space. *Psychol Bull*, **124**(2), 123–64.

Pridmore, S., Garry, M.I., Karst, M., Rahe-Meyer, N., & Rybak, M., 2006. Tickling healthy subjects. *German J Psychiatr*, **9**(3), 107–10.

Proulx, M. J., Stoerig, P., Ludowig, E., & Knoll, I., 2008. Seeing "where" through the ears: effects of learning-by-doing and long-term sensory deprivation on localization based on image-to-sound substitution. *PLoS One*, **3**(3), e1840.

Proust, J., 1997. *Perception et intermodalité. Approches actuelles de la question de Molyneux*. Presses Universitaires de France (F), 1–303.

Provine, R.R., 2004. Laughing, tickling, and the evolution of speech and self. *Curr Dir Psychol Sci*, **13**(6), 215–8.

Provine, R.R., 2001. *Laughter: A Scientific Investigation*. New York: Penguin USA.

Putnam, H., 1975. *Mind, Language, and Reality: Philosophical Papers*. Cambridge: Cambridge University Press.

Putzar, L., Hötting, K., & Röder, B., 2010. Early visual deprivation affects the development of face recognition and of audio-visual speech perception. *Rest Neurol Neurosci*, **28**(2), 251–7.

Qureshy, A., Kawashima, R., Imran, M.B., Sugiura, M., Goto, R., Okada, K., et al. 2000. Functional mapping of human brain in olfactory processing: a PET study. *J Neurophysiol*, **84**, 1656–66.

Radeau, M. & Bertelson, P., 1974. The after-effects of ventriloquism. *Q J Exp Psychol*, **26**(1), 63–71.

Radocy, R.E. & Boyle, J.D., 2012. *Psychological Foundations of Musical Behavior* (5th ed.). Springfield (IL): Charles C. Thomas Publisher, Ltd.

Ramachandran, V.S., 1993. Behavioral and magnetoencephalographic correlates of plasticity in the adult human brain. *Proc Natl Acad Sci USA*, **90**, 10413–20.

Ramachandran, V.S. & Altschuler, E.L., 2009. The use of visual feedback, in particular mirror visual feedback, in restoring brain function. *Brain*, **132**(Pt 7), 1693–710.

Ramachandran, V.S. & Azoulai, S., 2006. Synesthetically induced colors evoke apparent-motion perception. *Perception*, **35**(11), 1557–60.

Ramachandran, V.S. & Hubbard, E.M., 2001. Psychophysical investigations into the neural basis of synaesthesia. *Proc Biol Sci*, **268**(1470), 979–83.

Ramachandran, V.S. & Hubbard, E.M., 2001. Synaesthesia—a window into perception, thought and language. *J Consciousness Stud*, **8**(12), 3–34.

Ramachandran, V.S. & Rogers-Ramachandran, D., 1996. Synaesthesia in phantom limbs induced with mirrors. *Proc Biol Sci*, **263**(1369), 377–86.

Ramachandran, V.S., Rogers-Ramachandran, D., & Cobb S. 1995. Touching the phantom limb, *Nature* **377**, 489–90.

Rao, R.P. & Ballard, D.H., 1999. Predictive coding in the visual cortex: a functional interpretation of some extra-classical receptive-field effects. *Nature Neurosci*, **2**(1), 79–87.

Reales, J.M. & Ballesteros, S., 1999. Implicit and explicit memory for visual and haptic objects: Cross-modal priming depends on structural descriptions. *J Exp Psychol Learn Mem Cogn*, **25**(3), 644–63.

Recanzone, G.H., 2003. Auditory influences on visual temporal rate perception. *J Neurophysiol*, **89**(2), 1078–93.

Redding, G.M. & Wallace, B., 2008. Intermanual transfer of prism adaptation. *J Mot Behav*, **40**(3), 246–62.

Redding, G.M. & Wallace, B., 2009. Asymmetric visual prism adaptation and intermanual transfer. *J Mot Behav*, **41**(1), 83–94.

Redding, G.M., Rossetti, Y., & Wallace, B., 2005. Applications of prism adaptation: a tutorial in theory and method. *Neurosci Biobehav Rev*, **29**(3), 431–44.

Renier, L., Bruyer, R., & De Volder, A. G., 2006. Vertical-horizontal illusion present for sighted but not early blind humans using auditory substitution of vision. *Percept Psychophys*, **68**(4), 535–42.

Renier, L., Laloyaux, C., Collignon, O., Tranduy, D., Vanlierde, A., Bruyer, R., et al., 2005. The Ponzo illusion with auditory substitution of vision in sighted and early-blind subjects. *Perception*, **34**(7), 857–67.

Rensink, R.A., O'Regan, J.K., & Clark, J.J., 1997. To see or not to see: The need for attention to perceive changes in scenes. *Psychol Sci*, **8**(5), 368–73.

Reynolds, R.F. & Bronstein, A.M., 2003. The broken escalator phenomenon. Aftereffect of walking onto a moving platform. *Exp Brain Res*, **151**(3), 301–8.

Rigato, S., Bremner, A.J., Mason, L., Pickering, A., Davis, R., & van Velzen, J., 2013. The electrophysiological time course of somatosensory spatial remapping: vision of the hands modulates effects of posture on somatosensory evoked potentials. *EurJ Neurosci*, **38**(6), 2884–92.

Rihs, S., 1995. The influence of audio on perceived picture quality and subjective audiovisual delay tolerance. Paper presented at: *MOSAIC Workshop: Advanced Methods for the Evaluation of Television Picture Quality, Eindhoven. Sep 18, 1995.*

Rizzolatti, G. & Arbib, M.A., 1998. Language within our grasp. *Trends Neurosci*, **21**(5), 188–94.

Rizzolatti, G. & Fabbri-Destro, M., 2010. Mirror neurons: from discovery to autism. *Exp Brain Res*, **200**(3-4), 223–37.

Rizzolatti, G., Camarda, R., Fogassi, L., Gentilucci, M., Luppino, G., & Matelli, M., 1988. Functional organization of inferior area 6 in the macaque monkey. II. Area F5 and the control of distal movements. *Exp Brain Res*, **71**(3), 491–507.

Rizzolatti, G., Fadiga, L., Matelli, M., Bettinardi, V., Paulesu, E., Perani, D., & Fazio, F., 1996. Localization of grasp representations in humans by PET: 1. Observation versus execution. *Exp Brain Res*, **111**(2), 246–52.

Rizzolatti, G., Scandolara, C., Matelli, M., & Gentilucci, M., 1981. Afferent properties of periarcuate neurons in macaque monkeys. I. Somatosensory responses. *Behav Brain Res*, **2**(2), 125–46.

Robinson, D. & Podoll, K., 2000. Macrosomatognosia and microsomatognosia in migraine art. *Acta Neurol Scand*, **101**(6), 413–16.

Rock, I. & Victor, J., 1964. Vision and touch: an experimentally created conflict between the two senses. *Science*, **143**, 594–6.

Rock, I., 1985. *The Logic of Perception*. Cambridge (MA): MIT Press, Bradford books.

Rode, G., Charles, N., Perenin, M.T., Vighetto, A., Trillet, M., & Aimard, G. 1992. Partial remission of hemiplegia and somatoparaphrenia through vestibular stimulation in a case of unilateral neglect. *Cortex*, **28**(2), 203–8.

Röder, B., Rösler, F., & Spence, C., 2004. Early vision impairs tactile perception in the blind. *Curr Biol*, **14**(2), 121–4.

Rogers, S.K. & Ross, A.S., 1975. A cross-cultural test of the Maluma-Takete phenomenon. *Perception*, **4**(1), 105–6.

Rohe, T. & Noppeney, U. 2016. Distinct computational principles govern multisensory integration in primary sensory and association cortices. *Curr Biol*, **26**(4), 509–14.

Rolls, E.T. & Baylis, L.L., 1994. Gustatory, olfactory, and visual convergence within the primate orbitofrontal cortex. *J Neurosci*, **14**(9), 5437–52.

Romano, D., Gandola, M., Bottini, G., & Maravita, A., 2014. Arousal responses to noxious stimuli in somatoparaphrenia and anosognosia: clues to body awareness. *Brain*, **137**(Pt 4), 1213–23.

Romano, D., Caffa, E., Hernandez-Arieta, A., Brugger, P., & Maravita, A., 2015. The robot hand illusion: inducing proprioceptive drift through visuo-motor congruency. *Neuropsychologia*, **70**, 414–20.

Romanski, L.M., 2007. Representation and integration of auditory and visual stimuli in the primate ventral lateral prefrontal cortex. *Cereb Cortex*, 17 Suppl 1, i61–9.

Roper, S.D., 2013. Taste buds as peripheral chemosensory processors. *Semin Cell Dev Biol*, **24**(1), 71–9.

Rorden, C., Heutink, J., Greenfield, E., & Robertson, I.H., 1999. When a rubber hand "feels" what the real hand cannot. *Neuroreport*, **10**(1), 135.

Rosenbaum, D.A., 1991. *Human Motor Control*. New York: Academic Press.

Rossetti, Y., Desmurget, M., & Prablanc, C., 1995. Vectorial coding of movement: vision, proprioception, or both. *J Neurophysiol*, **74**(1), 457–63.

Rossetti, A., Romano, D., Bolognini, N., & Maravita, A., 2015. Dynamic expansion of alert responses to incoming painful stimuli following tool use. *Neuropsychologia*, **70**, 486–94.

Rousseau, L. & Rousseau, R., 1996. Stop-reaction time and the internal clock. *Percept Psychophys*, **58**(3), 434–48

Rouw, R. & Scholte, H.S., 2007. Increased structural connectivity in grapheme-color synesthesia. *Nat Neurosci*, **10**(6), 792–7.

Rouw, R., Scholte, H.S., & Colizoli, O., 2011. Brain areas involved in synaesthesia: a review. *J Neuropsychol*, **5**(2), 214–42.

Rozin, P., 1982. "Taste–smell confusions" and the duality of the olfactory sense. *Percept Psychophys*, **31**, 397–401.

Ruggieri, V. & Milizia, M., 1983. Tickle perception as micro-experience of pleasure: its phenomenology on different areas of the body and relation to cerebral dominance. *Percept Mot Skills*, **56**(3), 903–14.

Runeson, S. & Frykholm, G., 1981. Visual perception of lifted weight. *J Exp Psychol Hum Percept Perform*, **7**(4), 733–40.

Runeson, S., 1977. On the possibility of "smart" perceptual mechanisms. *Scand J Psychol*, **18**(1), 172–9.

Sambo, C.F., Gillmeister, H., & Forster, B., 2009. Viewing the body modulates neural mechanisms underlying sustained spatial attention in touch. *Eur J Neurosci*, **30**(1), 143–50.

Samuelkamaleshkumar, S., Reethajanetsureka, S., Pauljebaraj, P., Benshamir, B., Padankatti, S.M., & David, J.A., 2014. Mirror therapy enhances motor performance in the paretic upper limb after stroke: a pilot randomized controlled trial. *Arch Phys Med Rehabil*, **95**(11), 2000–5.

Sanabria, D., Correa, A., Lupiáñez, J., & Spence, C., 2004. Bouncing or streaming? Exploring the influence of auditory cues on the interpretation of ambiguous visual motion. *Exp Brain Res*, **157**(4), 537–41.

Sanabria, D., Soto-Faraco, S., Chan, J., & Spence, C., 2005. Intramodal perceptual grouping modulates multisensory integration: evidence from the crossmodal dynamic capture task. *Neurosci Lett*, **377**(1), 59–64.

Santangelo, V., Fagioli, S., & Macaluso, E., 2010. The costs of monitoring simultaneously two sensory modalities decrease when dividing attention in space. *NeuroImage*, **49**(3), 2717–27.

Santangelo, V. & Macaluso, E., 2012. Spatial attention and audiovisual processing, in B. E. Stein (Ed.), *The New Handbook of Multisensory Processes*. Cambridge, MA: MIT Press, pp. 359–70.

Santangelo, V., Olivetti-Belardinelli, M., Spence, C., & Macaluso, E., 2009. Interactions between voluntary and stimulus-driven spatial attention mechanisms across sensory modalities. *J Cogn Neurosci*, **21**(12), 2384–97.

Santangelo, V. & Spence, C., 2007. Multisensory cues capture spatial attention regardless of perceptual load. *J Exp Psychol Hum Percept Perform*, **33**(6), 1311–21.

Santangelo, V., Van der Lubbe, R.H., Belardinelli, M.O., & Postma, A., 2006. Spatial attention triggered by unimodal, crossmodal, and bimodal exogenous cues: a comparison of reflexive orienting mechanisms. *Exp Brain Res*, **173**(1), 40–8.

Santangelo, V., Olivetti-Belardinelli, M., & Spence, C., 2007. The suppression of reflexive visual and auditory orienting when attention is otherwise engaged. *J Exp Psychol Hum Percept Perform*, **33**(1), 137–48.

Santello, M. & Soechting, J.F., 1998. Gradual molding of the hand to object contours. *J Neurophysiol*, **79**(3), 1307–20.

Sathian, K. & Zangaladze, A. 2002. Feeling with the mind's eye: contribution of visual cortex to tactile perception. *Behav Brain Res.* **135**(1-2):127–32.

Sato, A. & Yasuda, A., 2005. Illusion of sense of self-agency: discrepancy between the predicted and actual sensory consequences of actions modulates the sense of self-agency, but not the sense of self-ownership. *Cognition*, **94**(3), 241–55.

Sauvageot, F. & Chapon, M., 1983. La couleur d'un vin (blanc ou rouge) peut-elle etre identifée sans l'aide de l'oeil? *Les Cahiers de l'ENS. BANA*, **4**, 107–15.

Schacter, D.L., 1994. Priming and multiple memory systems: Perceptual mechanisms of implicit memory, in D.L. Schacter & E. Tulving (Eds.), *Memory Systems 1994*. Cambridge (MA): MIT Press, pp. 233–68.

Schauder, K.B., Mash, L.E., Bryant, L.K., & Cascio, C.J., 2015. Interoceptive ability and body awareness in autism spectrum disorder. *J Exp Child Psychol*, **131**, 193–200.

Scheier, C.R., Nijhawan, R., & Shimojo, S., 1999. Sound alters visual temporal resolution. *Invest Ophthalmol Vis Sci*, **40**, S792

Schilder, P., 1935. *The Image and Appearance of the Human Body*, New York: International Universities Press.

Schiltz, K., Trocha, K., Wieringa, B.M., Emrich, H.M., Johannes, S., & Munte, T.F., 1999. Neurophysiological aspects of synesthetic experience. *J Neuropsychiatry Clin Neurosci*, **11**(1), 58–65.

Schmelz, M., Schmidt, R., Bickel, A., Handwerker, H.O., & Torebjörk, H.E., 1997. Specific C-receptors for itch in human skin. *J Neurosci*, **17**(20), 8003–8.

Schmidt, R.A., & Lee, T.D., 1999. *Motor Control and Learning*. Champaign (IL): Human Kinetics.

Schmitt, M., Postma, A., & de Haan, E., 2000. Interactions between exogenous auditory and visual spatial attention. *Q J Exp Psychol A*, **53**(1), 105–30.

Schmitt, M., Postma, A. & de Haan, E.H.F., 2010. Cross-modal exogenous attention and distance effects in vision and hearing. *Eu J Cogn Psychol*, **13**(3), 343–68.

Schott, G.D., 1993. Penfield's homunculus: a note on cerebral cartography. *J Neurol, Neurosurg, Psychiatry*, **56**(4), 329–33.

Schumacher, R., 2003. What are the direct objects of sight? Locke on the Molyneux question. *Locke Stud*, **3**, 41–62.

Scwoebel, J. & Coslett, H.B., 2005. Evidence for multiple, distinct representations of the human body. *J Cognitive Neurosci*, **17**, 543–53.

Segond, H., Weiss, D., & Sampaio, E., 2005. Human spatial navigation via a visuo-tactile sensory substitution system. *Perception*, **34**(10), 1231–49.

Seitz, A.R. & Dinse, H.R., 2007. A common framework for perceptual learning. *Curr Op Neurobiol*, **17**(2), 148–53.

Seitz, A.R., Kim, R., & Shams, L., 2006. Sound facilitates visual learning. *Curr Biol,* **16**(14), 1422–7.

Sekuler, R., Sekuler, A.B., & Lau, R., 1997. Sound alters visual motion perception. *Nature*, **385**(6614), 308.

Selden, S.T., 2004. Tickle. *J Am Acad Dermatol*, **50**(1), 93–7.

Semenza, C., 2001. Disorders of body representation, in R.S. Bemdt (Ed.) *Handbook of Neuropsychology*, vol. **3**, 2a ed., Amsterdam: Elsevier Science, pp. 285–302.

Senden, M. von, 1932. *Raum- und Gestaltauffassung bei operierten Blindgeborenen*. Barth, German.

Senkowski, D., Senkowski, D., Saint-Amour, D., Gruber, T., & Foxe J.J., 2008. Look who's talking: the deployment of visuo-spatial attention during multisensory speech processing under noisy environmental conditions. *Neuroimage*, **43**(2), 379–87.

Sereno, M.I. & Huang, R.-S., 2006. A human parietal face area contains aligned head-centered visual and tactile maps. *Nature Neurosci*, **9**(10), 1337–43.

Serino, A., Annella, L., & Avenanti, A., 2009. Motor properties of peripersonal space in humans. *PLoS ONE*, **4**(8), p.e6582.

Serino, A., Bassolino M, Farnè A, Làdavas E., 2007b. Extended multisensory space in blind cane users. *Psychol Sci*, **18**(7), 642–8.

Serino, A., Canzoneri, E., & Avenanti, A., 2011. Fronto-parietal areas necessary for a multisensory representation of peripersonal space in humans: an rTMS study. *J Cogn Neurosci*, **23**(10), 2956–67.

Serino, A., Farnè, A., Rinaldesi, M.L., Haggard, P., & Làdavas, E., 2007a. Can vision of the body ameliorate impaired somatosensory function? *Neuropsychologia*, **45**(5), 1101–7.

Serino, A., Giovagnoli, G., de Vignemont, F., & Haggard, P., 2008. Spatial organisation in passive tactile perception: is there a tactile field? *Acta Psychol (Amst)*, **128**(2), 355–60.

Servos, P. 2000. Distance estimation in the visual and visuomotor systems. *Exp Brain Res*, **130**(1), 35–47.

Sforza, A., Bufalari, I., Haggard, P., & Aglioti, S.M., 2010. My face in yours: Visuo-tactile facial stimulation influences sense of identity. *Social Neurosci*, **5**(2), 148–62.

Shams, L. 2012. Early integration and Bayesian causal inference in multisensory perception, in M.M. Murray & M.T. Wallace (Eds.), *The Neural Bases of Multisensory Processes*. Boca Raton (FL): CRC Press/Taylor & Francis.

Shams, L., Kamitani, Y., & Shimojo, S., 2000. Illusions. What you see is what you hear. *Nature*, **408**(6814), 788.

Shams, L., Kamitani, Y., & Shimojo, S., 2002. Visual illusion induced by sound. *Brain Res. Cogn Brain Res*, **14**(1), 147–52.

Shams, L. & Kim, R., 2012. Cross-modal facilitation of unisensory learning, in B. E. Stein (Ed.), *The New Handbook of Multisensory Processes*. Cambridge, MA: MIT Press.

Shams, L. & Seitz, A.R., 2008. Benefits of multisensory learning. *Trends Cogn Sci*, **12**(11), 411–17.

Shams, L., Wozny, D.R., Kim, R., & Seitz, A., 2011. Influences of multisensory experience on subsequent unisensory processing. *Front Psychol*, **2**, 264.

Sherrington, C.S., 1906. *The Integrative Action of the Nervous System*. New Haven (CT): Yale University Press.

Shibasaki, H. & Hallett, M. 2006. What is the Bereitschaftspotential? *Clin Neurophysiol*, **117**(11), 2341–56.

Shimojo, S., Miyauchi, S., & Hikosaka, O., 1997. Visual motion sensation yielded by non-visually driven attention. *Vision Res*, **37**(12), 1575–80.

Shimojo, S. & Shams, L., 2001. Sensory modalities are not separate modalities: plasticity and interactions. *Curr Opin Neurobiol*, **11**, 505–9.

Shimojo, S., Scheier, C., Nijhawan, R., Shams, L., Kamitani, Y., & Watanabe, K., 2001. Beyond perceptual modality: auditory effects on visual perception. *Acoust Sci Technol*, **22**(2), 61–7.

Shomstein, S. & Yantis, S., 2004. Control of attention shifts between vision and audition in human cortex. *J Neurosci*, **24**(47), 10702–6.

Shopland, C. & Gregory, R.L., 1964. The effect of touch on a visually ambiguous three-dimensional figure. *Q J Exp Psychol*, **16**, 66–70.

Shore, D.I., Spry, E., & Spence, C., 2002. Confusing the mind by crossing the hands. *Brain Res Cogn Brain Res*, **14**(1), 153–63.

Shulman, G. L., Astafiev, S. V., McAvoy, M. P., d'Avossa, G., & Corbetta, M. 2007. Right TPJ deactivation during visual search: functional significance and support for a filter hypothesis. *Cereb Cortex*, **17**(11), 2625–33.

Simner, J., & Hubbard, E.M., 2006. Variants of synesthesia interact in cognitive tasks: evidence for implicit associations and late connectivity in cross-talk theories. *Neurosci*, **143**(3), 805–14.

Simons, D.J. & Chabris, C.F., 1999. Gorillas in our midst: sustained inattentional blindness for dynamic events. *Perception*, **28**(9), 1059–74.

Simons, D.J. & Levin, D.T., 1998. Failure to detect changes to people during a real-world interaction. *Psychonom Bull Rev*, **5**, 644–49.

Simons, D.J. & Rensink, R.A., 2005. Change blindness: Past, present, and future. *Trends Cogn Sci.* **9**, 16–20.

Sirigu, A., Daprati, E., Ciancia, S., Giraux, P., Nighoghossian, N., Posada, A., & Haggard, P., 2004. Altered awareness of voluntary action after damage to the parietal cortex. *Nat Neurosci*, **7**(1), 80–4.

Sirigu, A., Grafman, J., Bressler, K., & Sunderland, T., 1991. Multiple representations contribute to body knowledge processing. Evidence from a case of autotopagnosia. *Brain*, **114** (Pt 1B), 629–42.

Slater, M., Spanlang, B., Sanchez-Vives, M.V., & Blanke, O., 2010. First person experience of body transfer in virtual reality. *PLoS ONE*, **5**(5), p.e10564.

Slocombe, B.G., Carmichael, D.A., & Simner, J., 2016. Cross-modal tactile-taste interactions in food evaluations. *Neuropsychologia*, **88**, 58–64.

Slutsky, D.A. & Recanzone, G.H., 2001. Temporal and spatial dependency of the ventriloquism effect. *Neuroreport*, **12**(1), 7–10.

Smeets, J.B. & Brenner, E., 1999. A new view on grasping. *Motor Control*, **3**(3), 237–71.

Smeets, J.B., Brenner, E., & Biegstraaten, M., 2002. Independent control of the digits predicts an apparent hierarchy of visuomotor channels in grasping. *Behav Brain Res*, **136**(2), 427–32.

Smith, D.V., Van Buskirk, R.L., Travers, J.B., & Bieber, S.L., 1983a. Coding of taste stimuli by hamster brain stem neurons. *J Neurophysiol*, **50**(2), 541–58.

Smith, D.V., Van Buskirk, R.L., Travers, J.B., & Bieber, S.L., 1983b. Gustatory neuron types in hamster brain stem. *J Neurophysiol*, **50**(2), 522–40.

Sommer, R., 1959. Studies in personal space. *Sociometry*, **22**, 247–60.

Soto-Faraco, S. & Alsius, A., 2007. Conscious access to the unisensory components of a cross-modal illusion. *Neuroreport*, **18**(4), 347–50.

Soto-Faraco, S. & Azañón, E., 2013. Electrophysiological correlates of tactile remapping. *Neuropsychologia*, **51**(8), 1584–94.

Spector, F. & Maurer, D., 2013. Early sound symbolism for vowel sounds. *i-Perception*, **4**(4), 239–41.

Spence, C., 2010. Crossmodal spatial attention. *Ann N Y Acad Sci*, **1191**(1), 182–200.

Spence, C., 2011. Crossmodal correspondences: a tutorial review. *Atten Percept Psychophys*, **73**(4), 971–95.

Spence, C., 2014. Charles Spence. *Curr Biol, *, **24**(11), R506–8.

Spence, C., 2015. Cross-modal perceptual organization, in J. Wagemans (Ed.), *The Oxford Handbook of Perceptual Organization*. Oxford: Oxford University Press, pp. 639–54.

Spence, C., Baddeley, R., Zampini, M., James, R., & Shore, D.I., 2003. Multisensory temporal order judgments: when two locations are better than one. *Percept Psychophys*, **65**(2), 318–28.

Spence, C. & Deroy, O., 2012. Crossmodal correspondence: Innate or learned? *i-Perception*, **3**, 316–18.

Spence, C. & Driver, J., 1996. Audiovisual links in endogenous covert spatial attention. *J Exp Psychol Hum Percept Perform,*, **22**(4), 1005–30.

Spence, C. & Driver, J., 1997. Audiovisual links in exogenous covert spatial orienting. *Percept Psychophys*, **59**(1), 1–22.

Spence, C. & Driver, J., 2004. *Crossmodal Space and Crossmodal Attention*, Oxford: Oxford University Press.

Spence, C., Harrar, V., & Piqueras-Fiszman, B., 2012. Assessing the impact of the tableware an other contextual variables on multisensory flavour perception. *Flavour*, **1**(7), 1–12.

Spence, C., Levitan, C.A., Shankar, M.U., & Zampini, M. 2010. Does food color influence taste and flavor perception in humans? *Chemosen Percept*, **3**(1), 68–84.

Spence, C. & McDonald, J., 2004. The crossmodal consequences of the exogenous spatial orienting of attention, in G.A. Calvert, C. Spence, & B.E. Stein (Eds.), *The Handbook of Multisensory Processing*. Cambridge (MA): MIT Press, pp. 3–26.

Spence, C. & Parise, C., 2010. Prior-entry: a review. *Conscious Cogn*, **19**(1), 364–79.

Spence, C., Pavani, F., & Driver, J., 2004. Spatial constraints on visual-tactile cross-modal distractor congruency effects. *Cogn Affect Behav Neurosci. Neurosci*, **4**(2), 148–69.

Spence, C., Ranson, J., & Driver, J., 2000. Cross-modal selective attention: on the difficulty of ignoring sounds at the locus of visual attention. *Percept Psychophys*, **62**(2), 410–24.

Spence, C. & Read, L., 2003. Speech shadowing while driving: on the difficulty of splitting attention between eye and ear. *Psychol Sci*, **14**(3), 251–56.

Spence, C. & Santangelo, V., 2009. Capturing spatial attention with multisensory cues: a review. *Hear Res*, **258**(1-2), 134–42.

Spence, C., Shore, D.I., & Klein, R.M., 2001. Multisensory prior entry. *J Exp Psychol, Gen*, **130**(4), 799–832.

Spence, C., Velasco, C., & Knoeferle, K., 2014. A large sample study on the influence of the multisensory environment on the wine drinking experience. *Flavour*, **3**(8), 1–12.

Spence, C. & Ho, D.C., 2012. *The Multisensory Driver*, Aldershot (UK): Ashgate Publishing, Ltd.

Sperling, J.M., Prvulovic, D., Linden, D.E., Singer, W., & Stirn, A., 2006. Neuronal correlates of colour-graphemic synaesthesia: a fMRI study. *Cortex*, **42**(2), 295–303.

Spizzo, G. 1984. La regolare associazione come fonte di associazioni causali fenomeniche, in G. Kanizsa (Ed.), *Fenomenologia sperimentale della visione*. Milano: Franco Angeli, *Ricerche di Psicologia* monograph, *7*(26), 221–30.

Sposito, A., Bolognini, N., Vallar, G., & Maravita, A., 2012. Extension of perceived arm length following tool-use: clues to plasticity of body metrics. *Neuropsychologia*, **50**(9), 2187–94.

Stein, B.E. (ed.) 2012. *The New Handbook of Multisensory Processing*. Cambridge, MA: MIT Press.

Stein, B.E. & Clamann, H.P., 1981. Control of pinna movements and sensorimotor register in cat superior colliculus. *Brain BehavEvol*, **19**(3-4), 180–92.

Stein, B.E., London N, Wilkinson LK, & Price DD., 1996. Enhancement of perceived visual intensity by auditory stimuli: a psychophysical analysis. *J Cogn Neurosci*, **8**(6), 497–506.

Stein, B.E. & Meredith, M.A., 1993. *The Merging of the Senses*. Cambridge, MA: MIT Press.

Stein, B.E., Meredith, M.A., & Wallace, M.T., 1993. The visually responsive neuron and beyond: multisensory integration in cat and monkey. *Prog Brain Res*, **95**, 79–90.

Stein, B.E. & Stanford, T.R., 2008. Multisensory integration: current issues from the perspective of the single neuron. *Nature Reviews Neurosci*, **9**(4), 255–66.

Stein, B.E., Stanford, T.R., & Rowland, B.A., 2014. Development of multisensory integration from the perspective of the individual neuron. *Nature Rev Neurosci*, **15**(8), 520–35.

Stekelenburg, J.J. & Vroomen, J., 2007. Neural correlates of multisensory integration of ecologically valid audiovisual events. *J Cogn Neurosci*, **19**(12), 1964–73.

Stevenson, R.J. 2009. *The Psychology of Flavour*. Oxford: Oxford University Press.

Stevenson, R.J. & Boakes, R.A., 2004. Sweet and sour smells: Learned synaesthesia between the senses of taste and smell, in G.A. Calvert, C. Spence, & B.E. Stein (Eds.), *The Handbook of Multisensory Processing*. Cambridge (MA): MIT Press, pp. 69–83.

Stevenson, R.J., Boakes, R.A., & Wilson, J.P., 2000. Resistance to extinction of conditioned odor perceptions: evaluative conditioning is not unique. *J Exp Psychol Learn Mem Cogn*, **26**(2), 423–40.

Stevenson, R.J., Prescott, J., & Boakes, R.A., 1999. Confusing tastes and smells: how odours can influence the perception of sweet and sour tastes. *Chem Senses*, **24**(6), 627–35.

Stillman, J.A., 2002. Gustation: intersensory experience par excellence. *Perception*, **31**, 1491–500.

Störmer, V.S., McDonald, J.J., & Hillyard, S.A., 2009. Cross-modal cueing of attention alters appearance and early cortical processing of visual stimuli. *Proc Natl Acad Sci USA*, **106**(52), 22456–61.

Stratton, G.M. 1897. Vision without inversion of the retinal image. *Psychol Rev*, **4** (4), 341–60.

Stratton, G.M. 1899. The spatial harmony of touch and sight. *Mind*, **8**, 492–505.

Stratton, G.M., 1896. Some preliminary experiments on vision without inversion of the retinal image. *Psychol Rev*, **3**, 611–7.

Strelnikov, K., Rosito, M., & Barone, P., 2011. Effect of audiovisual training on monaural spatial hearing in horizontal plane. *PLoS ONE*, **6**(3), e18344–9.

Stricanne, B., Andersen, R.A., & Mazzoni, P., 1996. Eye-centered, head-centered, and intermediate coding of remembered sound locations in area LIP. *J Neurophysiol*, **76**(3), 2071–6.

Stroop, J.R., 1935. Studies of interference in serial verbal reactions. *J Exp Psychol*, **18**, 643–62.

Sugihara, T., Diltz, M.D,, Averbeck, B.B., & Romanski, L.M., 2006. Integration of auditory and visual communication information in the primate ventrolateral prefrontal cortex. *J Neurosci*, **26**(43), 11138–47.

Sumby, W.H. & Pollack, I., 1954. Visual contribution to speech intelligibility in noise. *J Acoust Soc Am*, **26**(2), 212–15.

Suzuki, K., Garfinkel, S.N,. Critchley, H.D., & Seth, A.K., 2013. Multisensory integration across exteroceptive and interoceptive domains modulates self-experience in the rubber-hand illusion. *Neuropsychologia*, **51**(13), 2909–17.

Tajadura-Jiménez, A. & Tsakiris, M., 2014. Balancing the "inner" and the "outer" self: interoceptive sensitivity modulates self-other boundaries. *J Exp Psychol Gen*, **143**(2), 736–44.

Tajadura-Jiménez, A., Grehl, S., & Tsakiris, M., 2012. The other in me: interpersonal multisensory stimulation changes the mental representation of the self. *PLoS ONE*, **7**(7), p.e40682.

Takada, M., 2013. *Synesthetic Metaphor: Perception, Cognition, and Language,* Saarbrücken: VDM Verlag.

Takeuchii, A.H. & Hulse, S.H., 1993. Absolute pitch. *Psychol Bull*, **113**(2), 345–61.

Talsma, D., 2015. Predictive coding and multisensory integration: an attentional account of the multisensory mind. *Front Integr Neurosci*, **9**, 19.

Talsma, D., Senkowski, D., Soto-Faraco, S., & Woldorff, M.G., 2010. The multifaceted interplay between attention and multisensory integration. *Trends Cogn Sci*, **14**(9), 400–10.

Talsma, D., Senkowski, D., Soto-Faraco, S., & Woldorff, M. G., 2012. Influence of top-down attention on multisensory processing, in B.E. Stein (Ed.), *The Handbook of Multisensory Processing.* Cambridge (MA): MIT Press, pp. 371–82.

Tarr, M.J., 1995. Rotating objects to recognize them: A case study on the role of viewpoint dependency in the recognition of three-dimensional objects. *Psychon Bull Rev*, **2**(1), 55–82.

Tarr, M.J. & Bülthoff, H.H., 1995. Is human object recognition better described by geon structural descriptions or by multiple views? Comment on Biederman and Gerhardstein (1993). *J Exp Psychol Hum Percept Perform*, **21**(6), 1494–505.

Tarr, M.J. & Pinker, S., 1989. Mental rotation and orientation-dependence in shape recognition. *Cogn Psychol*, **21**(2), 233–82.

Tastevin, J., 1937. En partent de l'experience d'Aristotle: Les déplacements artificiels des parties du corps ne sont pas suivis par le sentiment de ces parties ni pas les sensations qu'on peut y produire. *L'Encephale*, **32**, 57–84.

Taylor-Clarke, M., Jacobsen, P., & Haggard, P., 2004. Keeping the world a constant size: object constancy in human touch. *Nature Neurosci*, **7**(3), 219–20.

Taylor-Clarke, M., Kennett, S., & Haggard, P., 2002. Vision modulates somatosensory cortical processing. *Curr Biol*, **12**(3), 233–6.

Teerling, A., 1992. The colour of taste. *Chem Senses,* **17**, 886.

Teller, D.Y., 1984. Linking propositions. *Vision Res, 24*, 1233–46.

Teneggi, C., Canzoneri, E., di Pellegrino, G., & Serino, A., 2013. Social modulation of peripersonal space boundaries. *Curr Biol, 23*(5), 406–11.

Theeuwes, J., Atchley, P., & Kramer, A. F., 2000. On the time course of top-down and bottom-up control of visual attention, in S. Monsell, & J. Driver (Eds.), *Attention and Performance*, Cambridge (MA): MIT Press, pp. 104–24.

Thelen, E., 1986. Treadmill-elicited stepping in seven-month-old infants. *Child Dev, 57*(6), 1498–1506.

Thelen, A., Cappe, C., & Murray, M. M. 2012. Electrical neuroimaging of memory discrimination based on single-trial multisensory learning. *NeuroImage, 62*(3), 1478–88.

Thelen, E. & Cooke, D.W., 1987. Relationship between newborn stepping and later walking: a new interpretation. *Dev Med Child Neurol, 29*(3), 380–93.

Thelen, E. & Fisher, D.M., 1982. Newborn stepping: an explanation for a disappearing reflex. *Develop Psychol, 18*(5), 760–75.

Thelen, A., Matusz, P.J., & Murray, M.M., 2014. Multisensory context portends object memory. *Curr Biol, 24*(16), R734–5.

Thelen, A. & Murray, M.M., 2013. The efficacy of single-trial multisensory memories. *Multisens Res, 26*(5), 483–502.

Thelen, A., Talsma, D., & Murray, M. M. 2015. Single-trial multisensory memories affect later auditory and visual object discrimination. *Cognition, 138*, 148–60

Thomas, G.J., 1941. Experimental study of the influence of vision on sound localization. *J Exp Psychol, 28*, 163–77.

Thorpe, S., Fize, D., & Marlot, C., 1996. Speed of processing in the human visual system. *Nature, 381*(6582), 520–2.

Tipper, S.P., Lloyd, D., Shorland, B., Dancer, C., Howard, L.A., & McGlone, F., 1998. Vision influences tactile perception without proprioceptive orienting. *Neuroreport, 9*(8), 1741–4.

Tipper, S.P., Phillips, N., Dancer, C., Lloyd, D., Howard, L.A., & McGlone, F., 2001. Vision influences tactile perception at body sites that cannot be viewed directly. *Exp Brain Res, 139*(2), 160–7.

Titchener, E. B. 1908. *Lectures on the Elementary Psychology of Feeling and Attention.* New York: Macmillan.

Todorovic, D., 2011. What is the origin of the Gestalt principles? *Humana Mente, 17*, 1–20.

Todrank, J. & Bartoshuk, L.M., 1991. A taste illusion: taste sensation localized by touch. *Physiol Behav, 50*, 1027–31.

Trainor, L.J., Gao, X., Lei, J.J., Lehtovaara, K. & Harris, L.R., 2009. The primal role of the vestibular system in determining musical rhythm. *Cortex, 45*(1), 35–43.

Treisman, M., 1963. Temporal discrimination and the indifference interval. Implications for a model of the "internal clock". *Psychol Monogr, 77*(13), 1–31.

Trevena, J.A. & Miller, J., 2002. Cortical movement preparation before and after a conscious decision to move. *Conscious Cogn, 11*(2), 162–90.

Troje, N.F. & McAdam, M. 2010. The viewing-from-above bias and the silhouette illusion. *i-Perception, 1*, 143–8.

Tsakiris, M., 2008. Looking for myself: current multisensory input alters self-face recognition. *PLoS ONE, 3*(12), p.e4040.

Tsakiris, M. & Haggard, P., 2005. The rubber hand illusion revisited: visuotactile integration and self-attribution. *J Exp Psychol Hum Percept Perform, 31*(1), 80–91.

Tsakiris, M., Hesse, M.D., Boy, C., Haggard, P., & Fink, G.R., 2007. Neural signatures of body ownership: a sensory network for bodily self-consciousness. *Cereb Cortex, 17*(10), 2235–44.

Tsakiris, M., Tajadura-Jiménez, A., & Costantini, M., 2011. Just a heartbeat away from one's body: interoceptive sensitivity predicts malleability of body-representations. *Proc Biol Sci*, **278**(1717), 2470–6.

Tubaldi, F., Ansuini, C., Tirindelli, R., & Castiello, U. 2008. The grasping side of odours. *PLoS ONE*, **3**(3), e1795.

Tuomainen, J., Andersen, T.S., Tiippana, K., & Sams, M., 2005. Audio-visual speech perception is special. *Cognition*, **96**(1), B13–22.

Umiltà, M.A., Kohler, E., Gallese, V., Fogassi, L., Fadiga, L., Keysers, C., & Rizzolatti, G., 2001. I know what you are doing. a neurophysiological study. *Neuron*, **31**(1), 155–65.

Vallar, G. & Ronchi, R., 2009. Somatoparaphrenia: a body delusion. A review of the neuropsychological literature. *Exp Brain Res*, **192**(3), 533–51.

van Beers, R.J., Wolpert, D.M., & Haggard, P., 2002. When feeling is more important than seeing in sensorimotor adaptation. *Curr Biol*, **12**(10), 834–7.

van de Kamp, C., & Zaal, F.T., 2007. Prehension is really reaching and grasping. *Exp Brain Res*, **182**(1), 27–34.

Van der Burg, E., Olivers, C.N., Bronkhorst, A.W., & Theeuwes, J., 2008. Pip and pop: Nonspatial auditory signals improve spatial visual search. *J Exp Psychol Hum Percept Perform.*, **34**(5), 1053–65.

Van der Burg, E., Olivers, C.N., Bronkhorst, A.W., & Theeuwes J., 2009. Poke and pop: tactile-visual synchrony increases visual saliency. *Neurosci Lett*, **450**(1), 60–4.

Van der Burg, E., Talsma, D., Olivers, C.N., Hickey, C., & Theeuwes, J., 2011. Early multisensory interactions affect the competition among multiple visual objects. *Neuroimage*, **55**(3), 1208–18.

Van Doorn, G., Hohwy, J., & Symmons, M., 2014. Can you tickle yourself if you swap bodies with someone else? *Conscious Cogn*, **23**, 1–11.

van Ee, R. , van Boztel, J.J., Parker, A.L. & Alais, D. 2009. Multisensory congruency as a mechanism for attentional control over perceptual selection. *J Neurosci*, **29**(37), 11641–9.

van Eijk, R.L.J., Kohlrausch, A., Juola, J.F. & van de Par, S. , 2008. Audiovisual synchrony and temporal order judgments: Effects of experimental method and stimulus type. *Percept Psychophys*, **70**(6), 955–68.

van Ittersum, K. & Wansink, B., 2012. Plate size and color suggestibility: The Delboeuf illusion's bias on serving and eating behavior. *J Consumer Res*, **39**, 215–28.

van Leeuwen, T.M., Petersson, K.M., & Hagoort, P., 2010. Synaesthetic colour in the brain: beyond colour areas. A functional magnetic resonance imaging study of synaesthetes and matched controls. *PLoS One*, **5**(8), e12074.

Van Riper, C., 1935. An experimental study of the Japanese illusion. *Am J Psychol*, **47**, 252–63.

van Wassenhove, V., Buonomano, D.V., Shimojo, S., & Shams, L., 2008. Distortions of subjective time perception within and across senses.. *PLoS ONE*, **3**(1), e1437–13.

van Wassenhove, V., 2016. Temporal cognition and neural oscillations. *Curr Opinion in Behav Sci*, **8**, 124–30.

Vanrie, J., Willems, B., & Wagemans, J., 2001. Multiple routes to object matching from different viewpoints: mental rotation versus invariant features. *Perception*, **30**(9), 1047–56.

VanRullen, R. & Thorpe, S.J., 2001. Is it a bird? Is it a plane? Ultra-rapid visual categorisation of natural and artifactual objects. *Perception*, **30**(6), 655–68.

Vatakis, A., Ghazanfar, A.A., & Spence, C., 2008. Facilitation of multisensory integration by the "unity effect" reveals that speech is special. *J Vision*, **8**(9), 14.1–11.

Vatakis, A. & Spence, C., 2006. Audiovisual synchrony perception for speech and music assessed using a temporal order judgment task. *Neurosci Letters*, **393**(1), 40–4.

Vatakis, A. & Spence, C., 2006. Audiovisual synchrony perception for music, speech, and object actions. *Brain Res*, **1111**(1), 134–42.

Vatakis, A. & Spence, C., 2007. Crossmodal binding: evaluating the "unity assumption" using audiovisual speech stimuli. *Percept Psychophys*, **69**(5), 744–56.

Velasco, C., Jones, R., King, S., & Spence, C., 2013. Assessing the influence of the multisensory environment on the whisky drinking experience. *Flavour*, **2**(23), 1–11.

Vezzani, S., Marino, B.F.M., & Giora, E., 2012. An early history of the Gestalt factors of organisation. *Perception*, **41**, 148–167.

Vibell, J., Klinge, C., Zampini, M., Spence, C., & Nobre, A.C., 2007. Temporal order is coded temporally in the brain: early event-related potential latency shifts underlying prior entry in a cross-modal temporal order judgment task. *J Cogn Neurosci*, **19**(1), 109–20.

Vicario, G.B., 2005. *Il tempo: saggio di psicologia sperimentale.* Bologna: Il Mulino.

Violentyev, A., Shimojo, S., & Shams, L., 2005. Touch-induced visual illusion. *Neuroreport*, **16**(10), 1107–10.

Vitevitch, M.S., 2003. Change deafness: the inability to detect changes between two voices. *J Exp Psychol Hum Percept Perform* **29**(2), 333–42.

von Békésy, G., 1963. Interaction of paired sensory stimuli and conduction in peripheral nerves. *J Appl Physiol*, **18**, 1276–84.

von Holst, E.V. & Mittelstaedt, H., 1950. Das reafferenzprinzip. *Naturwissenschaften*, **37**, 464–76.

von Hornbostel, E.M., 1927. Die Einheit der Sinne. *Melos, Zeitschrift für Musik*, **4**, 290–97.

von Uexküll, J.J., 1957. A stroll through the worlds of animals and men: a picture book of invisible worlds, in C.H. Schiller (Ed.) *Instinctive Behavior: The Development of a Modern Concept*, New York: International Universities Press, Inc.

Vroomen, J. & Baart, M., 2009. Phonetic recalibration only occurs in speech mode. *Cognition*, **110**(2), 254–9.

Vroomen, J., Bertelson, P., & de Gelder, B., 2001. The ventriloquist effect does not depend on the direction of automatic visual attention. *Percept Psychophys*, **63**(4), 651–9.

Vroomen, J. & de Gelder, B., 2000. Sound enhances visual perception: cross-modal effects of auditory organization on vision. *J Exp Psychol Hum Percept Perform*, **26**(5), 1583–90.

Vroomen, J. & Keetels, M., 2006. The spatial constraint in intersensory pairing: no role in temporal ventriloquism. *J Exp Psychol Hum Percept Perform* , **32**(4), 1063–71.

Vroomen, J. & Keetels, M., 2009. Sounds change four-dot masking. *Acta Psychol*, **130**(1), 58–63.

Vroomen, J., Keetels, M., de Gelder, B., & Bertelson, P., 2004. Recalibration of temporal order perception by exposure to audio-visual asynchrony. *Brain Res Cogn Brain Res*, **22**(1), 32–5.

Vuillerme, N., Chenu, O., Pinsault, N., Moreau-Gaudry, A., Fleury, A., Demongeot, J., et al., 2007. Pressure sensor-based tongue-placed electrotactile biofeedback for balance improvement—biomedical application to prevent pressure sores formation and falls. *Conf Proc IEEE Eng Med Biol Soc, Suppl*, 6114–17.

Wade, N., Campbell, R.N., Ross,, H.E., & Linglbach, B., 2010. Necker in Scotch perspective. *Perception*, **39**, 1–4.

Wadhera, D. & Capaldi-Phillips, E.D., 2014. A review of visual cues associated with food on food acceptance and consumption. *Eat Behav*, **15**(1), 132–43.

Wagemans, J., Elder, J.H., Kubovy, M., Palmer, S.E., Peterson, M.A., Singh, M., & von der Heydt, R., 2012a. A century of gestalt psychology in visual perception: i. perceptual grouping and figure-ground organization. *Psychol Bull*, **138**(6), 1172–217.

Wagemans, J., Feldman, J., Gepshtein, S., Kimchi, R., Pomerantz, J.R., van der Helm, P.A., & van Leeuwen, C., 2012b. A century of gestalt psychology in visual perception: ii. conceptual and theoretical foundations. *Psychol Bull*, **138**(6), 1218–52.

Wallace, M.T., Meredith, M.A., & Stein, B. E. 1998. Multisensory integration in the superior colliculus of the alert cat. *J Neurophysiol*, **80**(2), 1006–10.

Walsh, V, 2003. A theory of magnitude: common cortical metrics of time, space and quantity. *Trends Cogn Sci*, **7**(11), 483–8.

Wandell, B.A., 1995. *Foundations of Vision*, Sunderland, MA: Sinauer Associates Incorporated.

Wang, J. & Stelmach, G., 1999. Temporal and spatial relationship between reaching and grasping. Commentary on "A new view on grasping". *Motor Control*, **3**(3), 307–11; discussion 316.

Wansink, B., 2004. Environmental factors that increase the food intake and consumption volume of unknowing consumers. *Annu Rev Nutr*, **24**, 455–79.

Warden, C.J. & Flynn, E.L., 1926. The effect of color on apparent size and weight. *Am J Psychol*, **37**, 398–401.

Warren, D.H., Welch, R.B., & McCarthy, T.J., 1981. The role of visual-auditory "compellingness" in the ventriloquism effect: implications for transitivity among the spatial senses. *Percept Psychophys*, **30**(6), 557–64.

Warren, W. H., Kay, B.A., Zosh, W.D., Duchon, A.P., & Sahuc, S. 2001. Optic flow is used to control human walking. *Nat Neurosci*, **4**(2), 213–6.

Watanabe, K. & Shimojo, S., 2001. When sound affects vision: effects of auditory grouping on visual motion perception. *Psychol Sci*, **12**(2), 109–16.

Watson, M.R., Akins, K.A., Spiker, C., Crawford, L., & Enns, J.T., 2014. Synesthesia and learning: a critical review and novel theory. *Front Hum Neurosci*, **8**, 98.

Watt, S.J., Bradshaw, M.F., & Rushton, S.K. 2000. Field of view affects reaching, not grasping. *Exp Brain Res*, **135**(3), 411–6.

Wayand, J.F., Levin, D.T., & Varakin, D.A., 2005. Inattentional blindness for a noxious multimodal stimulus. *Am J Psychol*, **118**(3), 339–52.

Wearden, J.H., Edwards, H., Fakhri, M., & Percival, A., 1998. Why "sounds are judged longer than lights": application of a model of the internal clock in humans. *Q J Exp Psychol B*, **51**(2), 97–120.

Weinstein, S., 1969. Neuropsychological studies of the phantom, in A.L. Benton (Ed.), *Contributions to Clinical Neuropsychology*. Chicago (IL): Aldine, pp. 73–107.

Weiskrantz, L., Elliott, J., & Darlington, C., 1971. Preliminary observations on tickling oneself. *Nature*, **230**(5296), 598–9.

Welch, R.B. & Warren, D.H., 1980. Immediate perceptual response to intersensory discrepancy. *Psychol Bull*, **88**(3), 638–67.

Wertheimer, M., 1923. Untersuchungen zur Lehre von der Gestalt. II. *Psychologichse Forschung*, **3**(4), 301–350.

Westbury, C., 2005. Implicit sound symbolism in lexical access: evidence from an interference task. *Brain Lang*, **93**(1), 10–19.

Wheatley, J. 1973. Putting colour into marketing. *Marketing*, October, 24–29, 67.

Wheatstone, C. 1838. Contributions to the physiology of vision: Part the first. On some remarkable, and hitherto unobserved, phenomena of binocular vision, *Phil Trans Soc R Lond*, **128**, 371–94.

Whitehead, W.E. & Drescher, V.M., 1980. Perception of gastric contractions and self-control of gastric motility. *Psychophysiology*, **17**(6), 552–8.

Whiteley, L., Kennett, S., Taylor-Clarke, M., & Haggard, P., 2004. Facilitated processing of visual stimuli associated with the body. *Perception*, **33**(3), 307–14.

Wilson, M. 2002. Six views of embodied cognition. *Psychon Bull Rev*, **9**(4), 625–36.

Witthoft, N. & Winawer, J. 2006. Synesthetic colors determined by having colored refrigerator magnets in childhood. *Cortex*, **42**(2), 175–83.

Wolfe, J.M., Kluender, K.R, Levi, D.M., Bartoshuk, L.M., Herz, R.S., Klatzky, R., et al. 2012. *Sensation and Perception, 4th edition*. New York: Sinauer Associates.

Wolpert, D. M.,1997. Computational approaches to motor control. *Trends Cogn Sci*, **1**, 209–16.

Wolpert, D.M. & Ghahramani, Z., 2000. Computational principles of movement neuroscience. *Nature Neurosci*, **3 Suppl**, 1212–17.

Wolpert, D.M., Goodbody, S.J., & Husain, M., 1998. Maintaining internal representations: the role of the human superior parietal lobe. *Nature Neurosci,* **1**(6), 529–33.

Woodworth, R.S. 1899. *The accuracy of voluntary movement*. Ph.D. thesis, Columbia.

Wu, C.T., Weissman, D.H., Roberts, K.C., & Woldorff, M.G., 2007. The neural circuitry underlying the executive control of auditory spatial attention. *Brain Res*, **1134**(1), 187–98.

Wu, C.-Y., Huang, P.C., Chen, Y.T., Lin, K.C., & Yang, H.W., 2013. Effects of mirror therapy on motor and sensory recovery in chronic stroke: a randomized controlled trial. *Arch Phys Med Rehabil*, **94**, 1023–30.

Wundt, W. 1908. *Grundzüge der physiologischen Psychologie*. (6th edition). Leipzig: Engelmann.

Xing, J. & Andersen, R.A., 2000. Models of the posterior parietal cortex which perform multimodal integration and represent space in several coordinate frames. *J Cognitive Neurosci*, **12**(4), 601–14.

Yamamoto, S. & Kitazawa, S., 2001. Sensation at the tips of invisible tools. *Nature Neurosci*, **4**(10), 979–80.

Yantis, S. & Jonides, J., 1984. Abrupt visual onsets and selective attention: evidence from visual search. *J Exp Psychol: Hum Percept Perf,* **10**(5), 601–21.

Yao, R., Simons, D., & Ro, T., 2009. Keep your eye on the rabbit: Cross-modal influences on the cutaneous rabbit illusion. *J Vision*, **9**, 705.

Yon, D. & Press, C., 2014. Back to the future: synesthesia could be due to associative learning. *Front Psychol*, **5**(702), 1–4.

Yonas, A. & Granrud, C.E., 1985. Development of visual space perception in infants: Beyond the blooming buzzing confusion, in J. Mehler & R. Fox (Eds.), *Neonate Cognition*. Hillsdale (NJ): Erlbaum, pp. 45–67.

Yue, Z., Gao, T., Chen, L., & Wu, J., 2016. Odors bias time perception in visual and auditory modalities. *Front Psychol*, **7**(143), 39.

Zakay, D. & Block, R. A. 1997. Temporal cognition. *Curr Dir Psychol Sci*, **6**, 12–16.

Zampini, M., Bird, K.S., Bentley, D.E., Watson, A., Barrett, G., Jones, A.K., & Spence, C., 2007. "Prior entry" for pain: attention speeds the perceptual processing of painful stimuli. *Neurosci Lett*, **414**(1), 75–9.

Zampini, M., Sanabria, D., Phillips, N., & Spence, C., 2007. The multisensory perception of flavor: assessing the influence of color cues on flavor discrimination responses. *Food Qual Prefer*, **18**, 975–84.

Zampini, M., Shore, D.I., & Spence, C., 2003. Audiovisual temporal order judgments. *Exp Brain Res*, **152**(2), 198–210.

Zampini, M., Shore, D. I., & Spence, C. 2005. Audiovisual prior entry. *Neurosci Lett*, **381**, 217–22.

Zampini, M., & Spence, C., 2004. The role of auditory cues in modulating the perceived crispness and staleness of potato chips. *J Sensory Stud*, **19**, 347–63.

Zarco, W., Merchant, H., Prado, L., & Mendez, J.C., 2009. Subsecond timing in primates: comparison of interval production between human subjects and rhesus monkeys. *J Neurophysiol*, **102**(6), 3191–202.

Zotterman, Y., 1935. Action potentials in the glossopharyngeal nerve and in the chorda tympani. *Skand Arch Physiol*, **72**, 73–7.

Author Index

Subject Index

Notes: Tables, figures and boxes are indicated by an italic *t*, *f* and *b* following the page number.
     vs. indicates a comparison
     Abbreviations used
        EEG—electroencephalography
        fMRI—functional magnetic resonance imaging